Rapid Review USMLE Step 2

Rapid Review Series

Series Editor
Edward F. Goljan, MD

Behavioral Science, Second Edition
Vivian M. Stevens, PhD; Susan K. Redwood, PhD; Jackie L. Neel, DO; Richard H. Bost, PhD; Nancy W. Van Winkle, PhD; Michael H. Pollak, PhD

Biochemistry, Second Edition
John W. Pelley, PhD; Edward F. Goljan, MD

Gross and Developmental Anatomy, Second Edition
N. Anthony Moore, PhD; William A. Roy, PhD, PT

Histology and Cell Biology, Second Edition
E. Robert Burns, PhD; M. Donald Cave, PhD

Microbiology and Immunology, Second Edition
Ken S. Rosenthal, PhD; James S. Tan, MD

Neuroscience
James A Weyhenmeyer, PhD; Eve A. Gallman, PhD

Pathology, Second Edition
Edward F. Goljan, MD

Pharmacology, Second Edition
Thomas L. Pazdernik, PhD; Laszlo Kerecsen MD

Physiology
Thomas A. Brown, MD

USMLE Step 2
Michael W. Lawlor, MD, PhD

USMLE Step 3
David Rolston, MD; Craig Nielsen, MD

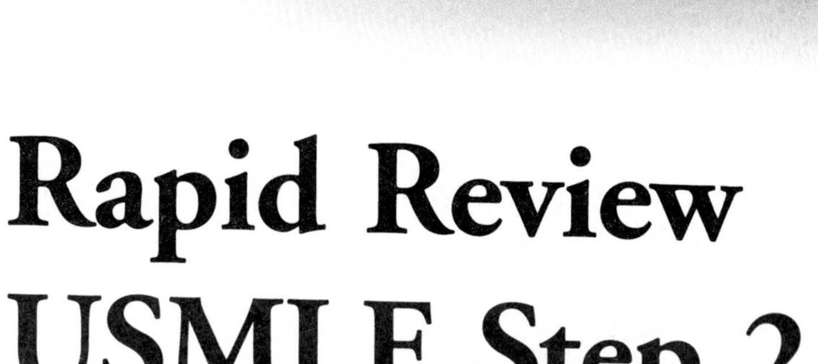

Rapid Review USMLE Step 2

Michael William Lawlor, MD, PhD

Resident in Pathology
Massachusetts General Hospital
Boston, Massachusetts

Clinical Fellow in Pathology
Harvard Medical School
Boston, Massachusetts

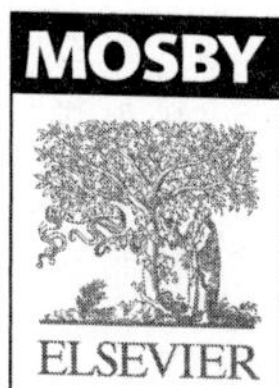

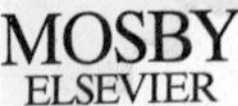

1600 John F. Kennedy Blvd.
Suite 1800
Philadelphia, PA 19103-2899

RAPID REVIEW USMLE STEP 2

ISBN 13: 978-0-323-02963-6
ISBN 10: 0-323-02963-9

NOTICE

Medicine is an ever-changing field. Standard safety precautions must be followed, but as new research and clinical experience broaden our knowledge, changes in treatment and drug therapy may become necessary or appropriate. Readers are advised to check the most current product information provided by the manufacturer of each drug to be administered to verify the recommended dose, the method and duration of administration, and contraindications. It is the responsibility of the licensed prescriber, relying on experience and knowledge of the patient, to determine dosages and the best treatment for each individual patient. Neither the publisher nor the author assumes any liability for any injury and/or damage to persons or property arising from this publication.

Library of Congress Cataloging-in-Publication Data

Lawlor, Michael William.
Rapid review USMLE step 2 / Michael William Lawlor.
p. ; cm.—(Rapid review series)
ISBN 0-323-02963-9
1. Medicine—Examinations, questions, etc. I. Title. II. Title: USMLE step 2. III. Series.
[DNLM: 1. Medicine—Examination Questions. WB 18.2 L418r 2007]
R834.5.L39 2007
610.76—dc22

2006044950

Printed in the United States of America.

Last digit is the print number: 9 8 7 6 5 4 3 2 1

Figure Credits

Albert R, Spiro S, Jett J: Clinical Respiratory Medicine, 2nd ed. Philadelphia, Mosby, 2004: Figures 13-1A–B and 13-1F

Andreoli T, Loscalzo J, Carpenter C, Griggs R: Cecil Essentials of Medicine, 6th ed. Philadelphia, Saunders, 2004: Figures 1-1A–D, 1-2A–P, and 1-4C–E

Armstrong P, Wilson A, Dee P, Hansell D: Imaging of Diseases of the Chest, 3rd ed. London, Mosby Ltd., 2000: Figure 6-2B

Behrman R, Kliegman R, Jensen H: Nelson Textbook of Pediatrics, 17th ed. Philadelphia, Saunders, 2004: Figures 6-2C–D and 11-2E

Brenner G: Pharmacology. Philadelphia, Saunders, 2000: Figure 5-2

Canale ST: Campbell's Operative Orthopaedics, 10th ed. St. Louis, Mosby, 2003: Figure 11-1D

Castro A, Neafsey E, Wurster R, Merchut M: Neuroscience. St. Louis, Mosby, 2002: Figure 8-6

Cohen J, Powderly W: Infectious Diseases, 2nd ed. Philadelphia, Mosby, 2004: Figures 6-1B, 6-2E, and 6-3C

Feldman M, Friedman L, Sleisenger M: Sleisenger and Fordtran's Gastrointestinal and Liver Disease, 7th ed. Philadelphia, Saunders, 2002: Figure 4-3

Fraser R, Muller N, Colman N, Pare P: Fraser and Pare's Diagnosis of Diseases of the Chest, 4th ed. Philadelphia, Saunders, 1999: Figures 6-3A and 13-1C–E

Gabbe S, Niebyl J, Simpson J: Obstetrics—Normal and Problem Pregnancies, 4th ed. Philadelphia, Churchill Livingstone, 2002: Figures 9-1A–C and 12-1B–C

Goldman L, Ausiello D: Cecil Textbook of Medicine, 22nd ed. Philadelphia, Saunders, 2004: Figures 1-4A, 3-1, 4-1, 5-1A–B, 5-1D, 5-4, 14-1C, and 14-2

Goldman L, Bennett JC: Cecil Textbook of Medicine, 21st ed. Philadelphia, Saunders, 2000: Figure 14-1A–B

Grainger R, Allison D, Dixon A: Grainger and Allison's Diagnostic Radiology: A Textbook of Medical Imaging, 4th ed. London, Churchill Livingstone, 2002: Figures 6-3B, 11-1A, 11-1C, 11-1E, and 11-1G

Green N, Swiontkowski: Skeletal Trauma in Children, 3rd ed. Philadelphia, Saunders, 2003: Figures 11-1B, 11-1F, and 11-1H

Guyton A, Hall J: Textbook of Medical Physiology, 10th ed. Philadelphia, Saunders, 2001: Figure 9-3

Haaga J, Lanzieri C, Gilkeson R: CT and MR Imaging of the Whole Body, 4th ed. Philadelphia, Mosby, 2003: Figures 8-2B–D and 8-3A–C

Habif T: Clinical Dermatology, 4th ed. St. Louis, Mosby, 2004: Figure 14-3C

Kumar V, Abbas A, Fausto N: Robbins and Cotran Pathologic Basis of Disease, 7th ed. Philadelphia, Saunders, 2005: Figures 5-1C, 5-1E–H, 5-3A–F, 14-3A, and 14-3E

Mandell G, Bennett J, Dolin R: Principles and Practice of Infectious Diseases, 5th ed. Philadelphia, Churchill Livingstone, 2000: Figure 6-4B

Marx J, Hockberger R, Walls R: Rosen's Emergency Medicine: Concepts and Clinical Practice, 5th ed. St. Louis, Mosby, 2002: Figure 6-2A

Morse S, Ballard R, Holmes K, Moreland A: Atlas of Sexually Transmitted Diseases and AIDS, 3rd ed. St. Louis, Mosby, 2003: Figure 6-4A

Murray J, Nadel J: Textbook of Respiratory Medicine, 3rd ed. Philadelphia, Saunders, 2000: Figure 6-1A

Porterfield S: Endocrine Physiology, 2nd ed. St. Louis, Mosby, 2001: Figure 3-2A–C

Regezi J, Sciubba J, Jordan R: Oral Pathology: Clinical Pathologic Correlations, 4th ed. St. Louis, Saunders, 2003: Figure 12-1A

Resnick D: Bone and Joint Imaging, 2nd ed. Philadelphia, Saunders, 1996: Figure 3-3B

Resnick D: Diagnosis of Bone and Joint Disorders, 4th ed. Philadelphia, Saunders, 2002: Figures 3-3A and 3-3C–D

Roberts J, Hedges J: Clinical Procedures in Emergency Medicine, 4th ed. Philadelphia, Saunders, 2004: Figure 2-1

Ruddy S, Harris E, Sledge C, Sergent J, Budd R: Kelley's Textbook of Rheumatology, 6th ed. Philadelphia, Saunders, 2002: Figures 14-3B, 14-3D, 14-3F–G, and 14-4

Taeusch HW: Avery's Diseases of the Newborn, 8th ed. Philadelphia, Saunders, 2005: Figure 11-1A–D

Townsend C, Beauchamp RD, Evers BM, Mattox K: Sabiston Textbook of Surgery, 17th ed. Philadelphia, Saunders, 2004: Figure 4-2

Young J, Bartholomew J: Peripheral Vascular Diseases, 2nd ed. St. Louis, Mosby, 1996: Figures 1-3A and 1-3B

Series Preface

The first editions of the *Rapid Review Series* have received high critical acclaim from students studying for the United States Medical Licensing Examination (USMLE) Step 1 and high ratings in *First Aid for the USMLE Step 1.* This volume provides a concise review for the USMLE Step 2 exam, summarizing most diseases' pathophysiology, presentation, diagnosis, and treatment in less than one page for efficient review.

SPECIAL FEATURES

Book

- **Outline format:** Concise, high-yield subject matter is presented in a study friendly format. In addition, key words and phrases appear in bold throughout.
- **High-yield margin notes:** Key content that is most likely to appear on the exam is reinforced in the margin notes.
- **High-quality visual elements:** Abundant two-color schematics, black and white images, and summary tables enhance your study experience.
- **Key points:** Boxed key points allow quick follow up and review of each chapter.
- **Two-color design:** The two-color design helps highlight important elements, making studying more efficient and pleasing.
- **Three practice examinations:** Two blocks of 50 and one block of 40 USMLE Step 2–type multiple-choice questions (including images where necessary) and complete discussions (rationales) for all options are included.

New! Online Study and Testing Tool

- **350 USMLE Step 2–type MCQs:** Clinically oriented, multiple-choice questions that mimic the current board format are presented. These include images where necessary, and complete rationales for all answer options. All the questions from the book are included so you can study them in the most effective mode for you!
- **Test mode:** Select from randomized 50-question sets or by subject topics for an exam-like review session. This mode features a 60-minute timer to simulate the actual exam, a detailed assessment report that can be printed or saved to your hard drive, and direct links either to all or only to incorrect questions. The links include your answer, the correct answer, and full rationales for all answer options, so you can fully analyze your test session and learn from your mistakes.
- **Study mode:** Like the test mode, in the study mode you can select from randomized 50-question sets or by subject topics to create a dynamic study session. This mode features unlimited attempts at each question, instant feedback (either on selection of the correct answer or when using the "Show Answer" feature), complete rationales for all answer options, and a detailed progress report that can be printed or saved to your hard drive.
- **Online access:** Online access allows you to study from an internet-enabled computer wherever and whenever it is convenient. This access is activated through registration on www.studentconsult.com with the pincode printed inside the front cover.

Student Consult

- **Full online access:** You can access the complete text and illustrations of this book on www.studentconsult.com.
- **Save content to your PDA:** Through our unique Pocket Consult platform, you can clip select text and illustrations and save them to your PDA for study on the go!
- **Free content:** An interactive community center with a wealth of additional valuable resources is available.

Preface

When I started this book it was with the same naïveté of my peers who said, "Studying for Step I takes 2 months, for Step II takes 2 weeks, and Step III takes 2 days." Faced with the upcoming USMLE Step II exam, I could not find a resource that was concise enough to cover the pertinent topics, yet had sufficient scope to prevent reference to larger textbooks. The lack of a complete single resource was especially frustrating because I had spent three years away from medical school following the Step I exam, to complete my graduate studies. Therefore, it was necessary to familiarize myself with the material at a more basic level than most third year medical students require, given their recent exposure to the Step I material.

This resource began as a compilation of notes, papers, and references I utilized during my third and fourth years of medical school. The final product is an amalgamation of material learned from my lectures, books, and peers. When possible, I have included schematics to accommodate visual learners, mnemonics to assist with the learning of lists, and mechanistic explanations for those few occasions where a deeper understanding will reproducibly bring a student to the correct answer. When the project was started, my goal was to create a short work that could easily be studied in two weeks. In my effort to be complete (as opposed to brief), this work became a larger undertaking than I had initially intended. Nevertheless, this work provides a concise review, while still incorporating sufficient detail to operate as a stand-alone resource. I sincerely hope that you, the reader, find it to be sufficient in this respect.

Thank you and good luck,
Michael William Lawlor, MD, PhD

Acknowledgments

This book never would have been possible without the support of my family, peers, and teachers. First and foremost, I want to acknowledge the role that my wife, Julie Tetzlaff, PhD, played through encouraging words and critical commentary of the book from its earliest form to the published edition. Without her support, I would have quit 100 times over, but she gave me the strength to push on even after I realized what a colossal undertaking this book was going to be. I also wish to thank my parents, Joe and Marilynn Lawlor, as well as my siblings, Melinda, Colleen, Margaret, Mary, and Joe, for a lifetime of good examples and for showing me the value of a good education in becoming successful. In addition, my friendships throughout college, medical school, and graduate school played a significant role in my comfort in the academic setting. Most notably, my close friendships with Robert Giachetti, Eric Gross, PhD, John Kinnison, MD, Michael Richards, and Chris Weber, MD, PhD provided me with excellent intellectual sounding-boards as I explored possible strategies for efficiently teaching complicated concepts. My current peers in the Pathology department at Massachusetts General Hospital have continued this generous tradition of listening to my ideas, and have been kind enough to inform me of their feasibility. My principal mentors throughout this period, Evan Stubbs, PhD, George DeVries, PhD, and Jim Maki, PhD, were instrumental in teaching me the art of organization and writing, and continue to be mentors and friends. My current mentors and peers at Loyola University Medical Center and Massachusetts General Hospital are, unfortunately, too numerous to name, despite the significant contribution that their teachings have made to this book. Finally, this book would not have been possible without extensive hard work and trust from the people working with Elsevier, including Susan Kelly, Tony Castro, PhD, Bill Schmitt, Ed Goljan, MD, Carla Holloway, and Jim Merritt, who have been encouraging and trusting enough to allow me to pursue this project, despite its broad scope and my youth.

Contents

CHAPTER 1

Cardiology

I. Arrhythmias/Electrocardiography (ECG)
   A. ECG Basics (Fig. 1-1)
   B. Diagnosis of Arrhythmias (Fig. 1-2)
   C. Principles of Arrhythmia Management
      1. Use antiarrhythmic medications (Table 1-1).
      2. Tachyarrhythmias may require carotid massage, adenosine, or verapamil to slow the heart and improve waveform resolution.
      3. First-line antiarrhythmic therapy usually involves the use of a beta-blocker or calcium channel blocker.
      4. Watch out for QT prolongation in all antiarrhythmics.
      5. Digoxin may work synergistically with beta-blockers or Ca^{++} channel blockers.
      6. Give anticoagulation for stroke prophylaxis (no anticoagulation is required if the patient is cardioverted within 48 hours of the onset of atrial fibrillation).
      7. Wide complex tachycardias (>0.12 sec) can be treated initially with the advanced cardiac life support (ACLS) protocol and more long-term with antiarrhythmics, radiofrequency ablation, or an implantable defibrillator.
         a. Cardioversion: Can be done via direct current (DC) or quinidine. Cardioversion is more likely to work if the onset is within 12 months. Patients with atrial fibrillation for >48 hours require anticoagulation or visualization of the left atrium by transesophageal echocardiography (TEE) to prevent stroke following cardioversion. Anticoagulation should be continued for 1 month following cardioversion. DC cardioversion is contraindicated in hyperkalemia and digoxin toxicity.
         b. Radiofrequency catheter ablation: Effective for arrhythmias caused by WPW syndrome, or for atrial fibrillation or flutter that is unresponsive to medical therapy.
         c. Implantable defibrillators: Provide rate control in patients at risk for tachyarrhythmias (especially if they have a history of unstable ventricular tachycardia or fibrillation).

II. Peripheral Vascular Disease/Atherosclerosis
   A. Risk Factors
      1. Diabetes
      2. Hypertension
      3. Dyslipidemia
      4. Family history of premature atherosclerosis
      5. Cigarette smoking

Text continued on p. 7

Owing to the potent negative inotropic interaction between beta-blockers and Ca^{++} channel blockers, it is better to switch to other drugs within these classes when switching medications rather than switch from one class to another.

Digoxin should not be used in the treatment of Wolff-Parkinson-White (WPW) syndrome, because it causes slowing of conduction through the atrioventricular (AV) node. In WPW syndrome, this could facilitate conduction through the alternate pathways and worsen the arrhythmia.

There is a 25% chance of stroke around the onset of atrial fibrillation, a 10% to 15% chance of stroke within the first year after onset of atrial fibrillation, and a 5% annual risk of stroke with atrial fibrillation without anticoagulation.

Indications for Pacemaker Placement (Mnemonic—SCCANT): Symptomatic **s**inus bradycardia, symptomatic **c**ongenital complete heart block, symptomatic **c**arotid sinus sensitivity, **a**cquired complete heart block, inus **n**ode dysfunction with life-threatening bradyarrhythmias, symptomatic **t**ype I heart block

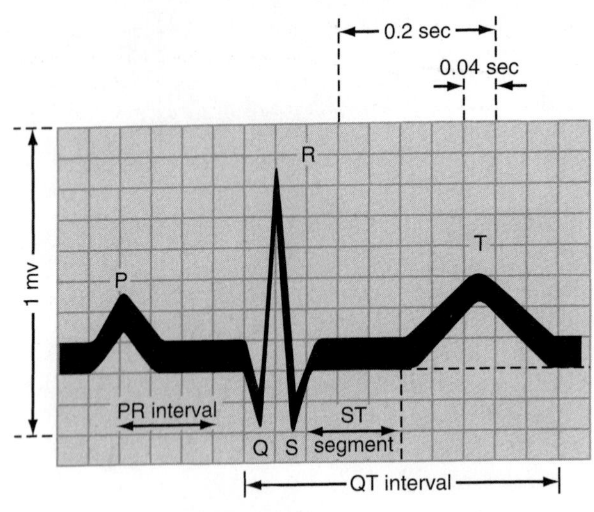
0.2 sec
0.04 sec
R
T
P
1 mv
PR interval
Q
S
ST
segment
QT interval

A

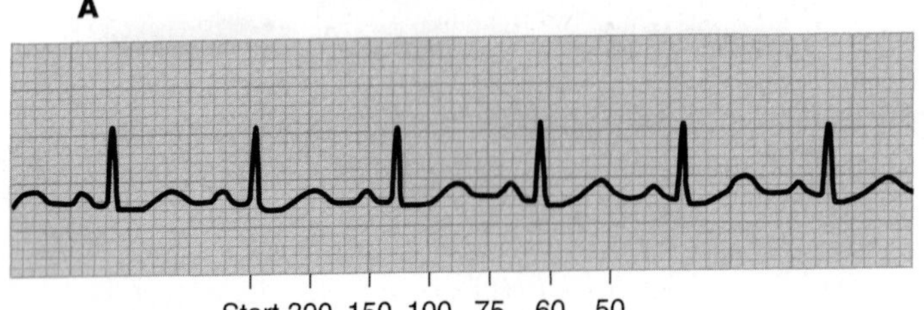
Start 300 150 100 75 60 50

B

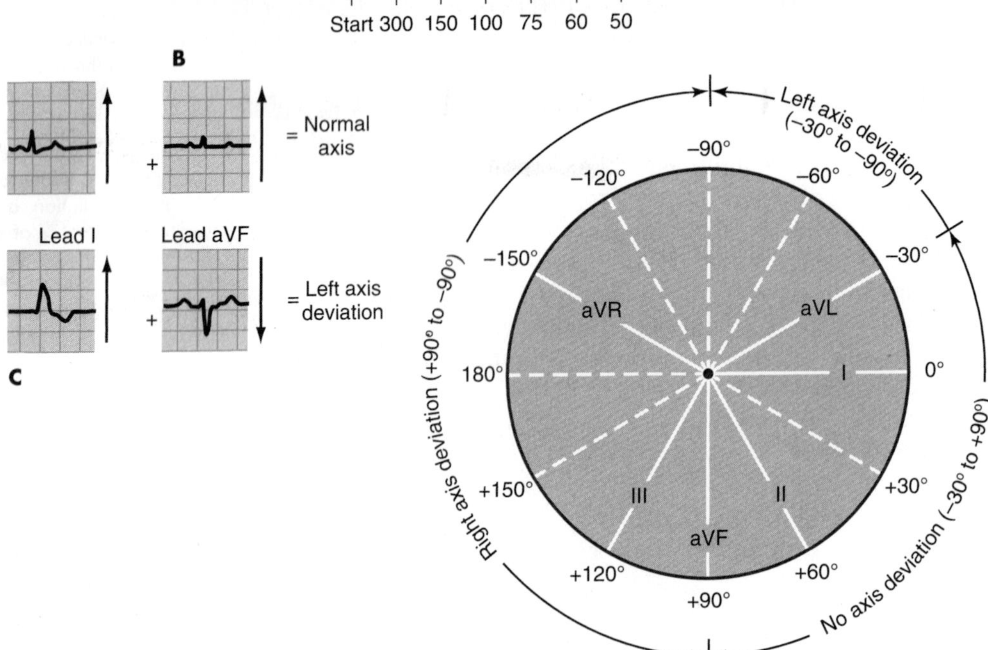
= Normal axis
Lead I
Lead aVF
= Left axis deviation
Left axis deviation (−30° to −90°)
−90°
−120°
−60°
−150°
−30°
aVR
aVL
180°
I
0°
+150°
III
II
+30°
aVF
+120°
+60°
+90°
Right axis deviation (+90° to −90°)
No axis deviation (−30° to +90°)

C

D

1-1: *A, Waves and intervals: The normal QT interval should be no longer than half the R-R interval and is taken from the beginning of the Q wave to the end of the T wave. Various medical conditions (electrolyte disturbances, hypothermia, myocardial ischemia) and drugs (classes I and III antiarrhythmics) can prolong the QT interval and predispose the patient to ventricular arrhythmias. B, Quick determination of heart rate: If the rate is regular, then you can estimate heart rate by dividing 300 by the number of large boxes per R-R interval. If the rate is irregular, you can use the hash marks at the bottom of the strip (which mark off 3-second intervals) and calculate the rate based on the number of beats through the whole strip. C, Quick determination of axis: Use your left hand for lead I and your right hand for aVF. If these leads have positive QRS complexes, point upward. If they have negative QRS complexes, point downward. If both hands are pointing up, then there is no axis deviation. If only the left hand is pointing up, then there is left axis deviation. If only the right hand is pointing up, then there is right axis deviation. D, To get a more precise approximation, look for the flattest (isoelectric) QRS, and you know that the axis is close to perpendicular to that value. The leads are located at the following angles (remember that the angles are positive below the horizontal).*

TABLE 1-1 Commonly Used Antiarrhythmic Medications

Class	Drugs	Indications and Side Effects
Class I (sodium channel blockers)	Quinidine (IA) Procainamide (IA) Disopyramide (IA) Lidocaine (IB) Mexiletine (IB) Flecainide (IC) Propafenone (IC)	(1) Class IA: Quinidine is indicated for supraventricular and ventricular arrhythmias. Procainamide and disopyramide are indicated for ventricular arrhythmias. They all can enhance atrioventricular conduction, so do not use them for atrial flutter. (a) Quinidine also causes hearing and vision problems, delirium, and hemolytic anemia. (b) Procainamide can cause drug-induced lupus syndrome and psychosis. (c) Disopyramide is anticholinergic with negative inotropic effects, so do not use it for patients with left ventricular dysfunction. (2) Class IB: These are not effective for supraventricular arrhythmias. Also, do not give during an acute myocardial infarction. In general, they cause CNS-related side effects (confusion, ataxia, paresthesias). (3) Class IC: Most useful for ventricular and supraventricular arrhythmias in structurally normal hearts. (a) Flecainide can cause ataxia and blurred vision. (b) Propafenone can cause a metallic taste sensation.
Class II (beta-adrenergic blockers)	Propranolol Metoprolol	Indicated for the prevention of supraventricular arrhythmias and the prevention of sudden death (due to ventricular ectopic depolarizations) following myocardial infarction. Side effects include fatigue, bradycardia, and impotence. Beta-blockers are contraindicated in patients with asthma, COPD, or heart block.

continued

TABLE 1-1 Commonly Used Antiarrhythmic Medications—cont'd

Class	Drugs	Indications and Side Effects
Class III (potassium channel blockers)	Amiodarone Ibutilide Sotalol Bretylium	(1) Amiodarone can be used for long-term suppression of both supraventricular and ventricular tachycardias. It is the drug of choice in patients with atrial fibrillation who have heart failure, and it is good for arrhythmia prevention following myocardial infarction. Amiodarone has the potential for liver, lung, and thyroid toxicity, as well as agranulocytosis. (2) Ibutilide is an intravenous agent that is good for chemical cardioversion in atrial fibrillation or flutter, but it can cause torsades de pointes, leading to ventricular arrhythmias. (3) Sotalol can be used for atrial fibrillation and ventricular arrhythmias, but it can cause torsades de pointes, leading to ventricular arrhythmias. (4) Bretylium is indicated in ventricular fibrillation, but its severe side effect profile (hypertension, tachycardia, worsening of arrhythmias) makes it a last-line agent.
Class IV (calcium channel blockers)	Diltiazem Verapamil	These drugs can be useful for supraventricular tachycardia, but they can exacerbate ventricular tachycardias. Verapamil and diltiazem can also cause hypotension, which can be treated with calcium gluconate.
Adenosine		Useful for acute treatment of supraventricular tachycardias and re-entrant atrioventricular tachycardias (including Wolff-Parkinson-White syndrome).
Digoxin		Useful in modulating the ventricular response to supraventricular tachycardia. Digoxin toxicity can cause bradycardia, arrhythmia, nausea, and confusion.

COPD, chronic obstructive pulmonary disease.

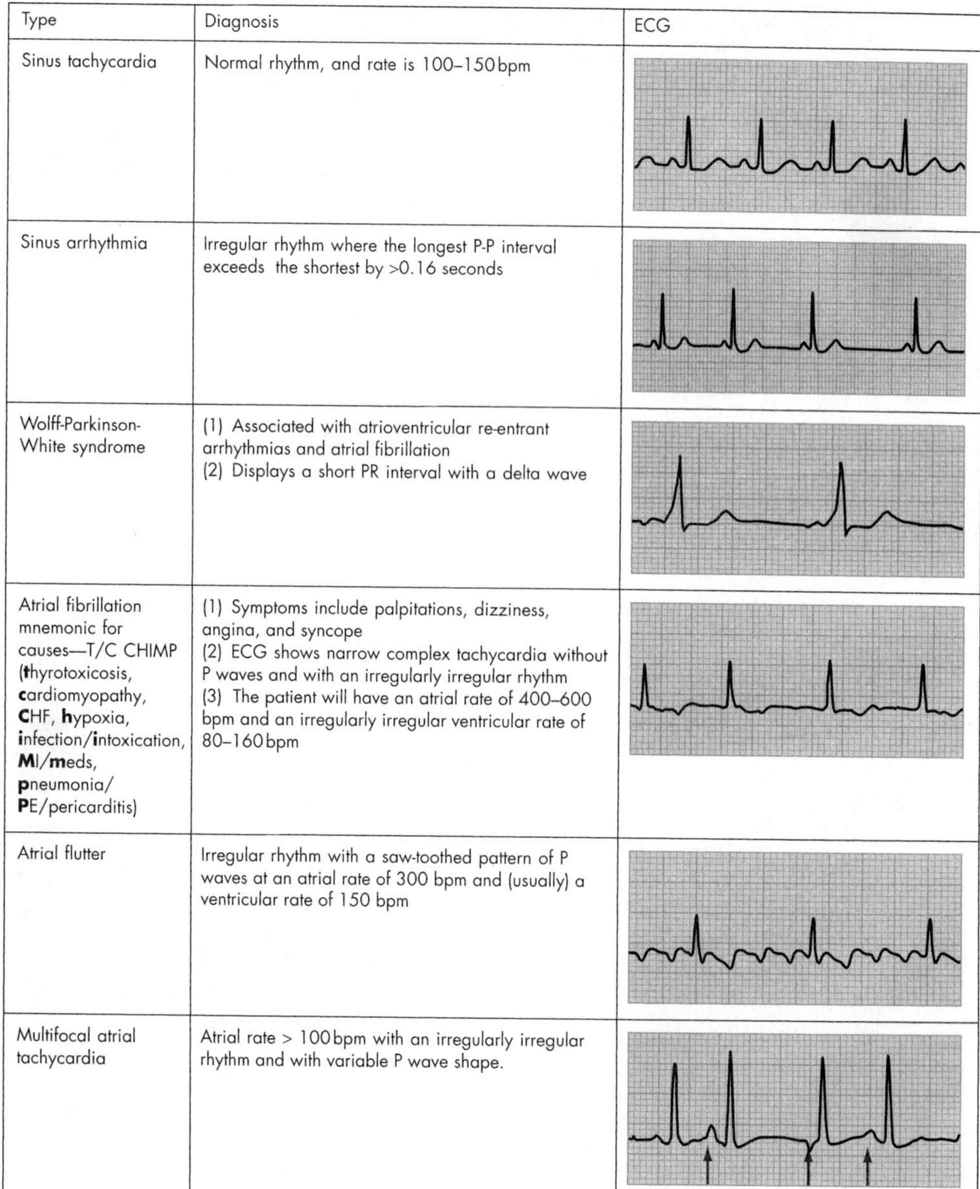

Type	Diagnosis	ECG
Sinus tachycardia	Normal rhythm, and rate is 100–150 bpm	
Sinus arrhythmia	Irregular rhythm where the longest P-P interval exceeds the shortest by >0.16 seconds	
Wolff-Parkinson-White syndrome	(1) Associated with atrioventricular re-entrant arrhythmias and atrial fibrillation (2) Displays a short PR interval with a delta wave	
Atrial fibrillation mnemonic for causes—T/C CHIMP (**t**hyrotoxicosis, **c**ardiomyopathy, **C**HF, **h**ypoxia, **i**nfection/**i**ntoxication, **MI**/**m**eds, **p**neumonia/**P**E/pericarditis)	(1) Symptoms include palpitations, dizziness, angina, and syncope (2) ECG shows narrow complex tachycardia without P waves and with an irregularly irregular rhythm (3) The patient will have an atrial rate of 400–600 bpm and an irregularly irregular ventricular rate of 80–160 bpm	
Atrial flutter	Irregular rhythm with a saw-toothed pattern of P waves at an atrial rate of 300 bpm and (usually) a ventricular rate of 150 bpm	
Multifocal atrial tachycardia	Atrial rate > 100 bpm with an irregularly irregular rhythm and with variable P wave shape.	

1-2: *Diagnosis of arrhythmias by electrocardiography. bpm, beats per minute; CHF, congestive heart failure; MI, myocardial infarction; PE, pulmonary embolism.*

continued

Type	Diagnosis	ECG
Ventricular tachycardia	(1) Ventricular tachycardia is defined as a run of three or more premature ventricular contractions (see below) (2) ECG shows atrioventricular dissociation and the QRS complex of all leads pointing in the same direction	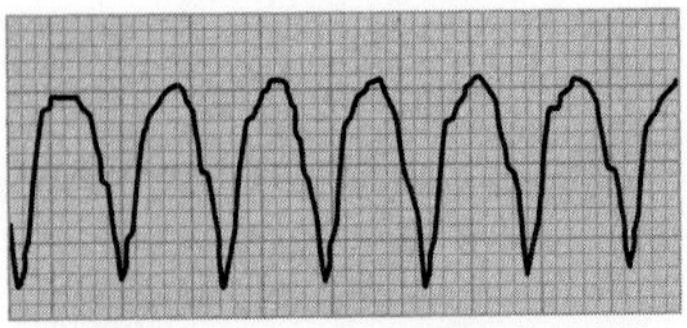
Ventricular fibrillation	Ventricular tachycardia can progress to ventricular fibrillation, which is a total lack of organized QRS complexes	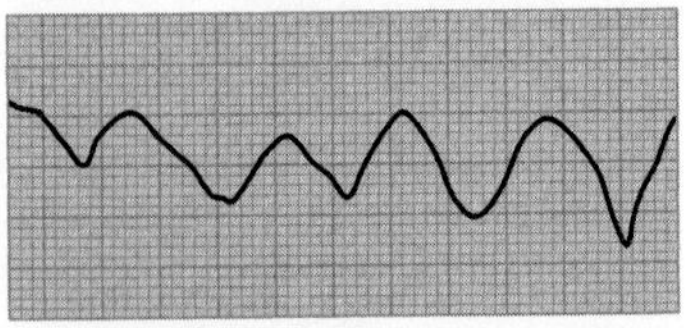
Premature atrial contractions	P wave occurs early with an unusual contour, but the QRS usually appears normal	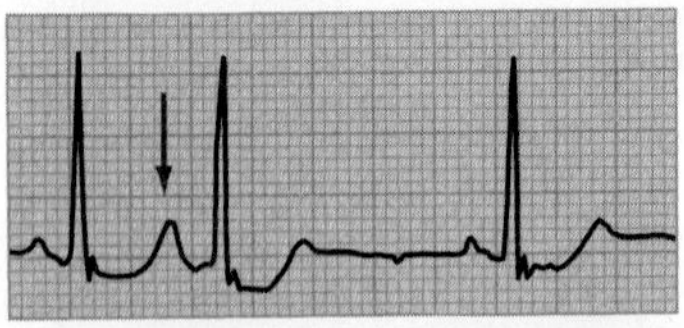
Premature ventricular contractions	(1) Premature beat with an absent P wave and a wide QRS complex (2) There is a compensatory pause so that the P-P interval is approximately two cycles, followed by a strong beat (3) Associated with bigeminal pulse, in which the pulse of the premature beat is decreased and the strong beat is increased	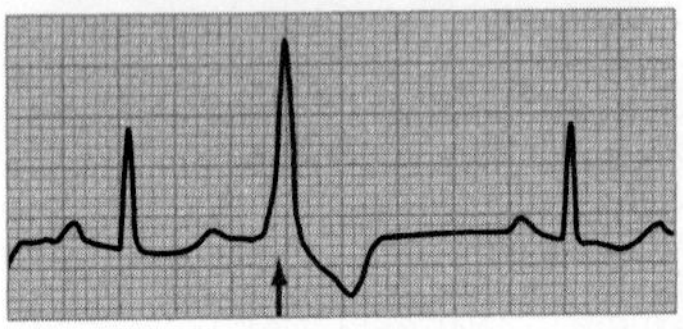
First-degree heart block	P-R interval is fixed and exceeds 0.2 seconds	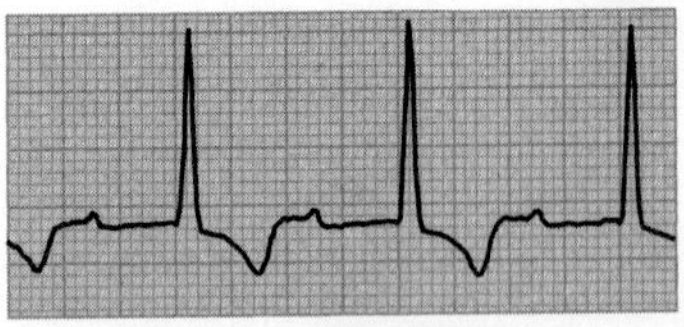
Second-degree heart block type I (Wenckebach)	Progressive P-R lengthening until a QRS complex drops out	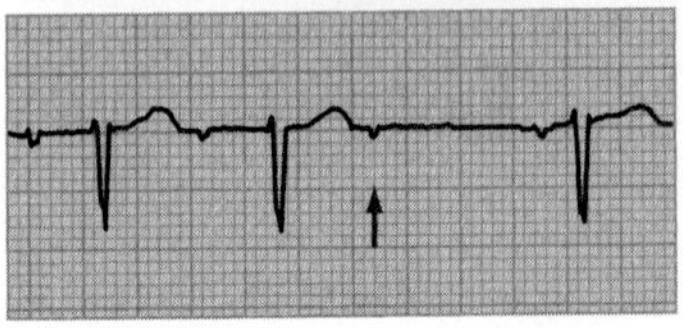

1-2, cont'd.

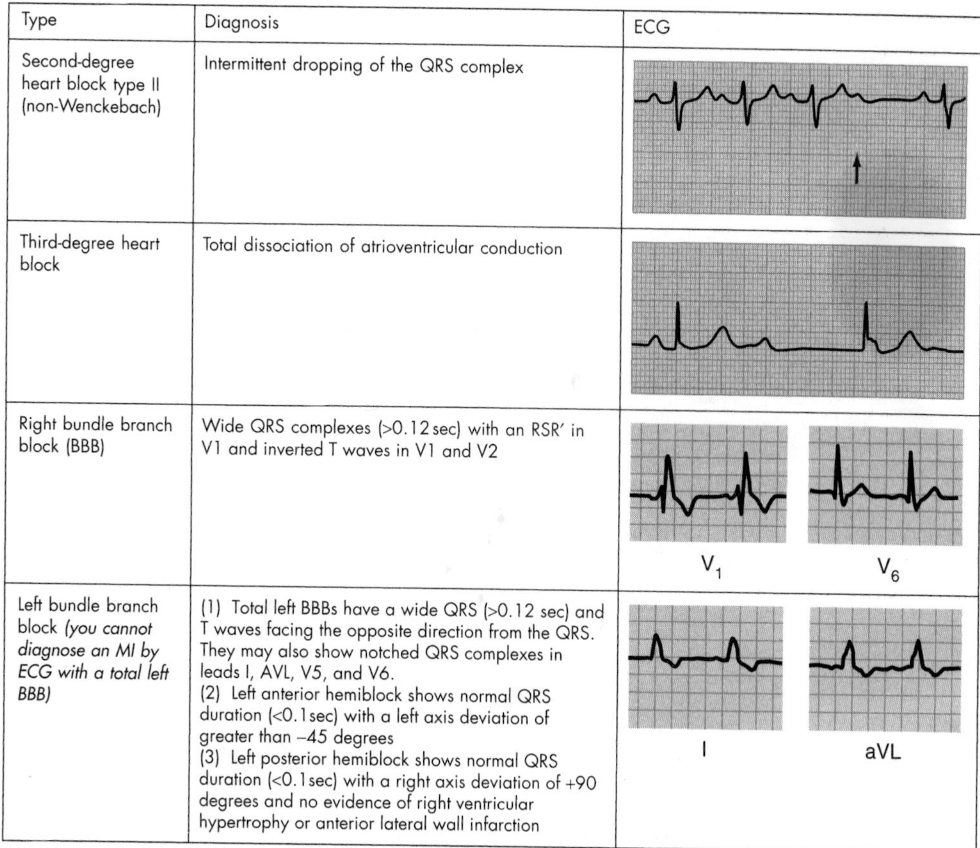

Type	Diagnosis	ECG
Second-degree heart block type II (non-Wenckebach)	Intermittent dropping of the QRS complex	
Third-degree heart block	Total dissociation of atrioventricular conduction	
Right bundle branch block (BBB)	Wide QRS complexes (>0.12 sec) with an RSR′ in V1 and inverted T waves in V1 and V2	V_1 V_6
Left bundle branch block *(you cannot diagnose an MI by ECG with a total left BBB)*	(1) Total left BBBs have a wide QRS (>0.12 sec) and T waves facing the opposite direction from the QRS. They may also show notched QRS complexes in leads I, AVL, V5, and V6. (2) Left anterior hemiblock shows normal QRS duration (<0.1 sec) with a left axis deviation of greater than –45 degrees (3) Left posterior hemiblock shows normal QRS duration (<0.1 sec) with a right axis deviation of +90 degrees and no evidence of right ventricular hypertrophy or anterior lateral wall infarction	I aVL

1-2, cont'd.

B. Symptoms and Signs
   1. Claudication: Exertion-induced pain within a muscle group that disappears after 1 to 5 minutes of rest. Claudication is usually described in terms of the distance traveled until onset of the pain.
   2. Rest pain: Constant pain at rest due to hypoperfusion. It is worst when lying down because of the lack of gravity-assisted blood flow.
   3. Leriche syndrome: Distal aortic occlusion due to atherosclerosis. Patients will have impotence (due to decreased flow to the hypogastric arteries), symmetric lower extremity muscle wasting, pallor of the legs and feet, claudication of the buttocks, and easy fatigability.
   4. Changes in the appearance of the extremities (dependent rubor, pallor on elevation, loss of hair, thinning of skin, muscle atrophy, arterial insufficiency ulcers, venous stasis ulcers). See Figure 1-3.
   5. Lack of distal pulses.
   6. Bruits over some arteries (femoral, renal).

C. Other Peripheral Vascular Syndromes (Table 1-2)

The most common site of atherosclerotic occlusion in the lower extremities is the superficial femoral artery in Hunter's canal, which can produce claudication in the calf.

Causes of Aneurysms: Atherosclerosis (95%), trauma, syphilis (thoracic aorta), congenital defects, Marfan syndrome (aortic root), pregnancy (splenic artery)

TABLE 1-2 Atherosclerotic Disorders

Type	Symptoms and Signs	Diagnostic Evaluation	Treatment
Carotid atherosclerosis	(1) Carotid bruit. (2) Transient ischemic attacks (TIAs)—Reversible neurologic deficits (see Chapter 8).	Carotid Doppler imaging	Perform carotid endarterectomy in asymptomatic patients with 70% occlusion or in patients with 50% occlusion and a history of stroke or TIA. Complications of surgery include MI, hematoma, infection, and hoarseness.
Subclavian steal syndrome	Ipsilateral arm movement will increase blood requirements to the arm and steal blood from the vertebral circulation, thereby causing upper extremity claudication, syncopal attacks, vertigo, confusion, ataxia, or blindness. Signs include a discrepancy in the blood pressure when comparing the upper extremities and the presence of a bruit above the clavicles.		Treat with surgical bypass.
Abdominal aortic aneurysm (AAA)	(1) Patient will have vague abdominal pain with a large pulsatile immobile mass, which is usually located above the umbilicus. Distal pulses may be diminished. (2) Risk factors for rupture include aneurysm size (negligible risk for <4 cm, 5% to 15% for 5–6 cm, 30% to 40% for >8 cm), hypertension, and chronic obstructive pulmonary disease. If rupture occurs, the pain will begin in the epigastrium and penetrate to the back. Tenderness will be present in the aneurysm area and in the flanks.	(1) People with first-degree relatives with AAA should get a screening ultrasound at the age of 55 (family history is a risk factor for AAA) (2) Aortography	Surgical repair: Surgery is indicated for low risk patients with aneurysms >4 cm and almost all patients with aneurysms >5 cm. It involves cross-clamping of the aorta, which can lead to the development of hypovolemia, acidosis, and electrolyte abnormalities.

TABLE 1-2 Atherosclerotic Disorders—cont'd

Type	Symptoms and Signs	Diagnostic Evaluation	Treatment
Mesenteric ischemia	(1) Weight loss, postprandial abdominal pain, abdominal bruit, and possibly occult blood–positive stool or nausea and vomiting. (2) Acute mesenteric ischemia: Can be due to digitalis treatment. Presents with a triad of acute onset of pain, vomiting, or diarrhea and a history of atrial fibrillation or heart disease.	Arteriogram: Two of the three mesenteric arteries will be occluded, and there will be narrowing of the third artery	Bypass, endarterectomy.
Renal artery stenosis	(1) Signs include headache, diastolic hypertension, flank bruits, and decreased renal function. (2) Suspect this in a young woman with hypertension that is unresponsive to pharmacologic treatment.	(1) Arteriogram: The gold standard test. (2) Intravenous pyelography (3) Captopril provocation test: Causes a drop in blood pressure	(1) Do not treat these patients with an ACE inhibitor, since it will cause renal insufficiency. (2) Percutaneous renal transluminal angioplasty (PRTA) and stent placement. (3) Surgery (resection, bypass, endarterectomy).

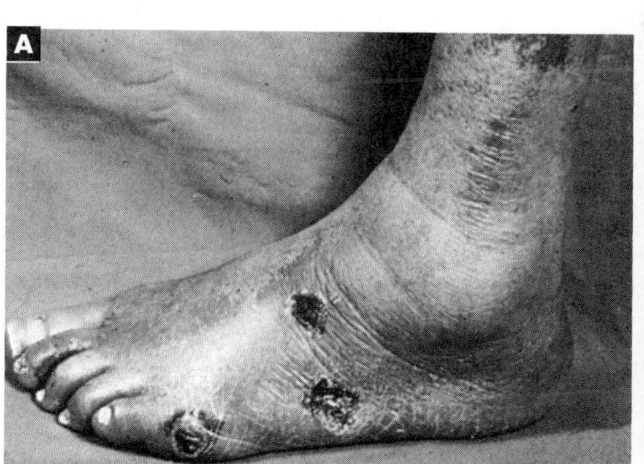

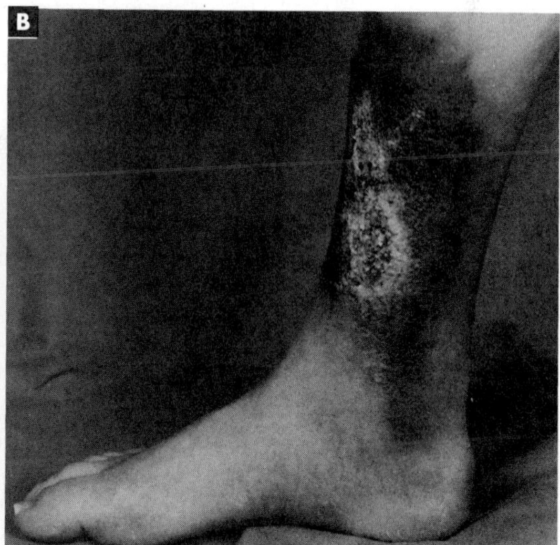

1-3: A, *Arterial insufficiency ulcer: Painful dry ulcers on pressure points can be seen, but discoloration is not a major feature.* B, *Venous insufficiency ulcer: Stasis, pigmentation, and large ulcers on the ankle and calf can be seen. The ulcers are not localized to pressure points.*

D. Evaluation
   1. Stress test: Electrocardiographic monitoring during exercise or chemical stressing (usually with dobutamine) may show signs of cardiac ischemia (ST segment depression) with increased demand. (See section III, Angina.)
   2. Doppler imaging: Can measure blood pressure at several points in the extremity. A difference of >20 mm Hg between two levels suggests significant occlusive disease. An ankle-brachial index (ABI) can also be calculated by dividing the systolic blood pressure measured in the ankle by the systolic blood pressure measured in the arm. An ABI below 0.95 is considered abnormal.
   3. Arteriogram: Maps anatomy and assists in the development of a treatment strategy.

E. Treatment
   1. Conservative: Quit smoking, start exercising, control hyperlipidemia.
   2. Bedside management: Sheepskin footrests, foot cradle, and skin lotion to avoid skin cracking and prevent infection.
   3. Procedures
      a. Can include vessel sewing, revascularization via conduit bypass, endarterectomy (removal of the diseased intima and media), or angioplasty.
      b. Postoperative management
         (1) Frequently assess graft patency.
         (2) Give prophylactic antibiotics (IV cefazolin).
         (3) Encourage walking.
      c. Lower extremity amputations: Indicated in cases of irreversible tissue ischemia, necrotic tissue, severe infection, or severe pain with no bypassable vessels.

F. Complications
   1. Perioperative myocardial infarction (MI): Most likely to occur at postoperative days 3–5. This may be due to fluid overload after 3rd spacing resolves. Mortality of postoperative MI is 20% to 50% (two to three times greater than a regular MI).
   2. Graft failure: Can be due to technical problems with the graft, intimal hyperplasia at the anastomosis, or progression of arterial disease.
   3. Thromboembolic complications.

III. Angina/Coronary Artery Disease

A. Symptoms and Signs
   1. Exertional substernal chest pressure that may radiate to the left jaw, shoulder, or arm.
   2. The pain worsens with activity, is relieved with rest or nitroglycerin, and lasts less than 30 minutes.

Classes of Angina—I: New-onset, severe, or accelerated angina without angina at rest, II: angina at rest in the past month, III: angina at rest or angina in the past 48 hours

B. Types of Angina (Table 1-3)

C. Evaluation
   1. Stress test: Can be done using an exercise protocol, medications (dobutamine, dipyridamole, or adenosine), and through imaging techniques (radionuclide scan or echocardiography).

TABLE 1-3
Types of Angina

Type	Cause	Timing	Diagnosis
Stable	A stable atherosclerotic plaque that is limiting blood flow to the heart	Occurs with exertion in a predictable pattern	ECG will show ST segment depression while the patient is symptomatic
Unstable	Formation of a thrombus on a plaque that causes a significant deficit of blood flow to the heart	Symptoms at rest, or new onset, or an increase in the frequency or severity of symptoms	ECG will show ST segment depression while the patient is symptomatic
Prinzmetal's	Mimics angina pectoris but is actually due to vasospasm rather than thrombotic occlusion of coronary vessels	Unrelated to activity	(1) ECG will show ST segment elevation (rather than depression) (2) Coronary angiography will be free of stenotic lesions and the arteries will spasm with administration of ergonovine. (3) Treat with vasodilators (nitroglycerin or Ca^{++} channel blockers)

a. Indications
   (1) Suspected coronary artery disease
   (2) Risk stratification following an MI
   (3) Documentation of progression of coronary artery disease (CAD)
b. Contraindications (mnemonic—UA ASS)
   (1) **U**nstable angina
   (2) **A**cute MI within 48 hours
   (3) **A**rrhythmias
   (4) **S**ymptomatic CHF
   (5) **S**evere aortic stenosis
c. Analysis of results
   (1) Heart rate and blood pressure: Must reach 85% of their predicted maximum in order for the test to be valid.
   (2) ECG: Abnormalities that are predictive of CAD include ST segment depressions or elevations.
   (3) Echocardiogram: Wall motion abnormalities are indicative of CAD.
   (4) Radionuclide scan: Filling defects are indicative of CAD.

2. Send blood for troponin measurement at the first presentation of angina to rule out MI.

D. Treatment
   1. Initially treat as an MI: Give aspirin, oxygen, beta-blocker, and heparin and track telemetry.
   2. Conservative management of risk factors for atherosclerosis.

3. Medical: Sublingual nitroglycerin, beta-blocker, aspirin, heparin, and maybe a calcium channel blocker (nifedipine or amlodipine).
4. Surgical: Coronary artery bypass graft (CABG) or angioplasty can be performed to increase oxygen delivery to cardiac muscle.
   a. Angioplasty is the treatment of choice in single vessel disease.
   b. Stents decrease the rate of angioplasty restenosis from 40% to 20%.
   c. Indications for CABG over angioplasty
      (1) Left main coronary artery occlusion >50%
      (2) Severe multivessel CAD
   d. Aspirin should be continued for at least 1 year after either surgery to reduce the restenosis rate.
   e. Half of saphenous vein grafts have restenosis at 10 years.

IV. Myocardial Infarction (MI)
   A. Symptoms
      1. Substernal pain or pressure similar to angina lasting longer than 30 minutes and that may radiate to the left jaw, arm, or shoulder. The pain does not resolve with nitroglycerin. Signs of acute-onset heart failure, including crackles in the lung and signs of increased jugular venous pressure (JVP), may also be present.
      2. Twenty percent are silent with mild or no symptoms.
   B. Q wave versus non Q wave MI: Q wave infarcts are usually transmural, whereas non Q wave infarcts are subendocardial and may subsequently progress further.
   C. Evaluation: A diagnosis of acute coronary syndrome involves the presence of two of the three following criteria for an MI:
      1. Clinical: By history and physical examination
      2. Electrical: By ECG (Fig. 1-4)
      3. Chemical: By cardiac enzymes
         a. CK-MB: Isozyme of creatine kinase that is fairly specific for cardiac muscle. This increases 4 to 6 hours post MI and peaks at 12 to 24 hours after MI. It usually disappears within 72 hours after MI.
         b. Troponin: Elevations are useful for detection of MI between 4 hours and 7 days after MI.

Treatment of MI (Mnemonic—MONA B): **M**orphine, **o**xygen, **n**itroglycerin, **a**spirin, **b**eta-blocker

Absolute Contraindications for Thrombolytic Therapy (Mnemonic—BP HAND): Active **b**leeding, acute **p**ericarditis, previous cerebral **h**emorrhage, cerebral **a**neurysm or arteriovenous malformation (AVM), intracranial **n**eoplasm, aortic **d**issection

   D. Treatment
      1. Supplemental O_2 and nitroglycerin to increase O_2 delivery.
      2. Aspirin and heparin to prevent further thrombosis.
      3. Morphine for pain control.
      4. Metoprolol and acetylcholinesterase inhibitors (ACE-Is): ACE-Is are indicated in patients with depressed ventricular function.
      5. Consider emergent angioplasty to restore blood flow: This procedure needs to be performed within 2 hours of MI.
      6. Thrombolysis can be attempted if the patient has a low risk of bleeding elsewhere and the MI has been happening for less than 12 hours (best results within 6 hours after MI).
   E. Complications
      1. Arrhythmias: Most common cause of death after MI.

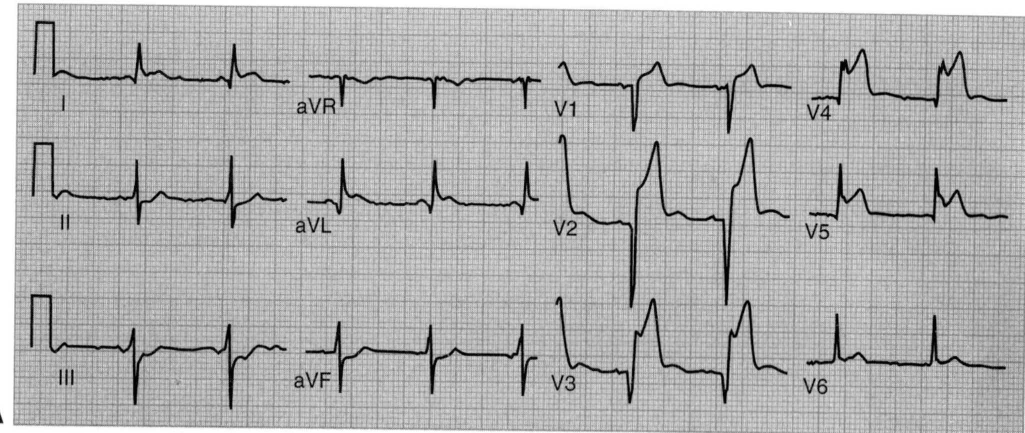

Location	ECG leads	Arterial supply
Anterior	V2–V4	Left anterior descending artery
Anteroseptal	V1–V4	Left anterior descending artery
Inferior	II, III, aVF	Right coronary artery
Lateral	I, aVL, V5–V6	Left circumflex artery
Posterior	V1 (will have large R wave)	Left circumflex and right coronary arteries
Right ventricle	Precordial leads must be rearranged.	Right coronary artery

B

C

D

E

1-4: Diagnosis of myocardial infarction (MI) by electrocardiography: A, Representative electrocardiogram of an acute anterior wall myocardial infarction, which is indicated by the ST segment elevations in leads V1–V5. B, Table clarifying the cardiac locations and arterial supplies involved when different leads show changes indicative of myocardial infarction. C–E, Depictions of the evolution of changes in the electrocardiogram following an MI. ST segment elevations are seen acutely at 2 hours after MI (C), which then progress to the presence of Q waves 24 hours later (D), and eventually progress to Q waves with T wave inversion by 8 days after MI (E).

2. Myocardial dysfunction: May be due to scarring, aneurysm formation, or valvular insufficiency.
3. Ventricular wall rupture.
4. Dressler's syndrome: Autoimmune disease with fever, pericarditis, and increased erythrocyte sedimentation rate (ESR) 2 to 4 weeks after MI.

V. Hypertension (HTN)

A. Causes

1. Essential (95%): Unknown etiology.
2. Renal (4%): Renal artery stenosis or parenchymal renal disease.

3. Endocrine (0.2%): Pheochromocytoma (headaches, sweating, and tachycardia), primary hyperaldosteronism (signs of hypokalemia), Cushing's syndrome.
4. Coarctation of the aorta.
5. Estrogen use (oral contraceptive pills or hormone replacement therapy).

B. Symptoms and Signs
1. More than two blood pressure measurements separated by more than 5 minutes that fit within the following categories (from the seventh report of the Joint National Committee on Prevention, Detection, Evaluation, and Treatment of High Blood Pressure [JNC 7] guidelines for the treatment of hypertension, which classify hypertension according to the following categories):
    a. Prehypertension: systolic BP 120–139, diastolic BP 80–89
    b. Stage 1 HTN: systolic BP 140–159, diastolic BP 90–99
    c. Stage 2 HTN: systolic BP > 160, diastolic BP greater than 100
2. Symptoms of congestive heart failure (see later discussion).
3. HTN due to renal artery stenosis may include renal bruits and symptoms of acute renal failure. HTN due to coarctation of the aorta will show decreased and delayed pulses in the lower extremities.
4. Hypertensive retinopathy
    a. Stage I: Arteriolar narrowing
    b. Stage II: Copper wiring and AV nicking
    c. Stage III: Hemorrhages, exudates
    d. Stage IV: Papilledema

C. Evaluation
1. Captopril renal scan or MR angiography (MRA): If renal artery stenosis is suspected.
2. Aortogram for coarctation of the aorta.
3. Renin activity: This should increase after ACE-I administration in bilateral renal artery stenosis.

D. Treatment
1. Lifestyle changes: Patients with moderate HTN can attempt these (quit smoking, increase exercise, lose weight, decrease alcohol consumption, and decrease Na^+ intake to <3 g/day) for 3 to 6 months if they want to avoid taking medications.
2. Medical therapies
    a. Frequently used medications (Table 1-4)
    b. Essential HTN
        (1) Diuretic and/or beta-blocker
        (2) Use an ACE-I if the patient is diabetic
        (3) Use beta-blocker if CAD is present
    c. Renal disease
        (1) Salt and fluid restriction if renal parenchymal disease is the cause
        (2) Angioplasty with stenting for renal artery stenosis
    d. Current recommendations for management
        (1) First-line: Beta-blocker and diuretic
        (2) In African Americans: Ca^{++} channel blocker and/or diuretic

TABLE 1-4 Common Antihypertensive Medications

Class	Mechanism	Contraindications	Side Effects
Diuretics	Reduce total volume and as a result lower blood pressure.	Thiazides and spironolactone are ineffective in renal insufficiency.	Most important adverse effects of diuretics are metabolic. Treat hypokalemia with potassium supplementation.
Beta-blockers	Reduce cardiac output and suppresses sympathetically mediated renin secretion.	Avoid use in COPD, asthma, or heart block.	Side effects include fatigue, bradycardia, and impotence.
Calcium channel blockers	Inhibition of calcium channels in vascular smooth muscle leads directly to reduction in peripheral vascular resistance.	Avoid use in heart block or systolic failure.	Adverse effects are highly dependent upon the class of calcium channel blocker. Nifedipine can cause tachycardia and peripheral edema. Verapamil and diltiazem may cause bradycardia, constipation, and (rarely) heart failure.
Angiotensin-converting enzyme (ACE) inhibitors	These agents block the conversion of angiotensin I to angiotensin II. The reduction in plasma angiotensin II levels removes vasoconstrictor influence from the vascular smooth muscle and also reduces angiotensin II–stimulated aldosterone, which may lead to natriuresis and reduction in circulating plasma volume.	Can worsen renal function in renal artery stenosis.	Cough, angioedema (rarely), and hyperkalemia (in patients with renal insufficiency).
Angiotensin receptor blockers	These agents have similar hemodynamics and metabolic effects to ACE inhibitors.	Can worsen renal function in renal artery stenosis.	Similar to ACE inhibitor side effects, but cough does not occur and angioedema is rare.
Clonidine	Decreases central sympathetic outflow.	None	Abrupt discontinuation will cause rebound hypertension.
Hydralazine	Is a direct vasodilator.	None	Can cause a lupus-like syndrome.

COPD, chronic obstructive pulmonary disease.

(3) Left ventricular (LV) systolic dysfunction: Diuretic and ACE-I
(4) Hypertensive urgencies: Treat with oral beta-blocker, Ca^{++} channel blocker, or ACE-I
(5) Hypertensive emergencies: IV nitroprusside or labetalol

Causes of Recurrent CHF (Mnemonic—FAILURE): **F**orgot meds, **a**rrhythmias/anemia, **i**schemia/infarct/infection, **l**ifestyle, **u**p-regulation (increased cardiac output), **r**enal failure, **e**mbolus

VI. Congestive Heart Failure (CHF; Box 1-1)
A. Symptoms and Signs
1. Low output
a. Left-sided: Presents with fatigue, crackles in lungs, orthopnea, dyspnea on exertion, paroxysmal nocturnal dyspnea, pleural effusions. The patient may have a history of MI and may have an enlarged heart on physical examination.
b. Right-sided: Presents with fatigue, exercise intolerance, and decreased peripheral perfusion. The patient may have peripheral edema, cold extremities, jugular venous distention (JVD), hepatomegaly, and ascites.
2. Severe disease can result in renal failure, confusion, and cardiogenic shock.
B. Classification (According to New York Heart Association)
1. Class I: Symptomatic with strenuous activity
2. Class II: Symptomatic with normal activity
3. Class III: Symptomatic with minimal activity
4. Class IV: Symptomatic at rest
C. Diagnostic Evaluation
1. Demonstrate hypoperfusion
a. Renal: Decreased urine output, increased blood urea nitrogen (BUN) and creatinine, hyponatremia
b. Hepatic: Abnormal liver function tests
2. Demonstrate ventricular dysfunction
a. Use echocardiography, radionuclide ventriculography, or cardiac catheterization.

BOX 1-1

MECHANISMS BY WHICH HTN OCCURS IN CHF

1. Renin-angiotensin-aldosterone (RAA) system: Decreased renal perfusion leads to renin release, which then causes the RAA system to increase sodium and water reabsorption.
2. Increases in circulating catecholamines: Cause positive inotropy with an increase in systemic vascular resistance.

Low cardiac output and decreased cardiac reserve will lead to organ hypoperfusion and venous congestion of both systemic and pulmonary circulations.

b. ECG changes include supraventricular and ventricular arrhythmias, Q waves, conduction block, and ST changes.
c. Chest radiograph may show cardiomegaly in left-sided CHF.

D. Treatment
1. Lifestyle changes
a. Low sodium diet (<2 g/day).
b. Restrict physical activity until the patient stabilizes, then start a regimen of gradual aerobic exercise to improve the patient's functional capacity.
c. Weight loss.
d. Fluid restriction less than 1.5 L/day.
2. For acute cardiogenic pulmonary edema
a. "LMNOP" regimen: **L**asix, **m**orphine, **n**itrates, **o**xygen, **p**osition.
b. ACE inhibitors: For patients who are intolerant of ACE-I, hydralazine and nitrates can be given.
c. Spironolactone: Decreases mortality by 30% in CHF when given with ACE-I, digoxin, and diuretics in patients with left-sided systolic dysfunction.
d. Inotropic agents: Digoxin has no effect on mortality, but may decrease symptoms of CHF if they persist despite ACE I and diuretic treatment. Do not use in patients with CHF due to restrictive cardiomyopathy.
e. Patients refractory to medications should be fitted with a mechanical assist device (intra-aortic balloon pump).
f. Do not use Ca^{++} channel blockers, because of their negative inotropic side effects.
g. For arrhythmias: Do not use class I antiarrhythmics, because they increase mortality. Amiodarone can be used for any atrial arrhythmias with CHF. Implantable defibrillators should be used for ventricular arrhythmias with CHF.

VII. Cardiomyopathies (Table 1-5)

VIII. Valvular Disease (Table 1-6)

IX. Pericardial Disease (Table 1-7)

Causes of Pericarditis *(Mnemonic—I MUNCH)*: **I**nfectious *(coxsackievirus B, echovirus, Streptococcus pneumoniae, Staphylococcus aureus)*/**I**diopathic, after **M**I, **u**remia, **n**eoplastic/radiation-induced, **c**ollagen vascular disease, **h**urt *(traumatic)*

X. Hyperlipidemia
A. Types
1. Acquired
a. High low-density lipoprotein (LDL).
(1) Diet, hypothyroidism, diabetes, nephrotic syndrome, and liver disease.
(2) Drugs (*mnemonic—PEST BAG*): **p**rogestins, **e**strogens, **s**teroids, **t**hiazides, **b**eta-blockers, **a**lcohol, **g**lucocorticoids.

Text continued on p. 22

TABLE 1-5
Cardiomyopathies

Type	Cause	Symptoms	Evaluation	Treatment
Dilated	(mnemonic—STIPE) (1) **S**tructural (ischemia, valvular disease, hypertension, tachycardia-induced) (2) **T**oxic (alcohol, adriamycin, cocaine) (3) **I**nfectious (Chagas disease, HIV) or *i*diopathic (4) **P**eripartum (5) **E**ndocrine (pheochromocytoma, hypothyroidism, acromegaly)	(1) CHF symptoms (2) Embolic events (3) Arrhythmias (4) Diffuse, laterally placed PMI (5) Third and fourth heart sounds (S_3, S_4), and regurgitation murmurs can be present if dilation has displaced the papillary muscles	(1) Chest X-ray: cardiomegaly (2) Echocardiogram: LV dilation, decreased EF, and hypokinetic ventricular walls	(1) Standard heart failure therapy (2) Anticoagulation if EF is <30% (3) Antiarrhythmics if necessary
Hypertrophic	Subaortic outflow obstruction	(1) Dyspnea, angina, and syncope (2) Associated with bisferiens pulse, with an increased systolic pulse with a double systolic peak	(1) Chest X-ray: cardiomegaly with a boot-shaped heart (2) ECG: LV hypertrophy (3) Echocardiogram: septal thickening and dynamic outflow obstruction	(1) Beta-blocker (2) Calcium channel blocker (verapamil or diltiazem) (3) Disopyramide (4) Can prevent sudden cardiac death using amiodarone or an implantable defibrillator (5) Rate control for atrial fibrillation (avoid digoxin, diuretics, and vasodilators)
Restrictive	(mnemonic—MERSA HS) (1) **M**etastatic disease (2) **E**ndomyocardial fibrosis (3) **R**adiation therapy (4) **S**cleroderma (5) **A**myloidosis (6) **H**emochromatosis (7) **S**arcoidosis	(1) Signs of right-sided heart failure (2) Unresponsiveness to diuretics (3) Thromboembolic events (4) Arrhythmias	(1) Chest X-ray: normal cardiac size (2) ECG: low-voltage QRS, possibly arrhythmias (3) Echocardiogram: Symmetric wall thickening	(1) Treatment of underlying disease (2) Gentle diuresis (3) Rate control

EF, ejection fraction; HIV, human immunodeficiency virus; LV, left ventricular; PMI, point of maximal impulse.

TABLE 1-6 Valvular Heart Disease

Condition	Signs and Symptoms	Evaluation	Treatment
Aortic stenosis	(1) Angina, syncope, heart failure (2) Systolic crescendo/ decrescendo murmur at the RUSB radiating to the sternal notch and apex (3) May hear an ejection click if the aortic valve is bicuspid (4) May have paradoxically split S_2, LV heave, S_4, and delayed carotid pulse (pulsus parvus et tardus)	(1) ECG: LVH, LAE, LBBB (2) Echocardiogram: valve morphology	(1) Patient should avoid vigorous exertion. (2) Give gentle diuresis for CHF and control the hypertension. (3) Repair valve in symptomatic or decompensated patients. An intra-aortic balloon pump can be placed as a bridge to surgery.
Aortic insufficiency	(1) Chronic: LV dilation causing CHF (2) Diastolic decrescendo murmur at LUSB; possible Austin Flint murmur (diastolic rumble at the apex) (3) Rapid rise and fall of pulse (water-hammer pulse) due to widened pulse pressure	(1) ECG: LVH, LAE (2) Chest X-ray: Cardiomegaly (3) Echocardiogram: Shows severity of the aortic insufficiency as well as the LV dilation	(1) Afterload reduction with nifedipine, ACE-I, and hydralazine. (2) Can also use diuresis and digoxin for CHF. (3) Surgery can be done for symptomatic aortic insufficiency.
Acute aortic regurgitation *(a medical emergency requiring immediate surgery)*	(1) Can be caused by infective endocarditis, rupture of the aortic leaflets, aortic root dissection, or acute prosthetic valve dysfunction (2) Patients will usually be in cardiogenic shock	Same as for aortic insufficiency (if possible)	Treat medically with vasodilators (IV nitroprusside and dobutamine) and diuretics, followed by urgent valve replacement.
Rheumatic heart disease *(occurs post-infection with group A beta-hemolytic streptococci)*	(mnemonic—C JoNES) (1) **C**arditis (2) **Jo**ints (polyarthritis) (3) **N**odules (subcutaneous) (4) **E**rythema marginatum (5) **S**ydenham's chorea	(1) Elevated ESR (2) Positive ASO antibody titer (3) Echocardiogram: To assess valvular dysfunction (4) Biopsy: Pericarditis with Aschoff bodies in the myocardium	(1) ASA. (2) Penicillin or erythromycin. (3) Antimicrobial prophylaxis during medical or dental procedures. (4) Prophylaxis for patients with a high risk for reinfection (health care, child care, military): Use penicillin G.

continued

TABLE 1-6 Valvular Heart Disease—cont'd

Condition	Signs and Symptoms	Evaluation	Treatment
Mitral stenosis *(most commonly caused by rheumatic heart disease)*	(1) Dyspnea and pulmonary edema (2) Atrial fibrillation, embolic events (3) Rumble in late diastole at the apex (4) Opening snap	(1) ECG: LAE (2) Chest X-ray: Dilated left atrium (3) Echocardiogram: Valve morphology and left atrial dilation	(1) Na^+ restriction, diuresis, beta-blockers. (2) Endocarditis prophylaxis. (3) Surgical repair if symptomatic.
Mitral valve prolapse *(most common congenital heart abnormality)*	(1) Usually asymptomatic, but patient may have history of syncope, panic attack, or stroke (2) Midsystolic click that may also have a late systolic murmur (3) Secondary mitral valve prolapse can be caused by connective tissue disorders (SLE, Marfan syndrome)	Echocardiogram	(1) Endocarditis prophylaxis if the click is audible. (2) Aspirin or anticoagulation if there is a history of embolic disease. (3) Beta-blockers for symptomatic patients.
Mitral regurgitation *(most commonly caused by degeneration of the valve due to mitral valve prolapse or rheumatic heart disease)*	(1) Acute regurgitation causes pulmonary edema and hypotension (2) Chronic regurgitation causes progressive dyspnea (3) Physical examination findings include a blowing holosystolic murmur at the apex that radiates to the axilla	(1) ECG: LVH, LAE (2) Echocardiogram: Characterizes anatomy and degree of regurgitation	(1) ACE-I, hydralazine/nitrates, digoxin. (2) Endocarditis prophylaxis. (3) Surgical repair for acute, symptomatic, or decompensated mitral regurgitation.

ASA, acetylsalicylic acid; CHF, congestive heart failure; ESR, erythrocyte sedimentation rate; LAE, left atrial enlargement; LBBB, left bundle branch block; LUSB, left upper sternal border; LV, left ventricular; LVH, left ventricular hypertrophy; RUSB, right upper sternal border.

TABLE 1-7
Pericarditis

Type	Signs and Symptoms	Evaluation	Treatment
Pericarditis	(1) Chest pain that radiates to the trapezius and lessens when the patient leans forward (2) Fever (3) Pericardial friction rub (4) Possible pericardial effusion (see below)	(1) ECG: ST elevations in all leads for the first few days, then T wave inversions (2) Pericardiocentesis: Check cytology, cultures, cell counts, etc.	(1) Anti-inflammatory: ASA or NSAIDs (2) Pericardial drainage and antibiotics for infectious effusions (3) Avoid anticoagulants
Pericardial effusion *(the pericardial space can accommodate up to 2 L of fluid)*	Heart sounds may be muffled	(1) Chest X-ray: Patient will have a flask-shaped cardiac silhouette (2) ECG: Electrocardiographic amplitudes may vary from beat to beat owing to increased mobility of the heart within the pericardium (3) Echocardiogram: Fluid	Therapeutic tap can be used if the patient has had the effusion for >2 weeks, has pericardial tamponade, or has suspected purulent pericarditis
Pericardial tamponade	(1) Beck's triad: Distant heart sounds, increased JVP, and hypotension (2) Dyspnea and fatigue (3) Pulsus paradoxus: Decrease in the systolic blood pressure by >10 mm Hg during inspiration	Echocardiogram: To visualize the heart and pericardium	(1) Volume resuscitation (not diuresis) (2) Pericardiocentesis (3) Vasopressors may be necessary if hemodynamic compromise is present (4) Pericardotomy if the effusion is loculated or recurrent
Constrictive pericarditis	(1) Symptoms of right-sided heart failure (Increased JVP with Kussmaul's sign, hepatosplenomegaly, ascites, peripheral edema) (2) Pericardial knock (3) PMI is not palpable (PMI is powerful in restrictive cardiomyopathy) (4) No pulsus paradoxus	(1) Chest X-ray: Pericardial calcification in the lateral view (2) Echocardiogram: Thickened pericardium and abnormal septal movement	Pericardectomy

ASA, acetylsalicylic acid; JVP, jugular venous pulse; NSAIDs, nonsteroidal anti-inflammatory drugs; PMI, point of maximal impulse.

b. Low high-density lipoprotein (HDL): Can be caused by hypertriglyceridemia, obesity, diabetes, cigarette smoking, lack of exercise, beta-blockers, progestin, and anabolic steroids.
c. Hypertriglyceridemia: Can be caused by obesity, diabetes, lack of exercise, alcohol intake, renal insufficiency, estrogen use, and beta-blockers.
2. Familial: Familial hypercholesterolemia, familial combined hyperlipidemia, dysbetalipoproteinemia, and polygenic hypercholesterolemia
B. Symptoms and Signs
1. Xanthomas, xanthelasmas.
2. Corneal arcus: Corneas lose their luster and the pupils become smaller.
3. Pupils may also become irregular in shape.
C. Lipoprotein Analysis
1. Patients with CAD or diabetes should have LDL levels less than 100 mg/dL.
2. Should be done after a 12-hour fast.
3. Can determine approximate LDL levels if the triglyceride levels are less than 400 mg/dL. LDL determinations are less reliable if the triglyceride levels are greater than 400 mg/dL.
D. Therapy
1. Diet control: Half of affected people can reduce lipids by greater than 10%. Patients can attempt diet control alone for 1 month. If this is unsuccessful, add a lipid-lowering agent and follow up after another month.
2. Exercise.
3. Discontinuation of offending drugs.
4. HMG-CoA reductase inhibitors (statins): Drugs of choice for lowering LDL.
a. Liver function tests should be checked for elevations every 6 weeks for 3 months, and then every 6 months. These changes are reversible.
b. Myopathy may occur, especially if the patient is also using cyclosporine, gemfibrozil, niacin, or erythromycin.
5. Bile acid sequestrant resins (cholestyramine, colestipol): These can raise triglycerides.
6. Nicotinic acid (niacin): Can lower triglycerides, raise HDL, and lower LDL but they can also lead to severe liver toxicity if used inappropriately.
7. Fibrates (gemfibrozil and fenofibrate): Drugs of choice for lowering triglyceride levels, but they can lead to gallstone formation.
8. HDL modification: HDL can be increased by lifestyle changes such as weight loss, exercise, and smoking cessation. Niacin, beta-adrenergic antagonists, androgenic compounds, and progestins can also increase HDL. Patients on niacin often experience flushing of the face, which can be decreased with aspirin or long-term use.

X. Endocarditis
A. Types
1. Acute: Infection of normal valves (*S. aureus*).
a. Can often happen as a result of IV drug abuse.

b. Tricuspid valve is the most commonly involved.

2. Subacute: Low-grade infection of abnormal valves (*S. viridans*), which may occur in rheumatic heart disease, in mitral valve prolapse, in bicuspid or calcified aortic valve, or with prosthetic valves.

B. Symptoms and Signs

1. Constitutional signs (anorexia, weight loss, fever) due to bacteremia.
2. Valvular murmurs.
3. Embolic lesions due to septic emboli.
   a. Janeway lesions: Hemorrhagic macules on palms or soles.
   b. Splinter hemorrhages on nail beds.
   c. Neurologic lesions in 30% of patients due to emboli.
4. Immunocomplex disease.
5. Acute endocarditis: Patients may have pleuritic chest pain followed by development of hemoptysis.

C. Evaluation

1. Blood cultures: Three sets from different sites to document bacteremia.
2. Transesophageal echocardiogram: Documents valve abnormalities and can show vegetations.

D. Treatment

1. Empiric therapies: Treat for 4 to 6 weeks.
   a. Acute bacterial endocarditis: Nafcillin + gentamycin. Use vancomycin instead of nafcillin in high methicillin-resistant *S. aureus* (MRSA) prevalence areas.
   b. Subacute bacterial endocarditis: Penicillin or ampicillin + gentamycin.
   c. Prosthetic valve infection: Vancomycin + gentamycin + rifampin.
2. Surgical repair: Indicated for prosthetic valves; persistent, refractory, or invasive infection fungal infection; or recurrent emboli. Antibiotic therapy may be used presurgically to minimize the risk of infection and maximize the chance of healing.
3. Endocarditis prophylaxis: Useful for patients with prosthetic valves or valvular disease. Usually involves the use of ampicillin or amoxicillin before or during a minor dental or surgical procedure. Vancomycin or clindamycin can be used if the patient is allergic to penicillin.

CHAPTER 2

Emergency Medicine Topics

Indications for Exploratory Laporotomy
-GSW to abdomen

CT Scan done in cases of blunt trauma to dx intra-abdominal bleeding and identify intra-abdominal injuries if patient is stable enough to go to Scanner

If there is concern for internal bleeding in unstable in unstable patient, investigate further with emergent ultrasound or diagnostic peritoneal lavage

I. Poisoning (Table 2-1)

II. Trauma

A. Primary Survey (Mnemonic—ABCDE: **a**irway, **b**reathing, **c**irculation, **d**isability, **e**xposure/**e**nvironment)

1. **A**irway: Evaluate airway patency and immobilize the cervical spine.

a. A patient who can speak has a patent airway. The airway is assumed to be nonpatent in an unconscious patient.

b. Maneuvers to establish a patent airway include a chin lift with jaw thrust, endotracheal intubation, nasotracheal intubation (this is contraindicated in patients with maxillofacial fracture), and cricothyroidotomy.

2. **B**reathing

a. Examination consists of inspection, auscultation, percussion (for hyperresonance or dullness), and palpation (for subcutaneous emphysema or flail segments).

b. Life-threatening conditions include

(1) Airway obstruction.

(2) Tension pneumothorax: Causes dyspnea, chest pain, decreased breath sounds, tracheal shift away from the affected side, and hyperresonance on the affected side. Treat with thoracostomy. (See Chapter 13.)

(3) Open pneumothorax.

(4) Flail chest: Occurs with some chest wall fractures when a segment of chest wall will move paradoxically and results in hypoventilation. Treat with positive pressure ventilation.

(5) Cardiac tamponade: Patients have Beck's triad (decreased heart sounds, jugular venous distension, and decreased blood pressure). Treat with immediate intravenous fluid bolus, pericardiocentesis, and subsequent surgical exploration.

(6) Massive hemothorax: Bleeding into the thorax can cause greater than 1500 mL of blood to be drained from the chest tube. Patients have hypotension, unilaterally decreased breath sounds, and dullness to chest percussion. Treat with volume replacement, tube thoracostomy, and exploratory thoracotomy if the bleeding exceeds 200 mL/hr.

TABLE 2-1 Recognition and Treatment of Poisoning

Poison	Symptoms	Antidote or Treatment
Acetminophen	Nausea, vomiting, delayed jaundice, and hepatic failure within 96 hours	N-acetyl cysteine
Anticholinergics (atropine, TCAs, antihistamines, phenothiazines)	Mania, delirium, dry mouth and eyes, tachycardia	(1) Physostigmine for atropine and antihistamines (in life-threatening situations) (2) Sodium bicarbonate and magnesium sulfate for TCAs.
Aspirin	Causes early alkalosis, late acidosis, and presents with tachypnea, fever, lethargy, and diaphoresis	Alkalinization of urine, dialysis, and supportive care
Cholinergics (organophosphates)	Miosis, salivation, urination, bronchospasm, weakness, and confusion	Pralidoxime chloride
Hydrocarbons	Ataxia, coma, and neuropathy	Prevent aspiration, and do not perform lavage
Iron	(1) Hematemesis, diarrhea, hypotension, and hepatic failure (2) Pills can be seen on the abdominal radiograph	Deferoxamine chelation
Opiates	Coma, respiratory depression, and pinpoint pupils	Naloxone
Benzodiazepines	Sedation	Flumazenil
Sympathomimetics (amphetamines, cocaine, theophylline)	Tachycardia, hypertension, psychosis, seizures, mydriasis, and diaphoresis	Benzodiazepines for agitation
Carbon monoxide	Headache, dizziness, coma, skin bullae, and cherry red discoloration of skin and blood	Hyperbaric O_2
Cyanide	Coma, convulsions, hyperpnea, and a bitter almond odor	Amyl nitrite, then sodium nitrite, then sodium thiosulfate
Ethylene glycol	Metabolic acidosis, hypocalcemia, and oxalate crystalluria "envelope-shaped" crystals	Dialysis with fomepizole or ethanol
Beta-blockers	Hypotension, dizziness	Glucagon
Calcium channel blockers	Hypotension, dizziness	Calcium chloride
Coumadin	Bruising or bleeding	Vitamin K

continued

TABLE 2-1 Recognition and Treatment of Poisoning—cont'd

Poison	Symptoms	Antidote or Treatment
Digoxin	Bradycardia	Digoxin-binding antibody fragments
Isoniazid	Possible peripheral neuritis, toxic encephalopathy, and seizures	Pyridoxine
Lead	Lead >20 μg/dL causes developmental delay and behavior problems	Dimercaprol, EDTA, and oral succimer

TCA, tricyclic antidepressant.

3. **C**irculation
   a. Check pulses: A palpable radial pulse means that the systolic blood pressure (SBP) is greater than 80 mm Hg. A palpable femoral or carotid pulse means that the SBP is greater than 60 mm Hg.
   b. Assess heart rate: Many patients with blood loss have tachycardia, but tachycardia may not be present with hypovolemic shock if the patient has an injured spinal cord or is taking beta-blockers.
   c. Evaluate peripheral perfusion and blood pressure to help determine volume status.
   d. Gain intravenous access using two large-bore lines in the upper extremities. For initial volume resuscitation, infuse 3 L of lactated Ringer's solution for every 1 L of blood loss.
   e. Determine class of blood loss (Table 2-2).
4. **D**isability: Evaluate mental status and basic neurologic function.
   a. Grade overall mental status using the Glasgow Coma Scale (GCS). See Table 2-3.
   b. Observe pupils, motor and sensory function, and level of consciousness to characterize the immediate neurologic effects of the injury.
   c. Determine whether a patient with a progressive decline in mental status is experiencing increasing intracranial pressure from hematomas or brain edema.
5. **E**xposure/**E**nvironment: Disrobe and examine patient for other injuries, and keep the patient in a warm environment.

B. Secondary Survey: Consists of a complete physical examination. Common findings in trauma are described in Table 2-4.

C. Decompression of the stomach and bladder can be accomplished with a nasogastric (NG) tube and Foley catheter.
   1. The NG tube is contraindicated in patients with maxillofacial fracture. Use an oral-gastric tube in these cases.
   2. A Foley catheter can only be placed following a normal rectal examination and genital examination. A high-riding prostate or other signs of urethral tear (periscrotal hematoma, blood at the urethral meatus) are contraindications for

TABLE 2-2 Classes of Blood Loss and Associated Symptoms

Class	Volume of Blood Lost	Symptoms and Signs
I	<750 mL	No symptoms.
II	750–1500 mL	Heart rate will be >100, respiratory rate will range from 20 to 30, but blood pressure will be normal.
III	1500–2000 mL	Heart rate will be >120, respiratory rate will range from 30 to 40, urine output will be markedly decreased, the patient will be confused, and blood pressure will be low.
IV	>2000 mL	Heart rate will be >140, respiratory rate will be >35, the patient will be confused and lethargic and will have negligible urine output.

catheter placement. If the examination is questionable, patency of the urethra can be established by a retrograde ureterogram.

D. Diagnostic Evaluation
   1. Send blood for type and cross-match, complete blood count (CBC), liver function tests (LFTs), lactic acid level, and coagulation tests (PT, PTT, and INR).
   2. Send urine for urinalysis.
   3. Radiography should be done of the chest (AP chest film), cervical spine (lateral cervical spine film), and pelvis (AP pelvis film). If spinal injury is

A cervical collar should not be removed until cervical fracture has been ruled out, which usually involves both clinical and radiographic evaluation.

TABLE 2-3 The Glasgow Coma Scale*

Category	Score	Behavior
Eye opening (4 eyes)	4 3 2 1	Spontaneous To voice To pain Never
Motor (6-cylinder motor)	6 5 4 3 2 1	To commands Localizes to pain Withdraws from pain Decorticate posturing (arms flexed) Decerebrate rigidity (arms extended) None
Verbal	5 4 3 2 1	Appropriate Confused Inappropriate words Incomprehensible sounds No sounds

*Each of these scores is tabulated and then added for a total Glasgow coma scale (GCS) score. The verbal score is not measured in intubated patients (a T is used to indicate intubation). The maximum score is 15 for a nonintubated patient and 10T for an intubated patient. GCS of ≤8 is consistent with coma in a nonintubated patient.

TABLE 2-4
Common Findings on Physical Examination in Trauma

Location	Findings
Face	Signs of facial or basilar skull fracture (raccoon eyes, Battle's sign)
Ears	Hemotympanum and otorrhea
Eyes	Direct injuries or traumatic hyphema (blood in the anterior chamber of the eye)
Nose	Rhinorrhea, nasal septal hematoma (can cause pressure necrosis of the nasal septum)
Mouth	Assess jaw alignment for mandibular fracture
Neck	(1) Crepitus or subcutaneous emphysema may be present with tracheobronchial disruption or pneumothorax (2) Tracheal deviation may be present in pneumothorax (3) Jugular venous distention may be present in cardiac tamponade (4) Carotid bruits will be present in carotid artery injury
Back	(1) Remember to examine the back for additional sites of injury. (2) Vertebral column injury can often be diagnosed with radiography. Specific types of injury include Jefferson's fracture (fracture through the arches of C1), hangman's fracture (fracture through the pedicles of C2 due to hyperextension), odontoid fracture (fracture through the odontoid process of C2), and clay shoveler's fracture (fracture of the spinous process of C7).
Chest	(1) Perform a lateral and anteroposterior compression of the ribs to assess for broken ribs or sternum. (2) Widened mediastinum (usually recognized radiographically) may be present with aortic injury. (3) Any injury below T4 may also involve the abdomen.
Abdomen	(1) The patient must be alert and oriented for an abdominal assessment to be adequate. (2) Assess intestines, liver, and spleen for injury. Assess for peritonitis and fluid collections.
Spleen	(1) The spleen may rupture at the time of trauma, or at a later time with a rupture of a subcapsular hematoma. (2) Signs of splenic rupture include hemoperitoneum, Kehr's sign (referred pain to the left shoulder), and pain with a mass in the abdominal left upper quadrant. (3) Treat a spleen rupture with splenectomy or splenorrhaphy (partial splenectomy). Complications of splenectomy include thrombocytosis, subphrenic abscess, and overwhelming postsplenectomy sepsis (OPSS). OPSS involves sepsis and coma due to infection with encapsulated organisms (*S. pneumoniae, Meningococcus, H. influenzae, E. coli*) with a high mortality.
Rectum	Assess sphincter tone/anal wink reflex (for spinal cord function), presence of blood (for colorectal trauma), and prostate position (for urethral injury).
Pelvis	(1) Perform a lateral compression of the iliac crests and greater trochanters and an anterior compression of the symphysis pubis to test for fractures. (2) Pelvic bleeding from the sacral veins can be dangerous. This can be treated with military anti-shock (MAST) trousers and subsequent embolization of the arteries supplying the bleeding site.
Extremities	(1) Assess fractures, joint injuries, open wounds, motor and sensory function, and pulses. (2) Absent pulses may be found in the presence of a dislocated or broken bone.

suspected, AP spine, open mouth odontoid, and a "swimmer's view" will allow greater visualization of the vertebral column.
4. Aortic injury can be assessed with thoracic aortograms and transesophageal ultrasound.
5. Abdominal injury can be assessed using ultrasonography, CT, and peritoneal lavage. Peritoneal lavage can be performed following decompression of the stomach and bladder, and a positive result includes an RBC count greater than 100,000/mm^3, or a WBC count greater than 500/mm^3.
6. A chest tube can be placed if hemothorax is suspected. Drainage and positive pressure ventilatory support can be used in cases of massive hemothorax.

III. Burn Injuries
A. Determination of Burn Area
1. The "rule of 9s" can be used to quickly characterize the involved body surface area in a burn injury (Fig. 2-1).
a. Head = 9%
b. Arms = 9% each

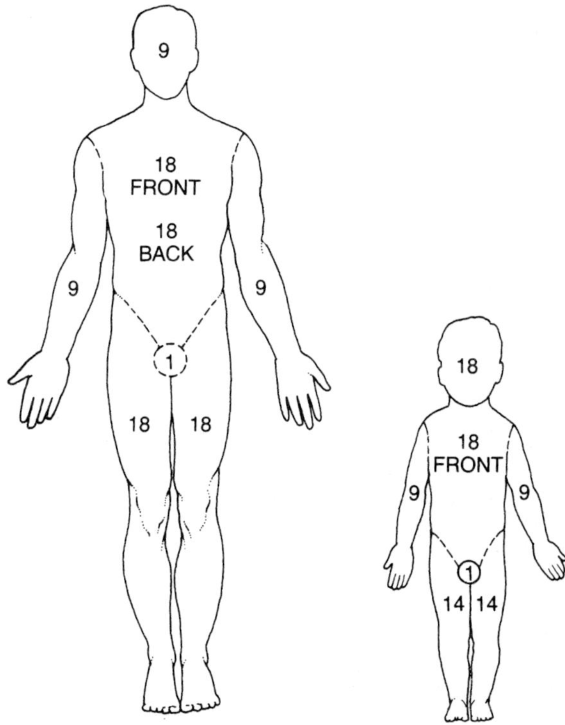

2-1: *Calculation of surface area involvement in burn injury. According to the "rule of 9s," most portions of the body will account for either 9% or 18% of the total body surface area. The proportions are slightly different in children, who proportionally have more area in their heads and less area in their legs.*

c. Front and back of the torso = 18% each
d. Perineum = 1%

2. Alternatively, the "rule of the palm" can be used to characterize discontinuous burns. In this method, the area of the patient's palm is approximately 1% of the patient's body surface area.

B. Types of Burns
1. Thermal: Due to heat and will display skin involvement in areas of exposure.
2. Electrical: May show only minimal skin involvement at the entry and exit sites. However, significant muscle and nerve damage could occur. Cardiac arrhythmias are common, and fascial compartment syndromes and myoglobinuria can be indicators of muscle injury.
3. Steam: Moist air has a higher heat capacity than dry air, so steam will cause burns more quickly and severely than dry air of the same temperature.
4. Chemical: Alkali burns are more serious than acid burns owing to the lack of buffering for alkali in the blood.

Compartment syndromes involve an increase in tissue pressures in tissue compartments that are incapable of expansion, such as the fascial compartments of the arm or leg. They present with neurologic deficits in the affected limb and can lead to necrosis in the affected limb if left untreated. Treatment consists of a fasciotomy, which allows decompression of the compartment.

C. Severity of a Burn Injury
1. First degree: Superficial burn that is red without blistering. Pain usually resolves in 2 to 3 days.
2. Second degree: Partial thickness burn that involves the epidermis and variable layers of the dermis. The patient will have blisters, and it may take weeks to heal.
3. Third degree: Full-thickness burn involving the entire dermis and epidermis, which prevents reepithelialization. Healing requires débridement or skin grafting. Skin will not have sensation.
4. Circumferential burns of the trunk or limbs can cause compression and vascular or respiratory compromise owing to circumferential swelling of the tissue. Decompression of the area through surgical incision of the burned tissue may be necessary to prevent impairment of the blood supply by circumferential swelling.

D. Inhalation Injury
1. Occurs most frequently in patients with a history of a burn injury in an enclosed space, facial burns, singed facial hair, hoarseness, coughing, wheezing, and carbonaceous sputum.
2. In cases of suspected inhalation injury, bronchoscopy and a carboxyhemoglobin test should be done to further characterize the severity of injury.
3. Patients will subsequently develop pulmonary insufficiency owing to carbon monoxide poisoning, bronchospasm, edema, and atelectasis. Pneumonia can occur 5 to 10 days after injury.
4. Carbon monoxide poisoning presents with cherry-red skin, hypoxemia, mental status changes, and persistent acidosis. Treatment is with hyperbaric oxygen.

E. Infection
1. Common organisms include *Staphylococcus aureus* and *Streptococcus, Pseudomonas, Escherichia coli, Enterococcus,* and *Candida* species.

2. More than 100,000 organisms per gram of tissue is diagnostic for invasive infection. Further evaluation can be done, if necessary, with a full-thickness skin biopsy.
3. Tetanus (due to *Clostridium tetani*) can also be a problem, so immunize all patients who have not had a tetanus shot in the last year. Also, administer antitetanus immune globulin if the patient has never been immunized.
4. Infection can cause tissue damage and upgrade a partial thickness injury to a full-thickness injury.

F. Criteria for Hospitalization of a Burn Patient (any of the following):
1. Second-degree burns—greater than 20% of body surface area.
2. Third-degree burns—greater than 10% of body surface area.
3. Any burns greater than 10% of body surface area in children or elderly persons.
4. Any burns involving the hands, face, feet, or perineum.
5. Any burns with inhalation injury.
6. Any burns with associated trauma.
7. Any electrical burns.

G. Treatment
1. Stop the burning process (remove burning clothes, flush away burning chemicals).
2. Address airway, breathing, and circulation issues.
3. Treat the patient immediately with humidified 100% O_2 for carbon monoxide poisoning.
4. Fluid resuscitation
   a. Calculate the required fluids for the first 24 hours: 4 mL of crystalloid per kilogram of body weight multiplied by the percentage of surface area that has the burn.

   $$\text{Required fluids} = 4\,\text{mL/kg} \times \%\ \text{body surface burned}$$

   b. Give half of this volume over the first 8 hours and the other half over the remaining 16 hours.
   c. Resuscitate using isotonic solutions that do not contain glucose.
   d. After 24 hours, capillary integrity returns to normal, so colloid solutions can be used. 5% colloid (albumin) solutions are often used at a volume of 0.3–0.5 mL/kg per percentage of surface area burned.
5. Wound care
   a. Cleanse burns with a topical antimicrobial and gently débride blisters initially.
   b. Antimicrobials used include
      (1) Sulfamylon: Broadest spectrum with best penetration, but it is painful when applied and can cause acidosis.
      (2) Silvadene: Does not penetrate as well, but it is not painful. It can cause neutropenia.
      (3) Silver nitrate: Bacteriostatic, but it stains the skin.
      (4) Betadine: Not used because it dries up the eschar.

c. After fluid resuscitation and pulmonary stabilization, excise any eschars and begin skin grafting. Early skin grafting and use of pressure dressings can prevent scarring.
d. Circumferential burns may require incision of the burned area to relieve pressure.

6. Treatment of other complications
a. Carbon monoxide poisoning: Use hyperbaric oxygen therapy.
b. Myoglobinuria: Hydrate aggressively and give mannitol, other diuretics, and bicarbonate to increase myoglobin excretion and prevent renal damage.
c. Curling's ulcer (a gastric or duodenal ulcer associated with burn injury): Give proton pump inhibitors.

IV. Shock

A. Types of Shock

1. Hypovolemic shock: Occurs as a result of decreased circulating blood volume following blood fluid loss. Patients have pale, cool, clammy skin; tachycardia; oliguria; and altered mental status. Patients often have a history consistent with vomiting, diarrhea, or bleeding from injury or gastrointestinal sources.
2. Distributive shock: Widespread vasodilation (both arterial and venous) will cause hypotension. Cardiac output can return to normal after volume resuscitation. One example is septic shock, where inflammatory cytokines cause widespread arterial and venous dilation.
3. Cardiogenic shock: Occurs owing to a dramatic reduction in cardiac functioning from a cardiac injury (usually an MI). Patients frequently have signs of peripheral hypoperfusion and symptoms consistent with an MI.
4. Extracardiac obstructive shock: Occurs owing to an obstruction in cardiovascular flow. Causes include pericardial tamponade, constrictive pericarditis, and massive pulmonary emboli. Pericardial tamponade and constrictive pericarditis will have equal pressures in the left and right sides of the heart, whereas pulmonary emboli will cause pulmonary hypertension and right-sided heart failure. Patients will have increased jugular venous pressure, causing jugular venous distention.
5. Neurogenic shock: Occurs following spinal cord trauma. Patients have bradycardia and loss of sympathetic tone to the extremities.

The systemic inflammatory response syndrome (SIRS) is a severe form of distributive shock that can be initiated by stresses including ischemia, pancreatitis, burns, and trauma. Large-scale cytokine release will produce hemodynamic manifestations of septic shock and the refractory catabolic state and tissue wasting seen in severe injury and infection. This can result in multisystem organ failure.

B. Evaluation

1. Can be strictly clinical or involve the use of a pulmonary artery (Swan-Ganz) catheter (Table 2-5).
2. ECG and echocardiography can identify cardiac and pericardial disease.
3. All standard blood tests should performed, but treatment should be administered immediately without waiting for the results.

Although the definition of hypotension is a mean arterial pressure less than 60 mm Hg, hypotension can actually occur at higher mean arterial pressures in patients who are chronically hypertensive.

C. Treatment

1. Start with fluid challenge of 500–1000 mL of IV fluids. Continue fluid resuscitation and transfuse blood (as needed) in patients with noncardiogenic shock.

TABLE 2-5 Use of Pulmonary Artery Catheter Measurements to Classify Shock

Cause	Pulmonary Capillary Wedge Pressure	Cardiac Output
Hypovolemic	Decreased	Decreased
Distributive (septic)	Decreased or normal	Increased or normal
Cardiogenic	Increased	Decreased
Obstructive (pericardial tamponade)	Increased	Decreased
Obstructive (pulmonary embolism)	Normal or decreased	Decreased

2. If the patient remains hypotensive, vasopressors (norepinephrine or dopamine) can be used.
3. Admit the patient to the intensive care unit.
4. Patients with cardiogenic shock can develop pulmonary edema if excessive fluids are administered. Definitive therapy involves surgery (either coronary revascularization, intra-aortic balloon pump placement, or corrective surgery for valvular abnormalities).
5. For septic shock, start antimicrobial therapy and restore the blood pressure and tissue perfusion using the principles described previously.

Low-dose dopamine does not cause vasoconstriction. For shock patients, use high doses (4–20 μg/kg/min) of dopamine.

CHAPTER 3

Endocrinology

I. Pituitary Disorders
   A. Hypopituitarism
      1. Symptoms and signs
         a. Patients generally have weakness, fatigue, headache, and hypotension. Visual field changes (bitemporal hemianopsia) may be present due to mass effects on the optic chiasm.
         b. Endocrine abnormalities may be present if specific hormones are deficient (Table 3-1).
      2. Diagnostic evaluation
         a. Head CT to evaluate for possible pituitary tumor.
         b. Target gland hormones will be low.
         c. Inability to elicit pituitary hormone release with appropriate stimuli (e.g., failure to elicit growth hormone [GH] release with hypoglycemia).
      3. Treatment
         a. Surgical removal of any tumor.
         b. Hormone replacement when available.
   B. Hyperpituitarism: Usually causes the overproduction of a single hormone, resulting in a variety of syndromes.
      1. Cushing's disease (increased adrenocorticotropic hormone [ACTH]): See later discussion.
      2. Hyperthyroidism (increased thyroid-stimulating hormone [TSH]): See later discussion.
      3. Hyperprolactinemia
         a. Patients can have amenorrhea, galactorrhea, impotence, and infertility.
         b. Can be caused by medications (antipsychotics), pregnancy, renal failure, and cirrhosis.
         c. Tests include MRI and prolactin level (>200 ng/mL).
         d. Treat with bromocriptine or cabergoline. If patients are unresponsive to treatment or have visual or neurologic abnormalities, then attempt surgery.
   C. Acromegaly: Caused by an overproduction of GH as an adult.
      1. Patients can have an increase in soft tissue, jaw, and tongue size accompanied by headache and arthralgias. Associated conditions such as impotence, amenorrhea, diabetes mellitus, and colonic polyps may also be present.
      2. Diagnostic evaluation
         a. GH measurement 3 hours after an oral glucose load.
         b. Increased somatomedin C.
         c. MRI to evaluate for tumor.
      3. Treatment includes transsphenoidal surgery, irradiation, and therapy with octreotide and dopamine agonists.

TABLE 3-1 Features of Pituitary Hormone Deficiency*

Hormone Insufficiency	Symptoms and Signs	Evaluation
Adrenocorticotropic hormone (ACTH)	Weakness, weight loss, nausea, and vomiting. Physical findings include hypotension and anorexia. Skin hyperpigmentation will not be present.	(1) Insulin tolerance test: IV insulin infusion and hypoglycemia will fail to elicit cortisol release. (2) Corticotropin-releasing hormone (CRH) infusion will fail to elicit ACTH release.
Thyroid-stimulating hormone (TSH)	Symptoms include weakness, fatigue, cold intolerance, constipation, depression, weight gain, hoarseness, and menstrual irregularities. Signs include dry, cold skin; nonpitting edema (myxedema); bradycardia; and hyporeflexia.	(1) Thyroid hormone and TSH levels will be low. (2) Thyrotropin-releasing hormone (TRH) infusion will fail to elicit TSH release.
Prolactin (PRL)	Inability to lactate postpartum.	TRH infusion will fail to elicit PRL release.
Growth hormone (GH)	Short stature since childhood, or adult onset of increased abdominal adiposity, weakness, and decreased exercise tolerance.	Insulin tolerance test: IV insulin infusion and hypoglycemia will fail to elicit GH release.
Antidiuretic hormone (ADH)	Severe polyuria and polydipsia.	Urine osmolality will be low but will increase in response to vasopressin administration.
Follicle-stimulating hormone (FSH) and Luteinizing hormone (LH)	Impotence, amenorrhea, infertility or decreased libido, with loss of pubic and body hair.	(1) Clomiphene test: FSH and LH will fail to rise after 5 days of oral clomiphene citrate. (2) Infusion of gonadotropin-releasing hormone (GnRH) will fail to elicit LH and FSH release.

*In most cases, patients will have a deficiency of multiple hormones and a combination of the associated symptoms.

II. Thyroid Disease
   A. Hypothyroidism
      1. Symptoms and signs
         a. Patients have complaints of weakness, fatigue, cold intolerance, constipation, depression, weight gain, hoarseness, and menstrual irregularities.
         b. Physical examination findings include dry cold skin, nonpitting edema (myxedema), bradycardia, and hyporeflexia.
      2. Causes (Table 3-2)
      3. Diagnostic evaluation

TABLE 3-2
Major Causes of Hypothyroidism

Condition	Description
Hashimoto's thyroiditis	(1) Chronic lymphocytic thyroiditis with antibodies to thyroglobulin. (2) Patients have neck enlargement with pain and tenderness. (3) Patients are usually euthyroid or hypothyroid. (4) Can be diagnosed by high-titer serum antithyroid antibodies. The most specific associated antibody is antithyroid peroxidase (antimicrosomal) antibody, but other antithyroid antibodies may also be present.
Reidel's struma	Chronic thyroiditis in which patients have profound irreversible thyroiditis with extensive fibrosis.
Iatrogenic	(1) Treatments for hyperthyroidism (such as surgery or radioiodine treatment) can leave patients with hypothyroidism. (2) Medications such as lithium and sulfonamides can impair thyroid hormone synthesis.
Congenital	See Chapter 11.
Thyroid neoplasia	(1) Papillary thyroid cancer is the most common type and usually occurs in patients with a history of irradiation. There are psammoma bodies on histologic examination, and the cancer is responsive to radioiodine. (2) Medullary thyroid cancer is composed of calcitonin-producing cells; it has an aggressive course and occurs as part of several familial neoplasia syndromes (including MEN IIA and IIB). (3) Follicular thyroid cancer is a well-differentiated variant that is responsive to radioiodine. (4) Hurthle cell thyroid cancer originates from follicular cells and is considered malignant only if it grows to greater than 4 cm in size. (5) Anaplastic thyroid cancer is an aggressive variant that occurs primarily in older people. Histologic examination shows undifferentiated cell types, and therapy does not improve survival.
Pituitary insufficiency (secondary hypothyroidism)	(1) Caused by neoplasia, surgery, irradiation, or postpartum pituitary necrosis. (2) Patients have low TSH and low thyroid hormone levels.

a. Fine-needle aspiration: To distinguish between cystic and solid lesions. It can also determine cellular characteristics to evaluate for the presence of certain cancers.
b. 24-Hour iodide uptake: Will be low in thyroiditis.
c. Ultrasound: To distinguish between cystic and solid lesions.
d. TSH level: TSH will be high in primary hypothyroidism (due to thyroid disease) and low in secondary hypothyroidism (due to pituitary disease and TRH deficiency). If TSH levels are borderline, then proceed to T_3 and T_4 level tests (Fig. 3-1).
e. Radioactive scans with I^{123} or Tc^{99m} can evaluate lesions as warm versus cold. Cold lesions suggest malignancy.

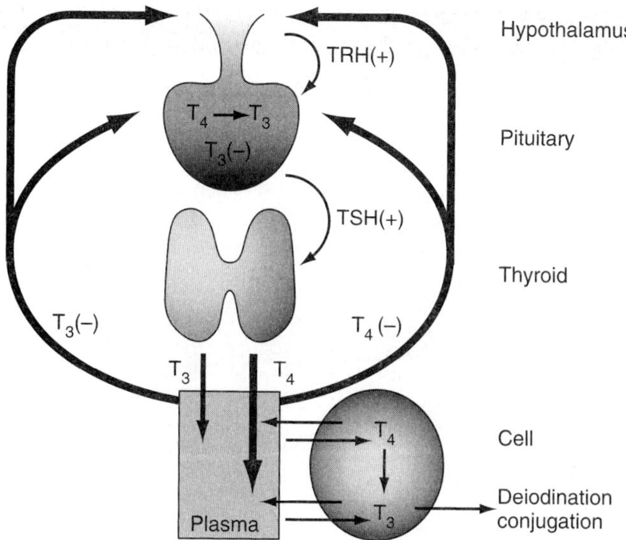

3-1: *Thyroid hormone physiology. Under normal conditions, thyrotropin-releasing hormone (TRH) is released from the hypothalamus, which causes the release of thyroid-stimulating hormone (TSH) from the anterior pituitary. TSH then causes the release of triiodothyronine (T_3) and thyroxine (T_4) by the thyroid gland, which act on various peripheral organs. T_3 and T_4 also regulate TRH and TSH secretion through negative feedback mechanisms. In primary hypothyroidism (due to thyroid dysfunction) T_3 and T_4 are low despite high TSH levels. In secondary hypothyroidism (due to pituitary or hypothalamic dysfunction), the levels of TSH, T_3, and T_4 all are low.*

4. Treatment is dependent on the cause of the hypothyroidism.
   a. Hashimoto's thyroiditis: Levothyroxine.
   b. Subacute thyroiditis: Aspirin and maybe cortisol.
   c. Myxedema coma: IV levothyroxine with or without hydrocortisone.
   d. Papillary thyroid cancer: Lobectomy with radioiodine adjuvant therapy. Levothyroxine must be given for life following total thyroidectomy to suppress TSH secretion. There is 95% survival to 20 years.
   e. Medullary thyroid cancer: Total thyroidectomy with a central node dissection for lesions confined to the thyroid. Unilateral modified radical neck dissection can be performed if metastatic disease is suspected. There is 80% survival to 10 years.

B. Hyperthyroidism (Thyrotoxicosis)
1. Symptoms and signs
   a. Patients may complain of heat intolerance, weight loss with increased appetite, emotional instability, insomnia, fatigue, muscle weakness, amenorrhea, and diarrhea.
   b. Physical examination findings include tachycardia, atrial arrhythmia, congestive heart failure, hyperkinetic behavior, and thyroid bruits.
2. Causes (Table 3-3)
3. Diagnostic tests
   a. Fine-needle aspiration
   b. 24-Hour iodide uptake: Will be high in Graves' disease.

TABLE 3-3 Causes of Hyperthyroidism

Condition	Description and Treatment
Graves' disease	(1) An autoimmune disease in which antibodies that bind to the TSH receptor cause thyroid stimulation. Additional antithyroid antibodies may be present. (2) Patients typically have an enlarged thyroid, skin thickening in the pretibial region (pretibial myxedema), and eye findings (proptosis, tearing, and rarely visual impairment). (3) Treat with antithyroid medications, radioiodine, and surgery. Surgery results in a more complete resolution of the eye abnormalities than does radioiodine.
De Quervain's disease (subacute thyroiditis)	(1) Patients experience thyroid pain and swelling with an elevated ESR but no antithyroid antibodies, with symptoms of hyperthyroidism. (2) Probably caused by a virus.
Toxic adenoma	(1) Patients have symptoms of hyperthyroidism with a solitary "hot nodule" on the thyroid scan. (2) Treat with radioiodine or thyroid lobectomy.
Toxic multinodular goiter	(1) Patients have hyperthyroidism and a thyroid scan that shows multiple foci of "hot nodules." (2) Treat with subtotal thyroidectomy or radioiodine.

c. Ultrasound: To distinguish between cystic and solid lesions.

d. TSH level: Will be low in primary hyperthyroidism (due to thyroid disease) and high in secondary hypothyroidism (due to pituitary disease and excess TRH). If TSH levels are borderline, then proceed to T_3 and T_4 level tests.

e. Radioactive scans with I^{123} or Tc^{99m} can evaluate lesions as warm versus cold. Cold lesions suggest malignancy.

4. Treatment

a. Benign lesions should be treated with suppressive doses of levothyroxine, and biopsy should be repeated in 3 to 6 months. The resultant decrease in TSH secretion following L-thyroxine therapy may shrink the lesion.

b. Thianomides (propylthiouracil, methimazole, carbimazole) can also be used for hyperthyroidism. Propylthiouracil is a preferred therapy for pregnant patients. Patients will need to take these for 1 to 3 years; the most significant side effect is agranulocytosis.

c. Iodine 131 treatment can shrink the thyroid gland as it accumulates radioactive iodine. Patients who undergo I^{131} therapy need to be medicated to euthyroid levels prior to I^{131} treatment in order to minimize the risk of excessive thyroid hormone release during treatment. Patients receiving I^{131} therapy should be informed that their eyes may become more proptotic.

d. Beta-blockers (e.g., propranolol) can be used for symptomatic relief of tachycardia, tremor, anxiety, and heat intolerance. They should not be used as the sole agents in therapy, however, because they act by decreasing sensitivity to thyroid hormones rather than by returning the patient to a euthyroid state.

e. Surgical interventions: Thyroid lobectomy or total thyroidectomy.

(1) Indications for surgery in thyroid disease include malignancy, nonmalignant lesions with significant mass, and compression symptoms due to the thyroid mass.

(2) Antithyroid drugs (propylthiouracil and methimazole) must be used before surgery to restore the euthyroid state. High doses of iodine are also administered because they paradoxically decrease iodine organification (through the Wolff-Chaikoff effect). Propranolol is used to decrease the heart rate.

5. Complications of therapy

a. Most patients receiving I^{131} therapy will have hypothyroidism following treatment.

b. Complications following surgery include hoarseness from recurrent laryngeal injury, transient hypoparathyroidism, hemorrhage, and hypothyroidism.

c. Thyroid storm is an acute adrenergic outburst that is augmented by the presence of thyroid hormone. It manifests clinically as hyperthermia, tachycardia, hypertension, and eventual hypotension and death. Treat the tachycardia with propranolol, and use oxygen and IV glucose to treat the hypermetabolic state. Use iodine and corticosteroids to prevent the development of adrenal insufficiency. Overall thyroid storm has a 10% mortality rate.

III. Parathyroid Disease

A. Hypoparathyroidism

1. Common causes include the surgical removal of the parathyroid glands and hypomagnesemia, which causes functional hypoparathyroidism by inducing resistance to PTH.

2. Symptoms and signs

a. Patients complain of perioral numbness, tingling of the fingers, intense anxiety, and involuntary muscle spasms.

b. Physical examination findings include Chvostek's sign (facial nerve contraction when cheek is tapped), Trousseau's sign (carpal spasm after occlusion of the brachial artery for 3 minutes), and spontaneous carpopedal spasm.

3. Diagnostic evaluation

a. Decreased serum Ca^{++} with concomitantly increased serum phosphorus and decreased or absent urinary Ca^{++}.

b. Parathyroid hormone levels: Will be low and will help differentiate hypoparathyroidism from other causes of hypercalcemia.

c. Human chorionic gonadotropin (hCG): Will be high in parathyroid carcinoma.

4. Treatment includes replacement of Ca^{++}, vitamin D, and Mg^{++} (if necessary).

Parathyroid hormone (PTH) stimulates osteoclastic bone resorption, increases tubular reabsorption of Ca^{++}, impairs renal tubular reabsorption of phosphate, and indirectly increases intestinal absorption of Ca^{++} by inducing renal hydroxylation of vitamin D. Calcitonin prevents osteoclastic bone resorption.

B. Hyperparathyroidism
1. Types (Table 3-4).
2. Patients usually have vague constitutional symptoms, and may have associated problems with renal stones, pancreatitis, and peptic ulcer disease due to hypercalcemia.
3. Diagnostic evaluation
a. Serum Ca^{++} will be high, and phosphorus will be low.
b. Radiography may show subperiosteal bone resorption (usually in the hands).
c. Bone densitometry may help when deciding whether to operate on apparently asymptomatic patients.
d. Localization studies can be performed using Tc^{99m} sestamibi. Localization is more important in patients who require reexploration.
4. Treatment
a. Treat acute hyperparathyroidism with volume repletion followed by furosemide to promote Na^+ and Ca^{++} diuresis. Mithramycin can inhibit bone resorption. Replace K^+ and Mg^{++} as needed. Operate when the patient is stable. In patients who cannot undergo surgery, treat long-term

TABLE 3-4
Types of Hyperparathyroidism

Condition	Definition	Symptoms and Signs
Primary hyperparathyroidism	Overproduction of parathyroid hormone (PTH) by the parathyroid gland in the absence of external stimulation.	(1) Patients have kidney stones, bone pain or fractures, pancreatitis, depression, anxiety, muscle pain, and weakness. (2) Mnemonic—stones, bones, groans, and psychiatric undertones. (3) Treat with surgical removal, sparing some parathyroid tissue.
Secondary hyperparathyroidism	(1) Reactive hyperparathyroidism of renal disease. (2) Renal disease prevents the hydroxylation of vitamin D and prevents intestinal Ca^{++} resorption. This will decrease plasma Ca^{++} and result in a need for higher PTH.	(1) Patients have bone pain or tenderness with pathologic fractures and proximal muscle weakness, severe pruritus, GI problems, and painful extraskeletal calcifications. (2) Treat with renal transplantation.
Tertiary hyperparathyroidism	Persistent high PTH after correction of secondary hyperparathyroidism.	(1) Patients continue to have hyperparathyroidism after receiving a renal transplant. (2) Remove all parathyroid glands and place 30 mg of thyroid tissue in the arm. Symptoms are unresponsive to medical management.

with oral phosphate, estrogens, or bisphosphonates to impair osteoclast function.

b. Treat secondary hyperparathyroidism by lowering phosphorus intake and increasing Ca^{++} intake.

c. Surgical treatments

(1) Surgery is indicated in all cases of symptomatic disease unless the operative risk is prohibitive.

(2) If one gland is clearly enlarged relative to the others, single removal is warranted. If all four parathyroids are enlarged, then hyperplasia has occurred and a subtotal parathyroidectomy (removal of three glands and part of the fourth) should be done.

5. Complications

a. Hungry bone syndrome (rebound hypoparathyroidism) can occur following surgical removal of the parathyroids. This occurs because the tissue left behind was most likely suppressed by the hypersecretion of PTH by the adenomatous tissue. Treat with Ca^{++} replacement until PTH secretion normalizes.

b. Persistent hypoparathyroidism or recurrent laryngeal nerve injury can also occur as postoperative complications.

IV. Adrenal Disease

A. Hyperaldosteronism (Conn's Syndrome)

1. Patients have hypertension (from hypovolemia) and hypokalemia (due to urinary K^+ wasting) with metabolic alkalosis. Secondary hyperaldosteronism can occur in cases of renal artery stenosis due to high renin levels.

2. Diagnostic evaluation

a. CT scan to evaluate for tumor.

b. Adrenal venous sampling for aldosterone.

c. Rule out renal artery stenosis.

d. Saline infusion test: Saline will decrease aldosterone levels in normal people but not in patients with adenoma.

e. Captopril test: Captopril will decrease aldosterone levels in healthy patients but not in patients with adenoma.

3. Treat preoperatively with spironolactone to suppress aldosterone secretion, and then remove the adenoma surgically.

B. Adrenal Insufficiency

1. Causes

a. Primary adrenal insufficiency

(1) Addison's disease: Autoimmune destruction of the adrenal gland. This is the most common cause of primary adrenal insufficiency in the United States.

(2) Tuberculosis: This is the most common cause of adrenal insufficiency in the world.

(3) Congenital adrenal hyperplasia.

(4) Medications (metyrapone, aminoglutethamide, trilostane, ketoconazole, mifepristone [RU486]).

b. Secondary adrenal insufficiency frequently occurs after discontinuation of glucocorticoid therapy, and symptoms can gradually improve over a year. It can be avoided by giving therapeutic glucocorticoids once every other day, rather than using daily dosing schedules.

2. Patients complain of weakness, weight loss, nausea, and vomiting. Physical findings include increased skin pigmentation, hypotension, and anorexia. In cases of secondary adrenal insufficiency, hyperpigmentation will not be present.

3. Evaluation (Fig. 3-2).

a. Addison's disease: Increased ACTH, low cortisol. Low cortisol response to ACTH administration.

b. Secondary adrenal insufficiency: Decreased ACTH, low cortisol. Increased cortisol levels in response to ACTH challenge.

c. Hyponatremia and hyperkalemia may also be present.

4. Treat with replacement of glucocorticoids and mineralocorticoids.

C. Glucocorticoid Excess (Cushing's Syndrome)

1. Frequently caused by steroid therapy, pituitary adenoma (Cushing's disease), or ectopic ACTH production by neuroendocrine tumors.

2. Fat deposits are mobilized to the face, neck, shoulders, and trunk, leading to a moon face, buffalo hump, and truncal obesity with relatively thin extremities.

3. Diagnostic evaluation (see Fig. 3-2).

a. Serum ACTH and cortisol: Adrenal tumors have high cortisol with low ACTH. Pituitary and ectopic tumors have high cortisol with high ACTH.

b. Dexamethasone suppression test: Should suppress ACTH secretion from the pituitary. A low dose (1 mg) of dexamethasone suppresses ACTH in normal subjects only. A high dose (2 mg) of dexamethasone suppresses ACTH production in normal subjects and most patients with pituitary tumors. Ectopic tumors are never suppressed by dexamethasone.

4. Treatment consists of surgical removal of the tumor once it has been identified. Presurgical suppression of cortisol with ketoconazole, mitotane, metyrapone, aminoglutethamide, mifepristone, or trilostane can be done when necessary. Recurrent tumors or inoperable situations can be treated with irradiation, but side effects such as panhypopituitarism are likely.

Remember the "rule of 10s" in pheochromocytoma: 10% are found outside the adrenal glands in the paravertebral ganglia, 10% have bilateral adrenal tumors, 10% are part of familial syndromes (e.g., MEN II), 10% are malignant, and 10% are found in children.

D. Pheochromocytoma

1. Patients have symptoms of **p**alpitations, **h**eadache, and **e**pisodic diaphoresis (mnemonic—PHE). Patients may also have urinary symptoms in cases of bladder pheochromocytoma.

2. Diagnostic evaluation

a. Measure urinary levels of catecholamines and their metabolites. Elevated metanephrine is the most specific test for pheochromocytoma. Vanilylmandelic acid and homovanillic acid will also be increased.

b. Imaging: CT scan is sensitive for tumors greater than 1 cm. I^{131}-MIBG scanning is less sensitive but useful for scanning the entire body and assessing recurrent tumor growth.

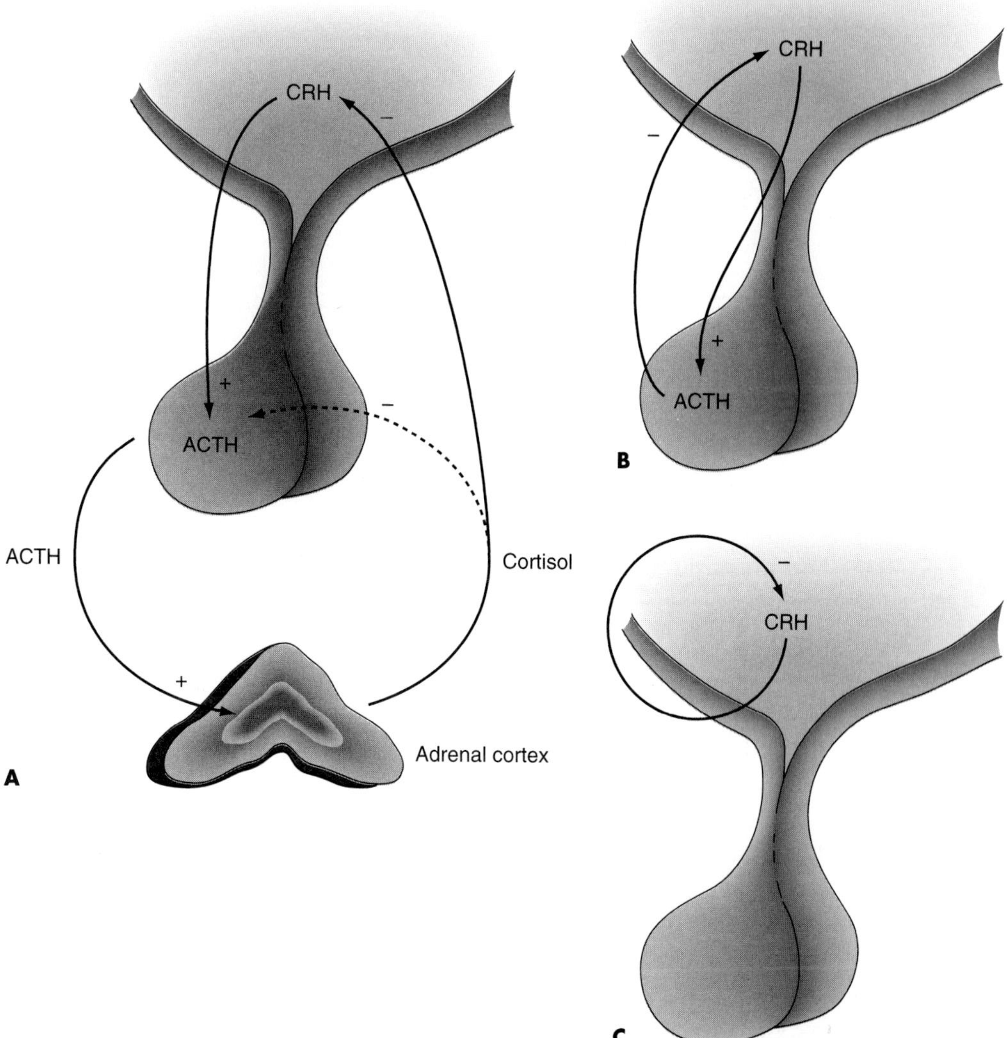

3-2: *A–C, Adrenocortical hormone physiology. Corticotropin-releasing hormone (CRH) is released from the hypothalamus, which stimulates the release of adrenocorticotropic hormone (ACTH) from the anterior pituitary gland. ACTH is released into the bloodstream, from which it can stimulate the production of cortisol from the adrenal cortex. Circulatory cortisol exerts a negative feedback inhibition on ACTH and CRH release. CRH secretion can also be inhibited by high circulatory levels of ACTH or CRH.*

3. Treatment
   a. Prior to surgery, the patient must be treated with antiadrenergic drugs to block the effects of a severe catecholamine crisis. Selective alpha-1 antagonists (phenoxybenzamine, prazosin, phentolamine) are preferred owing to their postsynaptic effects.

b. Surgical removal is performed using an anterior approach (this allows removal of the mass regardless of whether it is in the adrenal gland or on the paravertebral ganglia).

E. Multiple Endocrine Neoplasia (MEN) Syndromes

1. Syndromes with autosomal dominant inheritance that cause specific combinations of endocrine tumors in affected patients.

2. Types

a. MEN I (Wermer's syndrome): Patients have parathyroid gland hyperplasia, pancreatic islet cell tumor, and pituitary adenoma.

b. MEN IIA (Sipple's syndrome): Patients have pheochromocytoma, medullary thyroid cancer, and parathyroid gland hyperplasia.

c. MEN IIB: Patients have pheochromocytoma, medullary thyroid cancer, marfanoid body habitus, and cutaneous or mucosal neuromas. These patients commonly complain of constipation due to ganglioneuromatosis of the GI tract.

3. Treat specific endocrine abnormalities as described previously. For nonsecretory masses, remove any masses greater than 3 cm.

V. Diabetes Mellitus

A. Symptoms and Signs

1. Patients typically have a triad of polydipsia, polyuria, and polyphagia. They may also experience blurred vision and pruritus.

2. Patients with type 1 (insulin-dependent) diabetes mellitus tend to be young persons who experience rapid weight loss and the onset of diabetes following the autoimmune destruction of their pancreatic islets of Langerhans.

3. Patients with type 2 (insulin-independent) diabetes mellitus tend to be older, obese persons who have gradually become insensitive to circulating insulin.

B. Diagnostic Evaluation

1. Diagnostic criteria using blood glucose testing include any of the following.

a. Random plasma glucose greater than 200 mg/dL with the presence of classic clinical symptoms.

b. Fasting plasma glucose greater than 125 mg/dL.

c. Oral glucose tolerance test (using 75 g glucose) showing a 2-hour postprandial glucose of greater than 200 mg/dL.

2. Microalbuminuria can be tested using a dipstick test. An albumin/creatinine ratio less than 30 mg/g creatinine is normal, 30–300 is microalbuminuria, and greater than 300 is nephropathy.

3. Elevated hemoglobin A1c (Hb_{A1c}): Provides a long-term indicator of glucose control. It is recommended that Hb_{A1c} be as close to normal as possible with a goal of less than 7%. This corresponds to blood sugars consistently in the range of 80 to 140 mg/dL.

C. Complications (Table 3-5)

TABLE 3-5
Complications of Diabetes Mellitus

Condition	Description	Treatment
Diabetic ketoacidosis (type 1 only)	(1) Patients present with abdominal pain, vomiting, Kussmaul respirations (increased tidal volume), and fruity odor to breath. (2) Can be precipitated by infection, MI, medications (corticosteroids, thiazides), pancreatitis, or noncompliance with insulin. (3) Laboratory abnormalities include hyperglycemia, hypokalemia, and anion gap metabolic acidosis.	(1) Insulin infusion, with continued IV insulin management for glucose control. (2) Aggressive hydration. (3) Electrolyte repletion: Be careful not to correct Na^+ too quickly. (4) Bicarbonate therapy if the patient continues to have severe acidosis after fluid replacement. (5) Following stabilization and a return to eating by mouth, switch to subcutaneous insulin.
Hyperosmolar nonketotic syndrome (type 2 only)	Presentation is similar to diabetic ketoacidosis, but patients have higher hyperglycemia and no acidosis or ketonemia.	(1) Treat with fluid and electrolyte replacement over 36 to 72 hours. (2) Insulin treatment after rehydration has started. (3) Heparin prophylaxis.
Accelerated atherosclerotic disease	(1) Patients can experience severe coronary artery disease, as well as arterial insufficiency to organs and limbs (causing foot ulcers). (2) Because of this, the thresholds are lower for the management of other risk factors for coronary artery disease (the definition of hypertension in diabetics is blood pressure 130/85, and the upper limit of normal for LDL cholesterol is 100 mg/dL).	(1) The best option for treatment of hypertension in diabetics is the use of ACE inhibitors because of their renal protective effects. (2) Give one aspirin per day in diabetic patients over 30 years of age to prevent platelet aggregation.
Retinopathy	Focal hemorrhages, cotton wool exudates, neovascularization, retinal detachment, and blindness.	(1) Monitor with yearly visits to the ophthalmologist. (2) Treat with photocoagulation.
Nephropathy	(1) Microalbuminuria is the earliest sign, which can progress to end-stage renal disease 15 to 20 years later. (2) Usually occurs after retinopathy.	Control with strict blood pressure control, ACE inhibitors, low protein diet, dialysis, or transplantation.
Peripheral neuropathy	(1) Symmetrical peripheral polyneuropathy (mostly sensory). (2) Autonomic neuropathy: Can cause gastroparesis, neurogenic bladder, impotence, and orthostatic hypotension. (3) Mononeuropathy/entrapment syndromes. (4) See Chapter 8.	Try analgesics, tricyclic antidepressants (amitriptyline, imipramine), anticonvulsants (gabapentin, carbamazepine), or capsaicin cream.

D. Treatment
  1. Type 1 diabetics require insulin supplementation.
    a. Insulin can be administered in short-acting (e.g., regular, lispro), intermediate-acting (e.g., NPH, Lente), and long-acting (e.g., Ultralente, glargine) preparations.
    b. Standard insulin therapy usually consists of several injections per day of a mixture of different insulins.
    c. Combinations of short- and intermediate-acting insulins can provide good glycemic control when two-thirds of the dose is taken before breakfast and one third before dinner. An individual patient's dose is dependent on his or her responsiveness to insulin.
    d. Patients who have nightmares and sleep disturbances may be experiencing hypoglycemia while sleeping. In this case, have the patient change their evening dose to take the short-acting insulin before dinner and the intermediate-acting insulin before bedtime. This also counteracts the "dawn phenomenon," which involves a rise in glucose levels in the early morning hours.
    e. Continuous subcutaneous insulin infusion using an insulin pump device allows small amounts of insulin to be delivered according to the programming of the pump. The pump uses short-acting insulin (usually lispro) and allows flexibility and control over the varying insulin requirements during sleep, exercise, and meals. The disadvantage of these devices is that they require a significant amount of expertise by the clinician and frequent follow-up by the patient. Additionally, obstruction of the device can lead to an abrupt discontinuation of insulin infusion, which can cause hyperglycemia and ketoacidosis.
  2. Type 2 diabetics
    a. Diet/exercise modulation: Can decrease the degree of insulin resistance. Over 10% of type 2 diabetics can be controlled with diet alone.
    b. Classes of diabetic drugs (Table 3-6).

VI. Disorders of Bone
  A. Paget's Disease (Fig. 3-3A)
    1. Patients have pain, headache, skeletal deformity, neurologic compression symptoms, and bone tumors.
    2. Diagnostic evaluation
      a. Increased serum alkaline phosphatase and urinary hydroxyproline
      b. Bone scan
      c. Radiography to assess progression
    3. Treatment
      a. Aspirin or NSAIDs in patients with minimal symptoms
      b. Calcitonin, bisphosphonates (pamidronate or alendronate) in more severe cases
  B. Osteomalacia/Rickets: Failure to mineralize the newly formed matrix of bone
    1. Causes
      a. Vitamin D deficiency

TABLE 3-6
Oral Hypoglycemic Agents*

Class	Medications	Mechanism	Contraindications
Sulfonylureas	Glyburide, glipizide, glimepiride	Increase insulin secretion	Renal or liver disease
Meglitinides	Repaglinide	Increase insulin secretion	Liver disease
Biguanides	Metformin	Decrease glucose production and increase glucose consumption	(1) Renal insufficiency (will cause lactic acidosis) (2) May increase cardiovascular mortality
Alpha-glucosidase inhibitors	Acarbose, miglitol	Decrease glucose absorption	Liver disease or congestive heart failure
Thiazolidinedione derivatives	Troglitazone	Improve glucose consumption and insulin sensitivity	Liver disease (can cause fulminant hepatic failure)

*The two limbs of glycemic control involve the inability to secrete insulin and the inability to respond to circulating insulin. Metformin and troglitazone treat insulin resistance. Sulfonylureas, repaglinide, and insulin treat insulin secretory failure. If a patient fails to improve on one agent, it is better to add additional agents (especially if they act on the other limb of glycemic control) than to discontinue one and start another. If oral hypoglycemic agents provide insufficient glucose control, then insulin therapy can also be used.

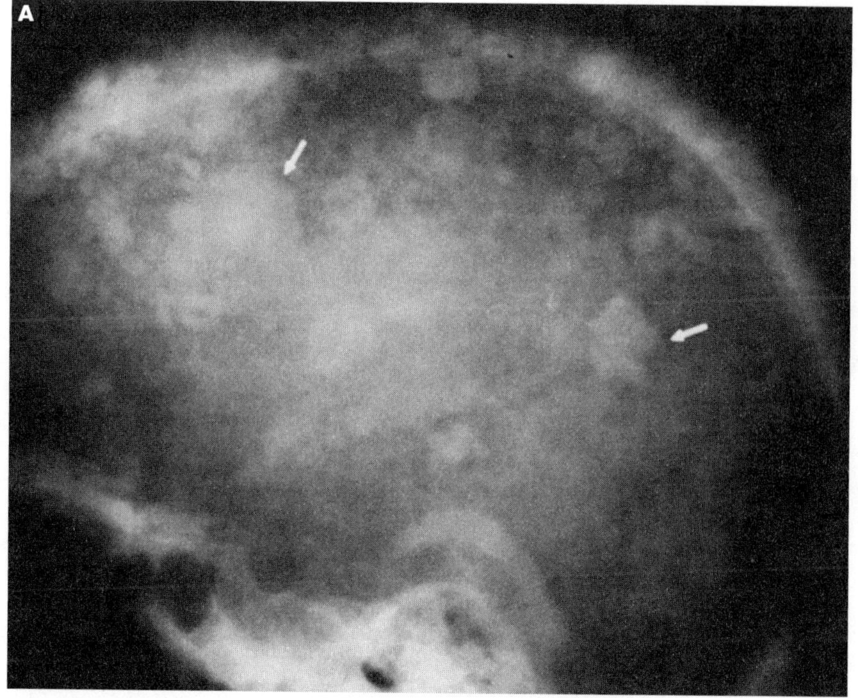

3-3: *Radiographic findings in endocrine bone disorders. A, In Paget's disease, thickening of the skull, indistinct bone edges, and a "cotton-wool" appearance* (arrows) *can be seen on radiography of the skull.* *Continued*

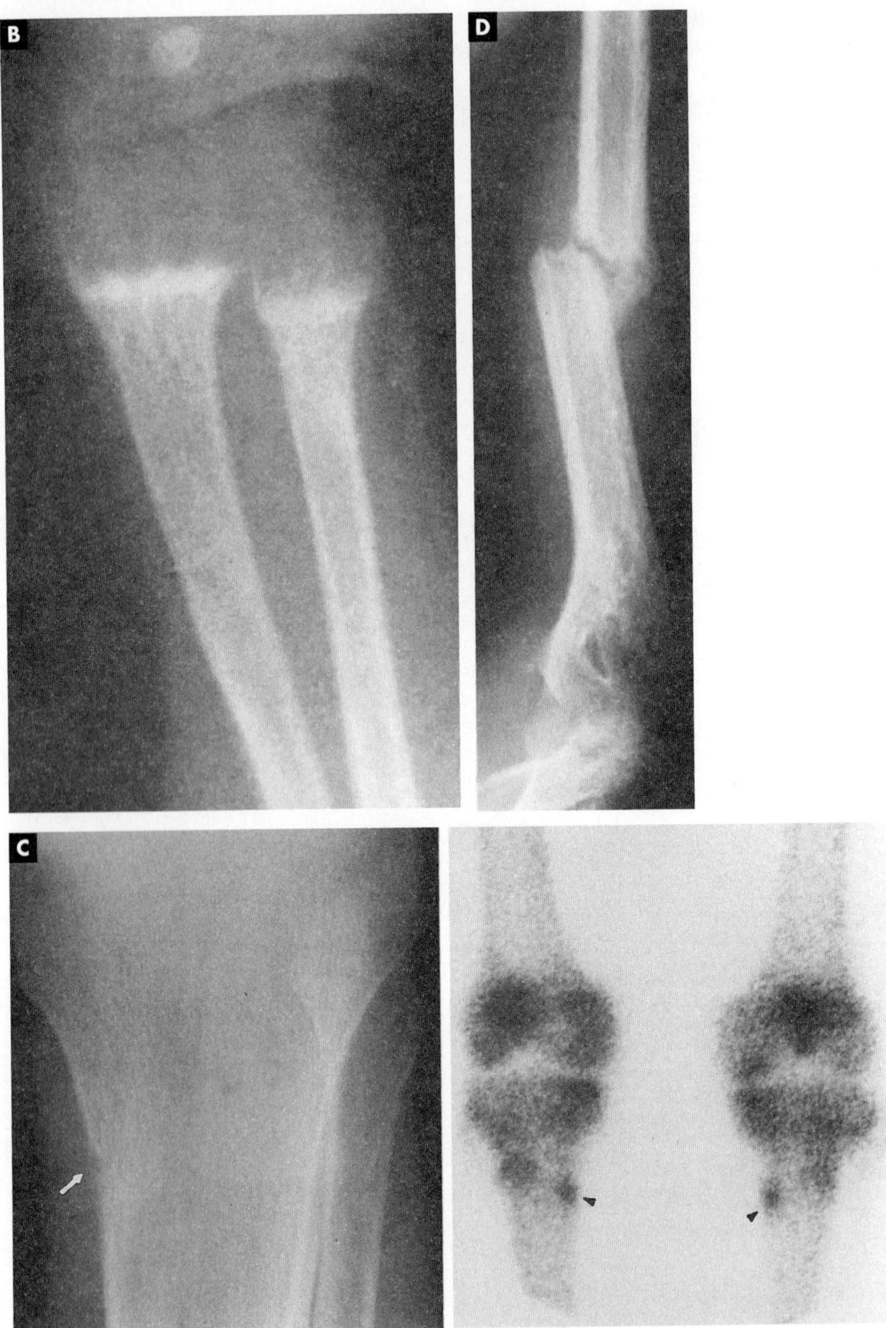

3-3, cont'd B, *In rickets, the metaphysis of the bone will show demineralization and disorganization, and the growth plate may enlarge.* C, *In osteomalacia, small fractures* (arrow) *related to insufficient mineralization can occur, as shown here in the iliopubic area* (arrowheads). D, *In osteoporosis, fractures may be present and bone may be radiolucent in areas due to demineralization.*

b. Chronic hypophosphatemia and/or hypocalcemia

c. Systemic acidosis: Stimulates osteoclast activity and directly dissolves bone

d. Inhibitors of mineralization (aluminum-containing antacids/dialysis fluids or high-dose bisphosphonates)

2. Symptoms and signs

a. In rickets, pediatric patients experience skeletal pain, deformity, fracture of abnormal bone, and growth disturbance. The patients are listless, weak, and hypotonic, and the enlarged epiphyses and costochondral junctions create a rachitic rosary (see Fig. 3-3B).

b. In osteomalacia, adult patients experience diffuse skeletal pain (particularly at the hips) and proximal muscle weakness, which can cause a waddling gait (see Fig. 3-3C).

3. Diagnostic evaluation

a. Electrolytes with calcium and phosphate levels.

b. Vitamin D levels will be low.

c. Chest radiograph will show pseudofractures (bilateral symmetrical lines perpendicular to the bone).

4. Treatment for patients with electrolyte or vitamin deficiencies is supplementation with Ca^{++}, vitamin D, or phosphate.

C. Osteoporosis

1. Symptoms and signs

a. Patients usually have symptoms of a vertebral compression fracture (back pain that occurs following an activity that may have been minimally stressful, and that is made worse by standing), or a hip fracture following a fall.

b. Patients experience height loss with dorsal kyphosis and cervical lordosis (dowager's hump).

2. Diagnostic evaluation (see Fig. 3-3D).

a. Radiography: Shows a loss of trabecular bone and may show collapse of bony structures.

b. Bone density scan: Dual-energy X-ray absorbitometry (DEXA) scan.

(1) Osteopenia: From 1 to 2.5 standard deviations below peak bone mass.

(2) Osteoporosis: In excess of 2.5 standard deviations below peak bone mass.

c. Treatment: Reversal is not possible, but the condition can be prevented or its progression can be stopped.

(1) Pain management.

(2) Exercise.

(3) Calcium and vitamin D supplementation.

(4) Bisphosphonates: Alendronate is the drug of choice, but it may cause esophagitis.

(5) Estrogen replacement therapy.

VII. Disorders of the Reproductive System (see Chapter 9)

CHAPTER 4

Gastroenterology

I. Oropharyngeal Motility Disorders
  A. Zenker's Diverticulum: Outpouching of the esophagus above the upper esophageal sphincter muscle that leads to saliva and food retention.
    1. Patients may experience aspiration or postprandial throat clearing with production of food particles.
    2. Evaluate with rapid-sequence cine-esophagography.
    3. Treat with surgical repair and section of the cricopharyngeus muscle.
  B. Achalasia: Occurs owing to impaired relaxation of the lower esophageal sphincter (Fig. 4-1).
    1. Patients regurgitate undigested material.
    2. Radiography shows a "bird beak" stricture.
    3. Treat with pneumatic dilation of the lower esophageal sphincter.

II. Esophageal Rupture
  A. Boerhaave's Syndrome: Postemetic esophageal rupture that tears through all layers of the esophagus but does not cause much bleeding.
    1. Patients experience postemetic pain, may have a left pneumothorax, and may display Hamman's sign (mediastinal crunch) produced by the heart beating against air-filled tissues.
    2. Test with radiography using water-soluble contrast.
    3. Treat with surgery within 24 hours to drain the mediastinum and repair the defect. Give broad-spectrum antibiotics.
  B. Mallory-Weiss Tear: Postemetic esophageal rupture of the mucosa (not the entire esophagus) that produces bright red hematemesis.
    1. Diagnosis is made by endoscopy.
    2. Bleeding can be stopped by localized epinephrine or electrocautery during endoscopy.

Common causes of upper GI bleeds include peptic ulcers, esophageal varices, Mallory-Weiss tears, hemorrhagic gastritis, and gastric cancer. Common causes of lower GI bleeds include diverticulosis, arteriovenous malformations, colitis, cancer, and upper GI bleeding.

III. Gastrointestinal Bleeding
  A. Symptoms and Signs
    1. Upper GI bleeding presents with hematemesis, coffee-ground emesis, and melena.
    2. Lower GI bleeding presents with hematochezia (bright red blood per rectum).
    3. Weight loss, anemia, dizziness, and weakness may be present, regardless of the source.
  B. Diagnostic Evaluation
    1. Nasogastric (NG) tube aspirate: Upper GI bleeding is blood (may look like coffee grounds), and lower GI bleeding has bilious fluid.
    2. Evaluate upper GI bleeds with esophagogastroduodenoscopy (EGD).

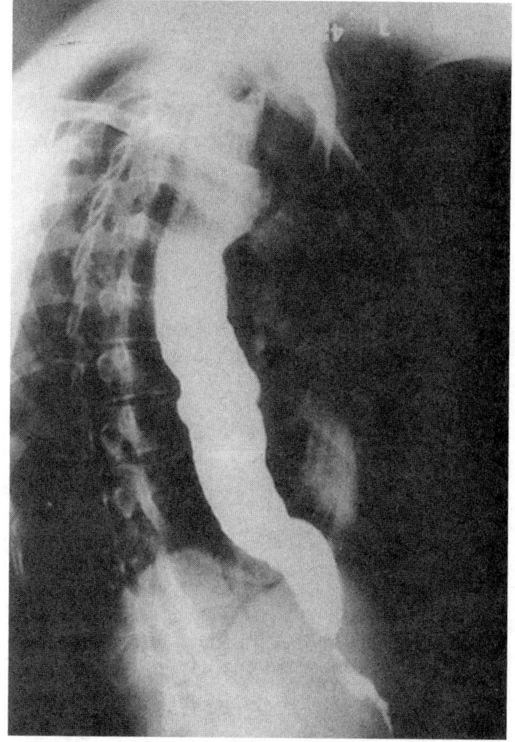

4-1: *Common radiographic abnormality in gastroenterology. The "bird beak" abnormality in achalasia.*

3. Evaluate lower GI bleeds with anoscopy and flexible sigmoidoscopy (in young healthy patients) or colonoscopy (in older patients).

C. Treatment

1. The patient should discontinue aspirin and NSAID use.
2. Start the patient on a proton pump inhibitor (PPI) or an H_2 (histamine receptor) blocker.
3. Upper GI bleed: During EGD, bleeding can be stopped by the local application of sclerotic agents, rubber banding, or cautery.

IV. Gastroesophageal Reflux Disease (GERD)

A. Symptoms and Signs

1. The patient experiences substernal chest pain (heartburn) and regurgitation that worsens when bending over or lying down. Other symptoms may include hoarseness, asthma, ear pain, loss of dental enamel, and dysphagia secondary to stricture.
2. The patient may also have a history of hiatal hernia or scleroderma.

B. Diagnostic Evaluation

1. EGD: Perform this first to evaluate for Barrett's esophagus (columnar metaplasia in the esophagus). Barrett's esophagus is a significant risk factor for the development of esophageal adenocarcinoma.

2. Barium esophagogram: Reveals structural abnormalities and motility dysfunction.
3. A pH probe in the lower esophagus: To detect acid reflux.
4. Barium study: Can demonstrate reflux and the presence of hiatal hernia.
5. Gastric emptying scan: To detect poor gastric emptying as a cause.
6. Manometry: To evaluate low esophageal sphincter (LES) pressure as the cause of reflux.
7. Tests to rule out angina and myocardial infarction as a cause of chest pain (ECG, stress test, cardiac enzymes, etc).

C. Treatment
1. Lifestyle changes: Changes in diet (low fat, low caffeine, low alcohol), sleeping position and time (raise head and sleep 3 to 4 hours after last meal), smoking cessation, and changing medications (Ca^{++} channel blockers lower the LES pressure) can alleviate symptoms.
2. Medications
a. Proton pump inhibitors (omeprazole, lansoprazole, and pantoprazole) are the most frequently used medications. They are well tolerated with minimal toxicity.
b. H_2 receptor blockers (ranitidine, cimetidine, nizatidine, and famotidine) can be effective alone or in combination with proton pump inhibitors. Cimetidine has numerous drug interactions owing to hepatic enzyme inhibition, and it may cause an increase in the serum concentrations of other medications.
c. Antacids can provide some relief, but are ineffective as long-term therapy.
d. Prokinetic agents (cisapride, metoclopramide, erythromycin) can improve symptoms by facilitating gastric emptying.
e. Sucralfate can provide a protective lining for the mucosa in an acid environment.
3. Procedures: Indications for surgery include failed medical therapy, complications of GERD (esophageal stricture, bleeding, or Barrett's esophagus), and unwillingness of the patient to take medications lifelong.
a. Antireflux procedures: Patients are usually surgically treated with a Nissen fundoplication, which involves wrapping a portion of the stomach around the lower esophagus to increase the lower esophageal sphincter pressure.
b. Antistricture procedures usually involve dilation of the esophagus to lyse strictures.

D. Complications of GERD include esophageal cancer, esophageal stricture, bleeding from esophagitis, and development of peptic ulcer disease.

Ninety percent of gastric ulcers and 80% of duodenal ulcers are associated with *Helicobacter pylori*.

V. Peptic Ulcer Disease (PUD)
A. Symptoms and Signs
1. Patients have epigastric or back pain that is relieved by antacids. The pain due to duodenal ulcers is frequently relieved by eating, whereas the

pain from gastric ulcers may be worsened by eating but relieved by vomiting. Nausea, anorexia, melena, and hematemesis may be present.

2. Risk factors include a history of smoking, aspirin ingestion, uremia, Zollinger-Ellison syndrome (tumor that secretes excessive gastrin), *H. pylori* infection, and trauma.

B. Diagnostic Evaluation

1. EGD: Confirms the diagnosis and defines the extent of disease. EGD will also rule out reflux, Barrett's esophagus, and gastritis. Biopsy must be performed for all gastric ulcers. EGD can also allow for localized stoppage of bleeding with heat or sclerosing agents.

2. Tests for *H. pylori* include a serologic antibody test, the urea breath test, and the CLO test (a test for urease in the gastric mucosa that is done during EGD).

3. If Zollinger-Ellison syndrome is suspected, the fasting serum gastrin level should be checked. The possibility of other endocrine tumors should also be investigated.

4. Tests to rule out other causes of chest and abdominal pain include ECG, liver function tests, and serum amylase levels.

C. Treatment

1. Medical treatment

a. Acute gastric ulcers are treated short term with omeprazole and discontinuation of NSAIDs.

b. Acute duodenal ulcers are treated short term with sucralfate.

c. Treat *H. pylori* infection with triple therapy (mnemonic—COM): **c**larithromycin, **o**meprazole, and **m**etronidazole.

2. Surgical treatment

a. EGD: Electrocautery, heat, and epinephrine can be used during endoscopy to stop the bleeding in an actively bleeding ulcer.

b. Indications for further surgical intervention (mnemonic—IHOP).

(1) **I**ntractability
(2) **H**emorrhage
(3) **O**bstruction
(4) **P**erforation

c. A Graham patch procedure oversews a duodenal ulcer with a patch made of viable omentum. This is often done in conjunction with a partial vagotomy and pyloroplasty.

d. In cases of Zollinger-Ellison syndrome, surgical removal of the gastrinomas should treat the gastrin hypersecretion.

D. Complications

1. GI hemorrhage: Treat endoscopically with a heat probe or injection therapy.

2. Perforated peptic ulcer: Will cause acute onset of abdominal pain with decreased bowel sounds, peritoneal signs, and tympany over the liver. Treat with NG tube decompression of the GI tract, fluid resuscitation, antibiotics, and corrective surgery.

Specific ulcer types include Cushing's ulcer (associated with CNS trauma or tumor), Curling's ulcer (associated with major burn injury), and Dieulafoy's ulcer (gastric mucosal defect bleeding from an underlying vascular malformation).

Visualization of a vessel in the ulcer crater is associated with a 90% rebleed rate following therapy. Clots with oozing blood indicate a visible vessel under the clot, and the clot should be washed away for further assessment and treatment.

Patients on proton pump inhibitors may have a falsely negative CLO test.

VI. Mesenteric Ischemia

A. Symptoms and Signs: Patients have postprandial periumbilical pain, early satiety, nausea, vomiting, absent bowel sounds, and abdominal pain out of proportion to the tenderness on examination.

B. Diagnostic Evaluation

1. Abdominal radiograph may show ileus.

2. Abdominal CT scan may show bowel wall thickening or pneumatosis of the bowel wall.

3. Angiography can be used to assess the vascular supply to the GI tract.

C. Treatment

1. Volume resuscitation and broad-spectrum antibiotics.

2. Anticoagulation or thrombolysis depending on the site of the occlusion.

3. Surgical embolectomy can be performed if the bowel is salvageable; otherwise, perform an intestinal resection to remove infarcted bowel.

VII. Pancreatitis

A. Symptoms and Signs

1. Patients have severe, stabbing epigastric abdominal pain radiating to the back, nausea, vomiting, anorexia, and fever. Steatorrhea may be present from intestinal malabsorption.

2. The patient may also have diabetes from endocrine insufficiency (depending on the extent of the pancreatic damage).

3. Risk factors include hypertriglyceridemia, gallstones, and alcohol ingestion.

Specialized signs of pancreatitis include Grey Turner's sign (ecchymosis in the flank), Cullen's sign (ecchymosis in the periumbilical area), and Fox's sign (ecchymosis of the inguinal ligament).

B. Diagnostic Evaluation

1. Elevated serum amylase or urinary amylase: Chronic pancreatitis may have normal serum amylase but usually will have high urinary amylase.

2. Abdominal radiograph may show pancreatic calcification in chronic pancreatitis. It may also show an ileus pattern with air/fluid levels in the small bowel.

3. Abdominal CT is required when infection is suggested (spiral CT is well suited for picking up abscess, pseudocyst, and pancreatic necrosis).

4. Ranson's criteria can be used to determine the prognosis from the abnormal test values.

a. At admission (mnemonic—GA LAW)

(1) Serum **g**lucose greater than 200 mg/dL

(2) **A**ge older than 55 years

(3) **L**actate dehydrogenase greater than 350 units/L

(4) **A**ST greater than 2250 units/L

(5) **W**BC greater than 16,000 cells/μL

b. During the initial 48 hours (mnemonic—C HOBBS)

(1) **C**a^{++} less than 8 units

(2) **H**ematocrit falling more than 10%

(3) Arterial p**0**$_2$ less than 60 torr

(4) **B**UN greater than 5 mg

(5) **B**ase deficit greater than 4

(6) **S**equestration of fluid greater than 6 L

c. Patients with less than 2 of these criteria have 1% mortality risk, patients with 3 or 4 of these criteria have 15% mortality risk, patients with 5 or 6 of these criteria have 40% mortality risk, and patients with more than 6 of these criteria have 100% mortality risk.

C. Treatment

1. Medical treatment

a. Acute pancreatitis: Give IV fluids and nutrition and keep the patient NPO ("nothing by mouth"). In the absence of infection, acute pancreatitis can be watched until it subsides. Surgery may be indicated in the presence of extensive pancreatic necrosis.

b. Chronic pancreatitis: Control the pain, tell the patient to avoid alcohol, and give pancreatic enzyme supplementation.

c. Prophylactic imipenem use decreases likelihood of infection.

d. If a pseudocyst occurs, radiology-guided percutaneous drainage can be performed.

2. Surgical treatment: For an infected or extensively necrotic pancreas.

a. Extensive débridement is done, and drains and a jejunostomy tube are placed. Several stages of débridement and packing of the abdomen may be required.

b. A Puestow (longitudinal pancreaticojejunostomy), a Duval (distal pancreaticojejunostomy), or a near-total pancreatectomy can be performed for chronic pancreatitis.

c. The gallbladder should be removed in patients with pancreatitis and cholelithiasis.

D. Complications (Table 4-1)

VIII. Appendicitis

A. Symptoms and Signs

1. Patients have periumbilical pain followed by anorexia, nausea, and vomiting. The pain will present before vomiting (opposite in gastroenteritis) and will migrate from the periumbilical region to the right lower quadrant of the abdomen.

2. Specialized signs of appendicitis (from peritoneal irritation)

a. Obturator sign: Pain elicited by internal rotation of the leg with the hip and knee flexed.

b. Psoas sign: Pain elicited by extending the hip with the knee in full extension or by flexing the hip against resistance.

c. Rovsing's sign: Palpation or rebound pressure of the left lower quadrant of the abdomen results in pain in the right lower quadrant.

B. Diagnostic Evaluation

1. Imaging studies: CT, abdominal radiography, and ultrasound can be performed.

2. Complete blood count may be consistent with active infection (high WBC, high neutrophils).

3. Tests to exclude other causes of abdominal pain (e.g., pancreatitis, pelvic inflammatory disease, cardiac disease, pyelonephritis) should be performed.

The patient will frequently localize the pain to McBurney's point, which is 2 inches medial to the anterior spinous process of the ileum.

Causes of appendicitis include lymphoid hyperplasia (60%), fecaliths (35%), foreign bodies (4%), and tumors (1%).

TABLE 4-1
Complications of Pancreatitis

Condition	Definition	Diagnostic Evaluation	Treatment
Pancreatic abscess	Infected peripancreatic purulent fluid collection.	Abdominal CT with needle aspiration	Give antibiotics and percutaneous drain placement, or operative débridement and placement of drains.
Pancreatic necrosis	Ischemia and death of a portion of the pancreas.	Abdominal CT with contrast	Débride surgically if the necrosis is infected. Otherwise, make the patient NPO and allow the necrosis to resolve on its own.
Pancreatic fistula	A leak can track along the retroperitoneum into the pleural cavities, mediastinum, or pericardium and may lead to effusions.	If an effusion is found, drain the fluid and test for amylase	Treat minor leaks with ERCP and stenting, and major ones with surgery. Make all patients NPO until leak resolves.
Pancreatic pseudocyst	Results from a contained pancreatic duct leak, which is often the result of proximal ductal obstruction. Suspect in a patient with a history of pancreatitis who has early satiety, abdominal distention, or an abdominal mass.	Confirm with abdominal ultrasound or CT	Can be internally drained to the stomach or jejunum, or externally drained with radiologic guidance. External drainage is always used for infected pseudocysts. Surgery is not indicated for small pseudocysts (<6 cm) because they will spontaneously resolve within 4–6 weeks after the pancreatitis resolves.
Splenic artery pseudoaneurysm	Due to inflammation of to pancreas in proximity to the splenic artery. May present as large blood loss in the left upper quadrant and a surgical abdomen.	CT scan	Surgical correction.
Pancreatic duct rupture	Presents with a sudden onset of severe abdominal pain and massive distention, causing respiratory distress. Ascites and pleural effusion can be present.	CT scan	If major disruption of the gland is noted, do a resection. If not, then stenting and external drainage may be sufficient.
Pancreatic duct stricture	Can be the result of scarring from recurrent pancreatitis.	CT scan	Treat with a distal pancreatectomy (if the stricture is proximal), or a Roux-en-Y pancreaticojejunostomy to reroute the flow.

ERCP, endoscopic retrograde cholangiopancreatography; NPO, "nothing by mouth."

C. Treatment: Surgical appendectomy by either an open or laparoscopic approach.

D. Complications: Appendiceal perforation is more common in the very young and very old. Risk of perforation is 25% after 24 hours of symptoms, 50% after 36 hours of symptoms, and 75% after 48 hours of symptoms. Give antibiotics for 1 day. If perforation occurs, obtain cultures and leave the wound open. Continue antibiotics for 5 to 7 days.

Risk of mortality is less than 1% in surgery for nonperforated appendicitis, but rises fivefold following perforation. Perforation also increases the likelihood of postoperative infection to 15% to 20%.

IX. Inflammatory Bowel Disease (IBD)

A. Symptoms and Signs (mnemonic—A PIE SACK)

1. **A**phthous ulcers: Ulcers found on mucous membranes.
2. **P**yoderma gangrenosum: An acute, purulent bacterial dermatitis that usually occurs on the trunk.
3. **I**ritis: May cause pain, photophobia, lacrimation, and visual field defects.
4. **E**rythema nodosum: Painful red nodules that usually occur on the legs.
5. **S**clerosing cholangitis
6. **A**rthritis, ankylosing spondylitis
7. **C**lubbing of fingers
8. **K**idney problems (amyloid deposits, nephrotic syndrome)

B. Crohn's Disease versus Ulcerative Colitis (Table 4-2)

C. Diagnostic Evaluation

1. Markers of inflammation are increased on blood tests.
2. Lesions can be visualized by colonoscopy.
3. Rule out *Clostridium difficile* and parasites by stool culture.
4. Abdominal radiograph will show the string sign in Crohn's disease (Fig. 4-2).

D. Treatment

1. Sulfasalazine: This is metabolized to its active form (5-ASA) by bacteria in the intestine and then acts as an anti-inflammatory.
2. Corticosteroids: Prednisone.

TABLE 4-2 Crohn's Disease versus Ulcerative Colitis

Disorder	Crohn's Disease	Ulcerative Colitis
Distribution by sex	Female > male	Male > female
Distribution of lesions	Involves area from mouth to anus with skip lesions (unaffected areas between affected ones)	Involves colon alone with no skip lesions
Biopsy findings	Granulomas and cobblestoning with lesions spanning the full thickness of the bowel wall	Crypt abscesses and pseudopolyps involving the mucosa and submucosa only
Complications	Anal fistula, enterocutaneous fistula, abscesses, toxic megacolon, obstruction, and colorectal cancer	Colorectal cancer, toxic megacolon, primary sclerosing cholangitis, colonic perforation, hemorrhage, strictures

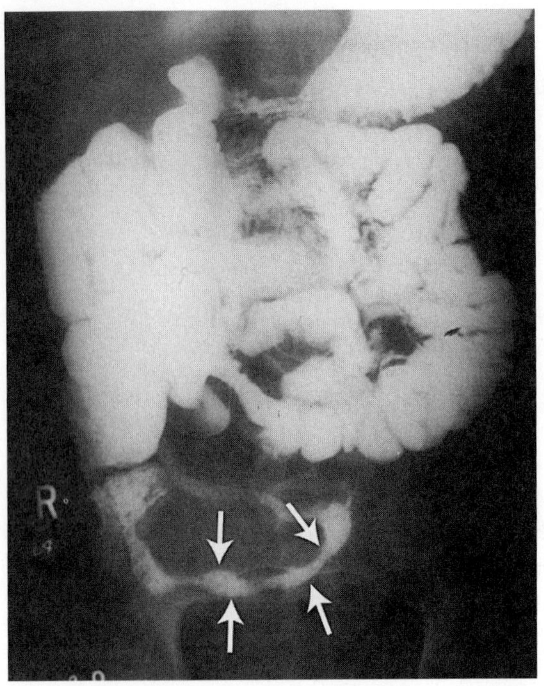

4-2: *Radiograph showing the "string sign" in inflammatory bowel disease. The arrows indicate the luminal narrowing that gives the radiograph a focal string-like appearance.*

3. Treat perianal Crohn's disease with oral metronidazole.
4. Treat long-term IBD with 6-mercaptopurine, azathioprine, or mesalamine.

X. Small Bowel Obstruction
   A. Symptoms and Signs
      1. Patients have crampy abdominal pain, nausea, and bilious vomiting. Emesis relieves the pain. On physical examination, the patient may have abdominal distention and hyperactive (early) or hypoactive (late) bowel sounds, depending on the duration of symptoms.
      2. The patient may show signs of dehydration and poor nutrition (lethargy, poor skin turgor, dry mucous membranes).
      3. Risk factors include previous abdominal surgery, hernias, and tumors.
   B. Diagnostic Evaluation
      1. Blood tests will be consistent with dehydration: Elevated hematocrit, BUN, Na^+.
      2. Vomiting will cause a hypochloremic, hypokalemic alkalosis due to the loss of HCl.
      3. Abdominal radiograph shows multiple loops of distended bowel in a stepladder pattern, air/fluid levels, and the absence of colonic air or stool (Fig. 4-3).

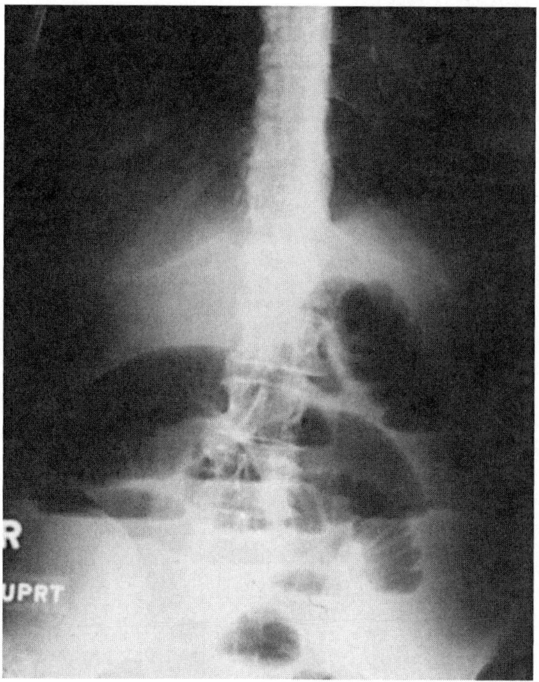

4-3: *Radiograph of dilated loops of bowel in small bowel obstruction.*

C. Treatment
   1. Decompress the GI tract with nasogastric suction, and resuscitate fluid status.
   2. Indications for surgery include
      a. Abdominal pain associated with fever, leukocytosis, acidosis, peritoneal signs, and shock.
      b. Unrelenting and increasing abdominal pain with obstipation and radiographic signs of small bowel obstruction.

D. Complications: Closed loop strangulation of the bowel, which presents with fever, pain, hematemesis, shock, peritoneal signs, acidosis, and abdominal free air.

XI. Diarrhea: In all subtypes, start fluid resuscitation with glucose-containing fluids.

A. Infectious (see Chapter 6).
   1. Toxin-induced: Usually lasts less than 24 hours.
   2. Invasive: Will have fecal blood and leukocytes.

B. Malabsorption
   1. Patients have diarrhea that improves with fasting. They may also have steatorrhea.
   2. Diagnostic evaluation
      a. Increased fecal fat and osmotic gap.

b. A positive D-xylose test indicates celiac sprue. Small bowel biopsy will show villous blunting in celiac sprue.
c. Check amylase and lipase to determine pancreatic function.
3. Treat enzyme insufficiencies with enzyme replacement (if possible). Treat celiac sprue with a gluten-free diet.

C. Osmotic
1. Patients have diarrhea that improves with fasting and may be associated with the use of antacids, lactulose, or sorbitol.
2. Diagnostic evaluation
a. Increased osmotic gap with normal fecal fat.
b. Lactose intolerance shows a positive lactose hydrogen breath test.

D. Inflammatory
1. Patients have fever, hematochezia, and abdominal pain.
2. Usually due to inflammatory bowel disease or irradiation.

E. Secretory
1. Usually due to laxative abuse, villous adenoma, or hormonal disorders (VIP, serotonin, calcitonin, gastrin, glucagon, substance P, or thyroxine).
2. The patient has large-volume diarrhea with no benefit from being NPO.
3. Osmotic gap is normal.
4. Perform colonoscopy to check for adenomas, and check hormone levels to determine the presence of secretory tumors.

F. Hypermotility: Can be due to irritable bowel syndrome (alternating constipation and diarrhea), scleroderma, diabetes, or hyperthyroidism.

XII. Hepatic Disease

A. Portal Hypertension and Esophageal Varices

Routes of collateral circulation in portal hypertension include the umbilical vein, the coronary vein to esophageal venous plexi, the retroperitoneal veins, the diaphragmatic veins, the splenic veins, and the hemorrhoidal veins.

1. Causes: The leading cause in North America is alcoholic liver disease but worldwide is extrahepatic obstruction and fibrosis due to schistosomiasis. Other causes include hepatic vein or vena cava obstruction (hepatic vein thrombosis = Budd-Chiari syndrome), and hypersplenism with portal hypertension due to increases in portal vein flow.
2. Symptoms and signs
a. Portal hypertension can cause ascites, hemorrhoids, splenomegaly, and caput medusae.
b. Esophageal varices occur as a result of portal hypertension causing dilation of the esophageal veins. These varices can bleed or rupture, causing hematemesis, hematochezia, and/or melena. Stabilization of this bleeding may be complicated by coagulopathy from liver disease.
c. Other symptoms that are indicative of liver disease or cirrhosis may also be present (see later discussion).
3. Diagnostic evaluation
a. CT and ultrasound can be used to assess the degree of ascites.
b. Liver function tests can be used to determine the cause of disease.
4. Treatment of bleeding varices
a. Beta-blockers can be used to prevent variceal hemorrhage by lowering the blood pressure.

b. Resuscitate the patient with fluids and blood products (fresh-frozen plasma and vitamin K to treat coagulopathy, if present.)

c. Control bleeding varices with octreotide or vasopressin/nitroglycerin in combination.

d. Surgical procedures

(1) Sclerotherapy: Agents include sodium morrhuate and ethanolamine oleate.

(2) Portocaval shunting: Better than sclerotherapy for esophageal varices.

(3) A Sengstaken-Blakemore tube can be placed in the stomach and esophagus and the large balloon inside can be inflated. The resultant pressure on the varices can facilitate hemostasis.

(4) TIPS (transjugular intrahepatic portosystemic shunting) procedure: Good for high-risk patients, but there is a postoperative risk of recurrent portal hypertension due to stent thrombosis or fibrosis.

(5) Liver transplantation is the only curative procedure for many underlying liver diseases.

5. Complications include Mallory-Weiss tears, which can cause post-retching hematemesis. Do not treat these tears with a Sengstaken-Blakemore balloon.

B. Liver Abscess: Occurs more commonly in the right lobe than in the left lobe.

1. Types

a. Bacterial: Most common cause in the United States.

(1) Causative organisms include ***P**roteus,* ***E**scherichia **c**oli,* and ***K**lebsiella* (mnemonic—PECK).

(2) Patients have constitutional symptoms, right upper quadrant pain, and signs of sepsis (hypotension, fever, etc.).

(3) Liver function tests are elevated, and CBC may be consistent with acute infection (increased WBCs, increased neutrophils).

(4) Treat with triple antibiotic therapy including metronidazole. The abscess can be drained percutaneously or surgically if medical therapy is insufficient.

b. Amebic: Most common cause outside the United States.

(1) Caused by *Entamoeba histolytica.*

(2) Patients have constitutional symptoms and right upper quadrant pain.

(3) "Anchovy paste pus" is present in the abscess if biopsy or drainage is attempted.

(4) Indirect hemagglutinin test for *Entamoeba* antibodies can confirm diagnosis.

(5) Treat with metronidazole.

C. Wilson's disease: Copper overload causes Kayser-Fleischer rings in the eyes and psychiatric problems.

1. Symptoms and signs (mnemonic—ABCD)

a. **A**sterixis

b. **B**asal ganglia deterioration
c. **C**eruloplasmin decreased/*c*irrhosis/*c*arcinoma/*c*horeiform movements
d. **D**ementia

2. Urinary copper will be increased, and serum ceruloplasmin will be decreased.
3. Treatment includes avoidance of copper-rich foods like shellfish, liver, and legumes. Also give penicillamine with pyridoxine, and oral zinc (to increase fecal copper chelation).

Hepatitis B (HBV) envelope antigen is the marker of ongoing viral replication. IgM hepatitis B core antigen indicates acute infection. IgG antibodies and anti–surface antigen antibodies can be seen in previously infected or immunized people.

D. Hepatitis
1. Types
a. Viral (Table 4-3).
b. Alcoholic: Patients have a history of alcohol use and symptoms of nausea, hepatomegaly, fever, and jaundice. WBC count will be very high.
c. Drug-induced (mnemonic—TIMS MAPS): Can be caused by **t**etracycline, **I**NH, **m**ethyldopa, **s**tatins, **m**ushrooms (toxic), **a**cetaminophen, **p**henytoin, and **s**ulfonamides.

TABLE 4-3 Diagnosis, Prevention, and Treatment of Viral Hepatitis

Virus	Route of Spread	Description	Evaluation	Treatment
Hepatitis A (HVA)	Fecal-oral, foreign travel/food (water and shellfish)	Not often fulminant	Test for anti-HVA IgM	(1) Vaccine is available but not often given (2) Immunoglobulin is available
Hepatitis B (HVB)	Parenteral, IV drugs, sex	(1) Can develop into chronic hepatitis (10%) (2) Risk factor for hepatocellular carcinoma	(1) Test for HBsAg or HBcAg (2) Biopsy should be done to evaluate for chronic disease	(1) Vaccine is used (2) Immunoglobulin is available (3) Interferon therapy for chronic hepatitis, if present
Hepatitis C (HVC)	Parenteral, IV drugs, sex	(1) Frequently develops into chronic hepatitis (80%) (2) Accounts for most cases of posttransfusion hepatitis	(1) Antibody testing is diagnostic with RNA to determine viral load (2) Biopsy should be performed in all patients	Aggressive therapy with interferon and ribavirin in patients with chronic hepatitis
Hepatitis D (HVD)	Parenteral, IV drugs, sex	Can be fatal if the patient is coinfected with HBV	IgM to HVD is diagnostic.	Supportive
Hepatitis E (HVE)	Fecal-oral, foreign travel	High mortality in pregnant women (especially in third trimester) and children	None	Supportive

d. Autoimmune: Causes chronic hepatitis, usually in young women.

e. Granulomatous: Can be caused by tuberculosis, sarcoidosis, and fungal infections. Diagnose with liver biopsy.

f. Ischemic: Following blood loss or surgery.

2. Symptoms and signs

a. Patients usually have malaise followed by jaundice and fatigue. They may complain of dark urine and/or pale stools.

b. Scleral icterus, tender hepatomegaly, and lymphadenopathy may also be present.

3. Diagnostic evaluation

a. Elevated liver function tests, bilirubin, and alkaline phosphatase.

(1) Aminotransferase levels (AST and ALT) that are both increased to an equivalent degree suggest viral hepatitis.

(2) Aminotransferases less than 500 units with AST/ALT ratio greater than 2 suggest alcoholic hepatitis.

(3) Aminotransferases in the thousands suggest ischemic hepatitis.

b. Hepatitis serologic tests (see Table 4-3).

4. Treatment: Depends on the cause of the hepatitis.

a. Interferon alpha for HBV and HCV to decrease the likelihood of chronic hepatitis.

b. Corticosteroids and drinking cessation for alcoholic hepatitis.

c. Liver transplantation, if possible, for chronic hepatitis.

d. N-acetyl cysteine if acetaminophen toxicity is the cause of the hepatitis.

e. Treat autoimmune hepatitis with prednisone, azathioprine, and transplantation, if possible.

f. Treat cases of sarcoidosis with prednisone.

E. Hepatic Cirrhosis

1. Causes (Table 4-4).

2. Symptoms and signs

a. Patients may have jaundice, telangiectasias, palmar erythema, Dupuytren's contractures, gynecomastia, testicular atrophy, and fetor hepaticus.

b. Portal hypertension may cause splenomegaly, ascites, and caput medusae.

c. The firm, nodular liver may be enlarged or shrunken depending on the disease stage.

d. Cirrhosis can progress to hepatocellular carcinoma, so patients may have symptoms or signs of metastatic disease.

3. Diagnostic evaluation

a. Elevated liver function tests (AST, ALT, GGT [gamma-glutamyltransferase]). The bilirubin and prothrombin time (PT) will also be elevated.

b. Albumin will be decreased.

c. Complete blood count will show anemia and thrombocytopenia.

d. Ultrasound can be used to detect small amounts of ascites.

TABLE 4-4 Causes of Hepatic Cirrhosis

Condition	Description
Alcoholic cirrhosis	Graded according to the Child classification. This takes into account the **a**scites, **b**ilirubin, **e**ncephalopathy, **a**lbumin, and **n**utrition of the patient (mnemonic—A BEAN). (1) Group a: bilirubin < 2, albumin > 3.5, no ascites or encephalopathy, and normal nutritional status. (2) Group b: bilirubin 2–3, albumin 3–3.5, controllable ascites, minimal encephalopathy, and adequate nutrition. (3) Group c: bilirubin > 3, albumin < 3, fixed ascites, significant encephalopathy, and prominent muscle wasting due to inadequate nutrition.
Hepatitis	See preceding section.
Primary biliary cirrhosis	(1) Autoimmune destruction of the intrahepatic bile ducts. (2) Starts with pruritus and progresses to steatorrhea, xanthomas, hyperpigmentation, and bone pain. (3) Patients have increased alkaline phosphatase, GGT, and bilirubin with a positive antimitochondrial antibody. (4) Treat with ursodeoxycholic acid, fat-soluble vitamins, cholestyramine, and liver transplantation.
Primary sclerosing cholangitis	(1) Fibrosis of intra- and extrahepatic bile ducts, possibly autoimmune in origin. (2) Associated with cholangiocarcinoma and ulcerative colitis. (3) Patients have elevated bilirubin and alkaline phosphatase with a positive p-ANCA antibody. (4) Multiple beaded bile duct strictures are seen on ERCP. (5) Treat by stenting bile ducts and with liver transplantation.
Hemochromatosis	(1) Iron overload causes bronzing of the skin, diabetes, arthritis, and heart failure (2) Patients have increased iron saturation and ferritin. (3) Treat with phlebotomy and deferoxamine.
Wilson's disease	See preceding section.
$Alpha_1$-antitrypsin deficiency	(1) Patients have liver failure with emphysema at a young age. (2) Liver biopsy shows PAS+ inclusions. (3) Treat with liver transplantation and enzyme replacement for the lungs.

ERCP, endoscopic retrograde cholangiopancreatography; GGT, gamma-glutamyltransferase.

e. Alpha-fetoprotein (AFP) can be elevated in cases that have progressed to hepatocellular carcinoma.

4. Treatment
   a. Ascites can be treated with diuresis (spironolactone and loop diuretics) or paracentesis. Shunt procedures can be performed to minimize ascites, if necessary.
   b. Treatment for specific causes are described in Table 4-4.

TABLE 4-5 Complications of Hepatic Cirrhosis

Condition	Comments
Spontaneous bacterial peritonitis	(1) Usually caused by infection due to enterobacteria or pneumococci. (2) Patients have fever, pain, and abdominal tenderness. (3) Ascitic fluid has a neutrophil count of >250/μL. (4) Treat with a third-generation cephalosporin for 5–7 days, and protect from further attacks using norfloxacin, ciprofloxacin, or trimethoprim/sulfamethoxazole.
Hepatic encephalopathy	(1) Caused by increased ammonia from medications (benzodiazepines, opiates, or tricyclic antidepressants), hypokalemia, GI bleeding, infection, or hepatic deterioration. (2) Acute cases occur in fulminant hepatic failure. Cerebral edema can cause coma and death. (3) Chronic cases are caused by chronic liver disease. Patients have cognitive deficits, neuromuscular dysfunction (hyperreflexia, myoclonus, asterixis), and disruption of the sleep/wake cycle. (4) Treat with dietary protein restriction, discontinuing causative medications, and bowel clearance if GI bleeding is present. Prevent bowel ammonia absorption with lactulose. Kill ammonia-producing bacteria with neomycin.
Hepatorenal syndrome	(1) Patients have oliguria, declining glomerular filtration rate (GFR), low urine sodium, normal urinary sediment, and azotemia. (2) Treat with volume expansion, low-dose vasopressin, octreotide, norepinephrine, and possibly liver transplantation. (3) Mortatity is 95%, usually due to sepsis.
Esophageal varices	See preceding sections.

c. Treatment for the complications of cirrhosis are described in Table 4-5.

5. Complications (see Table 4-5).

XIII. Biliary Disease

A. Types

1. Cholelithiasis: Gallstones in the gallbladder.
2. Choledocholithiasis: Gallstone in the common bile duct.
3. Cholecystitis: Inflammation of the gallbladder.
4. Cholangitis: Infection of the biliary tract. Necessary components include bacteriobilia, biliary stasis, and obstruction. Most common bacteria are *E. coli* and *Klebsiella.*

a. Acute nonsuppurative cholangitis: Milder variant caused by partial obstruction of the biliary tract.

b. Acute toxic cholangitis: Due to complete obstruction of biliary tract. Pus under pressure will be present, and the patient can rapidly deteriorate.

c. Sclerosing cholangitis: Progressive disease that causes inflammation and fibrosis of the bile ducts.

Acalculous cholecystitis is a motility disorder of the gallbladder or sphincter of Oddi, giving symptoms similar to cholelithiasis. Can detect with CCK-enhanced cholecystography. Usually occurs in critically ill patients owing to stasis of bile and subsequent injury to the submucosa of the gallbladder.

d. AIDS-related cholangiopathy: Cholangitis in AIDS patients, usually due to opportunistic infection.

5. Other bile duct obstructions

a. Klatskin's tumor: Cholangiocarcinoma of the bile duct at the junction of the right and left hepatic ducts.

b. Mirizzi's syndrome: Obstruction of the common bile duct or common hepatic duct due to contiguous inflammation of the gallbladder or compression of the common hepatic duct by an impacted stone in the neighboring cystic duct. This compression can lead to stricture.

c. Pancreatic cancer: If the tumor is in the head of the pancreas.

B. Symptoms and Signs

Courvoisier's law: If the common bile duct is obstructed by a stone, dilation of the gallbladder is rare. If it is obstructed via another way (e.g., cancer), dilation is common.

Painless jaundice should be suspected to be indicative of cancer of the pancreatic head until proved otherwise.

1. Patients initially have obstructive jaundice, with the symptoms of jaundice—dark urine, clay-colored stools, pruritus, anorexia, and nausea. The gallbladder may be dilated.

2. Most cases of cholelithiasis are asymptomatic, but patients can have episodic right upper quadrant abdominal pain, right subscapular pain (Boas' sign), epigastric pain, nausea, and vomiting.

3. Cholecystitis presents with unrelenting right upper quadrant pain, right subscapular pain, fever, nausea and vomiting, and positive Murphy's sign (pain during inspiration during right upper quadrant palpation).

4. Risk factors for cholelithiasis include being female, fat, forty, and fertile.

C. Diagnostic Evaluation

1. Liver function tests are elevated, with marked elevation of alkaline phosphatase and GGT.

2. Ultrasound is the test of choice for acute cholecystitis. It can identify stones (but not inflammation) and wall thickening and can differentiate between obstructive and nonobstructive lesions.

3. Hepato-iminodiacetic acid (HIDA) scan: Can establish the presence of acute cholecystitis using a radionuclide (HIDA) that is secreted into the bile. Failure to visualize the gallbladder at 1 hour makes acute cholecystitis highly likely. This test is less reliable in patients whose bilirubin is greater than 10 mg/dL, and it can give false results in patients on prolonged parenteral nutrition or those with acute pancreatitis.

4. Endoscopic retrograde cholangiopancreatography (ERCP).

5. CT scan: Can show dilated bile ducts and assess for nearby tumors.

D. Treatment

1. Medical treatments

a. Chenodeoxycholic acid, ursodeoxycholic acid: To dissolve cholesterol gallstones.

b. For cholangitis, antibiotics and hydration work in 85% of cases.

2. Extracorporeal shock wave lithotripsy (ESWL)

a. Usually combined with oral dissolution agents.

b. Useful for single stones less than 20 mm in diameter.

3. Surgical treatments

a. Indications for surgery include symptomatic biliary disease, or asymptomatic disease in patients who are children, have sickle cell disease, or have a calcified gallbladder.

b. Cholecystectomy can be performed through laparoscopic or open approaches.

c. Sphincterotomy with basket retrieval can be done during ERCP. ERCP is also the preferred modality for performing emergency bile duct decompressions.

E. Complications

1. Complications of untreated cholelithiasis include acute cholecystitis, obstructive jaundice, acute cholangitis, gallstone ileus, and gallstone pancreatitis. Hydrops (mucocele) can also develop and cause a palpable mass in the abdomen. Fistulas can form to the skin, duodenum, or pleura.

2. Complications of cholecystectomy include common bile duct injury, right hepatic duct/artery injury, cystic duct leak, and biloma formation.

XIV. Inguinal Hernia

A. Types

1. Direct: Protrusion of abdominal contents directly through the transversalis fascia and abdominal wall. The hernia will be medial to the inferior epigastric artery.

2. Indirect: Protrusion of abdominal contents through an enlarged internal ring and a patent processus vaginalis. The hernia will be lateral to the inferior epigastric artery.

3. Pantaloon: The hernia has both direct and indirect components (portions will be both medial and lateral to the inferior epigastric vessels).

4. Epigastric: In the midline above the umbilicus.

5. Spigelian: Along the lateral inferior border of the rectus muscle.

6. Richter's: Incarcerated or strangulated hernia that involves only one side wall of bowel.

The boundaries of Hasselbach's triangle include the inferior epigastric vessels, inguinal ligament, and the lateral border of the rectus sheath. The contents of the spermatic cord include the vas deferens, spermatic vessels, genital branch of the genitofemoral nerve, and the cremasteric vessels.

B. Symptoms and Signs

1. Patients can be asymptomatic or have abdominal pain, nausea, vomiting, or poor appetite. When strangulation of the bowel has occurred, patients may have a distended abdomen, peritoneal signs, and an area of painful swelling in the inguinal region.

2. Although most hernias are in the inguinal region, they can also be found in the femoral canal, at previous incision sites, and in the umbilical area.

3. Risk factors include previous abdominal surgery or injury, and frequent increases in intra-abdominal pressure (constipation, obesity, coughing from smoking or chronic bronchitis).

C. Treatment: Surgical techniques vary, but most currently employ a repair of the abdominal wall defect with the incorporation of a mesh for reinforcement. Uncomplicated cases can be repaired through laparoscopic herniorrhaphy.

D. Complications

1. Incarceration: Abdominal contents cannot be pushed back through the hernia ring. Incarceration is more likely to occur through small herniated rings than large ones. The omentum is the most commonly herniated structure.

2. Strangulation of small bowel: The blood supply is interrupted and necrosis of the bowel occurs, causing acute bowel obstruction.
3. Ischemic orchitis: Swollen painful scrotum with testicle high in the sac. This can be prevented by limiting the dissection of the spermatic cord.

XV. Bariatric Surgery
- A. Weight reduction surgery for the morbidly obese (>100 lb over ideal body weight, or body mass index [BMI] >35).
- B. Procedures: Focus on decreasing the size of the stomach to limit filling and provide early satiety.
  1. Gastric bypass: Stapling of small gastric pouch with a Roux-en-Y limb to the gastric pouch.
  2. Vertical banded gastroplasty: Vertical stapled small gastric pouch and placement of a Silastic ring band.
- C. Complications include gallstones, marginal ulcer, anastomotic leak, stenosis of the gastric pouch, and malnutrition.

5 CHAPTER

Hematology

I. Anemia

A. Definition: The definition of anemia is sex-dependent. In men, anemia occurs when the patient has a hematocrit (Hct) less than 41% or a hemoglobin (Hb) less than 13.5 g/dL. In women, anemia occurs when the patient has an Hct of less than 36% or an Hb less than 12 g/dL.

B. Symptoms and Signs

1. The patient may have general symptoms of fatigue and dyspnea on exertion (DOE) and may also have unusual behavior such as pica (eating dirt).

2. On physical examination, the patient may have pallor, orthostatic hypotension, and tachycardia.

3. Physical examination findings that suggest a cause for the anemia include glossitis (vitamin B_{12} deficiency, iron deficiency, or folate deficiency), jaundice (hemolytic anemia), splenomegaly (thalassemia or hemolytic anemia), and sensory nerve dysfunction or ataxia (vitamin B_{12} deficiency).

C. Types: Anemias are typically classified as microcytic, normocytic, or macrocytic, depending on the size of the patient's red blood cells (Tables 5-1 and 5-2).

Rarer forms of congenital macrocytic anemia with megaloblastosis include Diamond-Blackfan syndrome (an autosomal recessive pure red cell aplasia with short stature, web neck, cleft lip, shield chest, and triphalangeal thumb) and Fanconi's anemia (an autosomal recessive disorder with hyperpigmentation, café-au-lait spots, microcephaly, structural kidney problems, and absent thumbs).

D. Evaluation

1. Iron measurements

a. Total iron-binding capacity (TIBC): Characterizes the degree of iron absorption by transferrin.

b. Ferritin: Provides storage for nonheme iron. The level can rise during inflammatory processes.

c. Transferrin saturation = Serum iron/transferrin (usually >20%).

2. Complete blood count (CBC) with differential and analysis of red blood cell (RBC) parameters.

a. Hct and Hb will allow the diagnosis of anemia.

b. Mean corpuscular volume (MCV) will indicate whether the anemia is microcytic (small RBC), normocytic (normal-size RBC), or macrocytic (large RBC).

3. Peripheral blood smear (Fig. 5-1; see Tables 5-1 and 5-2).

4. Complete metabolic profile (CMP): Will detect an increased indirect bilirubin and an increased lactate dehydrogenase (LDH) in hemolytic anemia.

E. Treatment (see Tables 5-1 and 5-2)

II. Thrombocytopenia: Abnormally low platelet count.

A. Thrombotic Thrombocytopenic Purpura

1. Symptoms and signs (Mnemonic—FAT RN)

a. **F**ever

b. **A**nemia

TABLE 5-1
Types of Anemia*

Disorder (Type)	Symptoms and Signs	Evaluation	Treatment
Iron deficiency (microcytic)	(1) History of chronic bleeding, malnutrition, malabsorption, or pregnancy. Iron deficiency is also the most common cause of anemia in menstruating women. (2) Plummer-Vinson syndrome includes iron deficiency anemia with esophageal webbing and atrophic glossitis.	(1) Low iron and ferritin, increased total iron-binding capacity (TIBC). (2) Hypochromatic cells on peripheral blood smear.	Give supplemental iron.
Thalassemia (microcytic)	(1) More common in patients of Mediterranean ancestry. (2) Due to decreased synthesis of the alpha- or beta-globin chains of hemoglobin. (3) Alpha-thalassemia major is a lethal mutation resulting in a stillborn child or a neonate with hydrops fetalis. (4) Beta-thalassemia major requires homozygosity for the beta-thalassemia mutation. These patients have severe hemolytic anemia, splenomegaly, hemochromatosis, and eventually skeletal deformities (tower skull, frontal bossing, maxillary hypertrophy) from bone marrow hyperplasia.	(1) Peripheral blood smear has teardrop cells, Heinz bodies, and basophilic stippling. (2) Iron studies are normal. (3) Hemoglobin electrophoresis is abnormal and can distinguish between the types of thalassemia.	Give blood transfusions while preventing iron overload with deferoxamine.
Anemia of chronic disease (microcytic)	Occurs in the presence of chronic inflammatory disease. This may be caused by the inability to mobilize iron stores.	Decreased iron and TIBC, but ferritin may be increased due to systemic inflammation.	Treat the underlying disease. Iron is of no benefit, but erythropoietin may be beneficial in severe disease.
Sideroblastic anemia (microcytic)	Can be congenital, caused by drugs (lead alcohol, isoniazid, chloramphenicol), malignancy or collagen vascular disease.	Distinct population of microcytic, hypochromic RBCs with basophilic stippling and sideroblasts (nucleated RBCs with a perinuclear ring) due to abnormal iron metabolism.	Discontinue offending drugs.
Transient erythroblastopenia of childhood (normocytic)	(1) Presents at >6 months of age with gradual onset of anemia with a normal physical examination. (2) Caused by bone marrow suppression and pure red cell aplasia. Viral infection predisposes to development of this anemia.	None	Recovery is spontaneous, but symptomatic anemia may require transfusion.

TABLE 5-1 Types of Anemia*—cont'd

Disorder (Type)	Symptoms and Signs	Evaluation	Treatment
Hemolytic anemia	See Table 5-2.	See Table 5-2.	See Table 5-2.
Aplastic anemia (normocytic)	Anemia that can be caused by drugs, viruses, autoimmune disease, and a variety of congenital disorders. Drugs that can cause this include alkylating agents, antimetabolites, anthracyclines, chloramphenicol, sulfa drugs, and benzene.	Bone marrow biopsy shows acellular bone marrow and pancytopenia.	Treat with transfusion, immunosuppression, epoietin alfa, G-CSF, and bone marrow transplantation.
Myelophthisic anemia (normocytic)	Represents a reaction within the bone marrow to the invasion of tumor cells, granulomatous infections, or lipid deposition in Gaucher's disease.	(1) Fibrosis is present on bone marrow biopsy. (2) Peripheral blood smear findings consistent with extramedullary hematopoiesis.	Bone marrow replacement is indicated for patients with carcinoma, granuloma, or fibrosis.
Pure red cell aplasia (normocytic)	Associated with thymoma and viral infections.	Lack of erythroid precursors in the bone marrow.	Treat with thymectomy and/or immunosuppression.
Myelodysplastic anemias (normocytic)	Progressive pancytopenia that may present in a variety of ways, depending on which cell lineages are most deficient.	(1) CBC shows cytopenias with a hypercellular bone marrow and morphologic abnormalities in the cells. (2) Pelger-Huët cells can be seen on peripheral smear.	Treat with transfusions, epoietin, G-CSF, and bone marrow transplant.
Folate deficiency (macrocytic)	(1) Can be caused by malnutrition, malabsorption, pregnancy, hemolytic anemia, or carcinoma. (2) Patients will have megaloblastic anemia without neurologic deficits.	(1) Peripheral blood smear shows pancytopenia, macroovalocytes, and hypersegmented neutrophils. (2) Normal vitamin B_{12} and decreased folate levels.	Treat with folate supplementation.
Vitamin B_{12} deficiency (macrocytic)	(1) Can be due to malnutrition, malabsorption or pernicious anemia. (2) B_{12} deficiencies have megaloblastic anemia with neurologic symptoms including peripheral neuropathies, dementia, ataxia, and posterior column degeneration.	(1) Peripheral blood smear shows pancytopenia, macroovalocytes, and hypersegmented neutrophils. (2) Normal folate and decreased B_{12}.	(1) Treat with intramuscular vitamin B_{12}. Neurologic dysfunction may be reversible if the patient is treated within 6 months of symptom onset. (2) Do not treat vitamin B_{12} deficiency with folate because the anemia will be corrected but the neurologic problems will continue to progress.

*See Figure 5-1 for examples of abnormalities seen on peripheral smear.

TABLE 5-2 Hemolytic Anemias*

Disorder	Symptoms and Signs	Evaluation	Treatment
Hereditary spherocytosis	(1) Due to a defect in spectrin. (2) Patients may have aplastic crises after parvovirus B19 infection. (3) Chronic hemolysis predisposes patients to gallstones.	(1) Spherocytes on peripheral blood smear. (2) Positive osmotic fragility test.	Treat with splenectomy at 6 years of age.
Glucose-6-phosphate dehydrogenase deficiency (G6PD)	(1) X-linked recessive mutation that results in an inability to regenerate reduced glutathione (an antioxidant compound). (2) Hemolysis can be caused by infection, foods (fava beans), or medications (mnemonic—SAND: *s*ulfonamides, *a*ntimalarials, *n*itrofurantoin, *d*imercaprol).	Peripheral smear may show bite cells and Heinz bodies.	Stop the precipitant medications during a crisis. No long-term treatment needed.
Sickle cell anemia	(1) Caused by an autosomal recessive beta-globin substitution mutation. (2) Anemia develops at >4 months of age owing to the loss of RBCs containing fetal hemoglobin. (3) Clinical symptoms are the result of anemia, infection, or vaso-occlusion. (4) Medical emergencies can be caused by splenic sequestration (this will cause a functional splenectomy and predispose to *S. pneumoniae* and *H. influenzae* infection) and aplastic crisis following parvovirus B19 infection. (5) Hyperhemolytic crisis can occur in patients who also have G6PD deficiency.	(1) Sickle-shaped RBCs and Howell-Jolly bodies on peripheral blood smear. (2) Abnormal hemoglobin electrophoresis.	(1) Treat with hydroxyurea. (2) Treat crises with O_2, hydration, and analgesia. (3) Patients with functional splenectomy should be on penicillin prophylaxis.

TABLE 5-2 Hemolytic Anemias*—cont'd

Disorder	Symptoms and Signs	Evaluation	Treatment
Autoimmune hemolytic anemia (AIHA)	(1) Associated with lymphoproliferative disorders, autoimmune diseases, and infections. (2) IgG-mediated: Warm hemolytic anemia. Associated with autoimmune disease and drug reactions (quinidine, quinine, rifampin, methyldopa, procainamide). (3) IgM-mediated: Cold hemolytic anemia. Usually postinfectious (mycoplasma or Epstein Barr virus).	Spherocytes on peripheral blood smear	(1) IgG-mediated: Treat with prednisone, splenectomy, or immunosuppression. (2) IgM-mediated: Treat underlying disease. Can also treat with corticosteroids, plasmapheresis, or splenectomy.
Microangiopathic hemolytic anemia (MAHA)	Associated with disseminated intravascular coagulation, hemolytic uremic syndrome, thrombotic thrombocytopenic purpura, leukemia, and malignant hypertension.	Schistocytes are present on peripheral blood smear.	Treat the underlying abnormality.
Paroxysmal nocturnal hemoglobinuria	(1) The patient's RBCs are susceptible to lysis by complement. (2) Patients have iron deficiency anemia, abdominal pain, and venous thromboses.	Positive Ham's (acid) or sucrose hemolysis test.	Prednisone and cautious iron replacement (may cause more hemolysis).

*See Figure 5-1 for examples of abnormalities seen on peripheral smear.

c. **T**hrombocytopenia
d. **R**enal dysfunction
e. **N**eurologic abnormality (this will not be present in hemolytic-uremic syndrome)
f. Also, palpable purpura and splenomegaly

2. Evaluation
   a. CBC will display anemia with thrombocytopenia.
   b. Peripheral blood smear displays fragmented red blood cells (schistocytosis).
   c. CMP may display elevated indirect bilirubin and increased LDH.
   d. Coagulation laboratory tests (PT, PTT) will be normal.

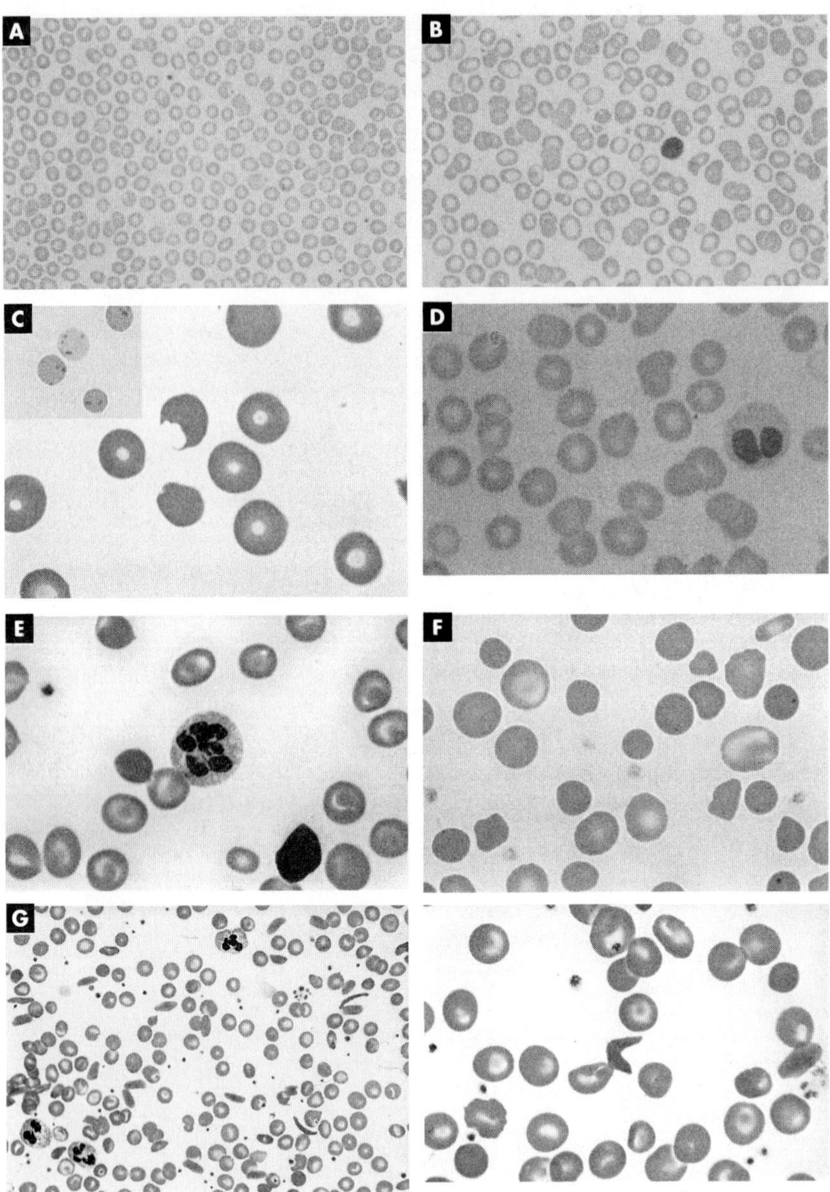

5-1: *Common abnormalities observed on peripheral blood smear in anemia.* A, *Normal.* B, *Hypochromic microcytic (iron deficiency).* C, *Heinz bodies and bite cells (thalassemia, glucose-6-phosphate dehydrogenase deficiency).* D, *Pelger-Huët cell (myelodysplastic anemia).* E, *Hypersegmented neutrophils (vitamin B_{12}, folate deficiency).* F, *Spherocytes (hereditary spherocytosis, autoimmune hemolytic anemia).* G, *Sickle cells (sickle cell anemia).*

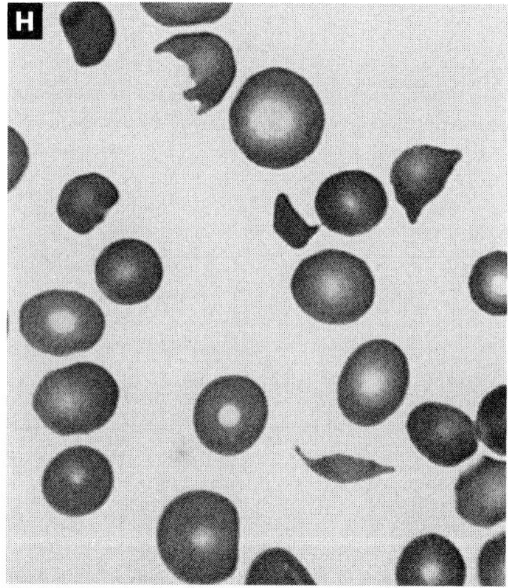

5-1, cont'd *H, Schistocytes (microangiopathic hemolytic anemia).*

3. Treat with plasmapheresis and a replacement infusion with normal plasma. Splenectomy may be useful if the symptoms are unresponsive to plasmapheresis.

B. Idiopathic Thrombocytopenic Purpura: Caused by autoimmune antibody formation against host platelets.
   1. Patients can have mucosal bleeding, petechiae, easy bruising, and purpura. They will be afebrile and will not have splenomegaly.
   2. Evaluation
      a. Very low platelets, but no anemia. This becomes dangerous if the platelet level drops below 20,000.
      b. No schistocytes on peripheral blood smear.
      c. Positive platelet-associated IgG test.
   3. Treatment: Most pediatric cases resolve spontaneously within 6 months, but most adults require treatment.
      a. Treat initially with corticosteroids.
      b. Intravenous immunoglobulin (IVIg) and splenectomy can be used in patients unresponsive to steroid treatment.
      c. Platelet infusions are indicated for severe, uncontrollable bleeding.

III. Coagulopathies
   A. The Coagulation Cascade (Fig. 5-2)
   B. Bleeding Disorders (Table 5-3)
   C. Hypercoagulable States
      1. Causes (Table 5-4).
      2. Symptoms and signs
         a. Patients most frequently have deep vein thrombosis (DVT) in early adulthood, but thrombosis at superficial veins or cerebral veins can also

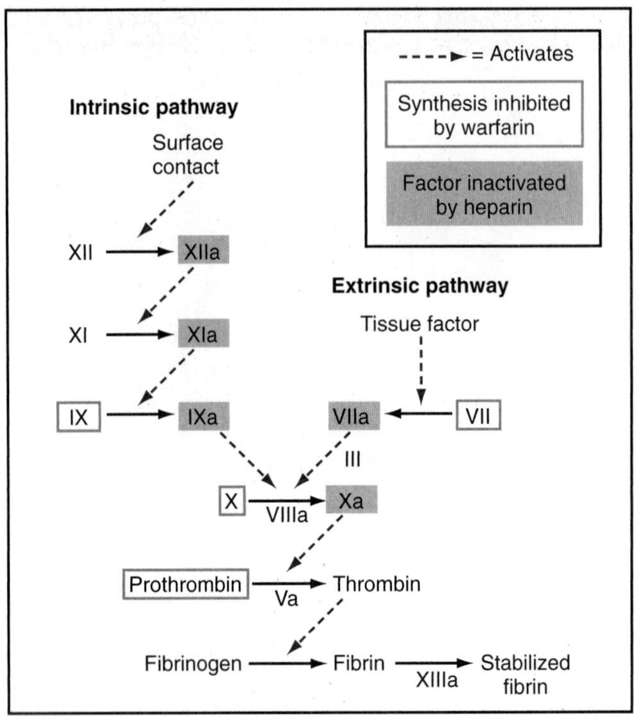

5-2: The coagulation cascade.

TABLE 5-3
Bleeding Disorders

Disorder	Description	Evaluation	Treatment
Von Willebrand's disease	Due to a deficiency of von Willebrand's factor (vWF), which interacts with factor VIII and protects it from clearance. This means that factor VIII deficiency may also be present.	(1) Decreased factor VIII, decreased vWF antigen, decreased ristocetin cofactor assay. (2) PT and PTT normal, bleeding time elevated.	DDAVP (a.k.a. desmopressin, a vasopressin analog that releases factor VIII from tissue stores) and either cryoprecipitates or factor VIII concentrates.
Vitamin K deficiency	(1) Vitamin K is needed for factors II, VII, IX, and X and proteins C and S. (2) Deficiency can occur in children as hemorrhagic disease of the newborn, or in adults owing to malnutrition, malabsorption, or warfarin therapy.	Increased PT, decreased factors II, VII, IX, and X.	Vitamin K with or without infusion of fresh-frozen plasma.

TABLE 5-3 Bleeding Disorders—cont'd

Disorder	Symptoms and Signs	Evaluation	Treatment
Disseminated intravascular coagulation	(1) Results from widespread coagulation (thrombin) and fibrinolysis (plasmin) during severe illness. Fibrin deposition in blood vessels can cause ischemia and clotting factor depletion. (2) Usually associated with massive trauma, malignancy, or obstetric complications.	(1) Increased PT, fibrin degradation products, and D-dimer. (2) Decreased fibrinogen and platelets.	Treat the underlying process and administer fresh-frozen plasma, cryoprecipitate, and platelets.
Hemophilia	(1) Hemophilia A: Factor VIII deficiency. X-linked recessive inheritance. (2) Hemophilia B: Factor IX deficiency. X-linked recessive inheritance.	(1) Both show normal PT. (2) Prolonged PTT that normalizes with a mixing study. (3) Decreased factor VIII or IX.	Factor VIII or IX concentrate and DDAVP.
Coagulation factor inhibitors	Antibodies present in the serum will inactivate specific portions of the coagulation cascade.	Increased PTT that does not normalize with a mixing study.	Porcine factor replacement, plasmapheresis, or immunosuppression.
Heparin use	History of recent heparin use.	Increases PTT.	(1) Cessation of heparin. (2) Protamine sulfate can be used.
Heparin-induced thrombocytopenia	(1) Due to an antibody response to unfractionated heparin and the binding of these antibodies on the Fc receptors of circulating platelets. (2) Patients may develop thrombotic complications.	Patients with these antibodies can develop thrombocytopenia (usually 50,000–100,000 platelets).	(1) Discontinue heparin and start lepirudin. (2) Also discontinue warfarin because of the risk of catastrophic limb thrombosis.
Thrombolysis	Patients should have a very recent history of thrombolytic therapy.	(1) Decreased fibrinogen. (2) Increased fibrin degradation products and D-dimer.	Cryoprecipitate or fresh-frozen plasma, if necessary.

TABLE 5-4 Hypercoagulable States

Type	Disorder	Description
Inherited	Protein C or S deficiency	(1) Cause impaired inactivation of factors VIIIa and Va in the coagulation cascade. (2) Patients usually have thrombosis between 20 and 40 years of age. (3) Tests are available to determine the activity and amount of protein C and S in the blood.
	Factor V Leiden mutation	(1) Causes activated protein C (APC) resistance. (2) Can be evaluated using a Factor V Leiden DNA assay.
	Hyperhomocysteinemia	(1) Homocysteine may damage the endothelial cells or interrupt their anticoagulant processes. (2) Can result in both venous and arterial thromboses. (3) Can be evaluated by measuring the fasting serum homocysteine level.
	Abnormalities of fibrinolysis	Leads to the inability to inactivate factor V, which results in increased thrombin generation.
	Prothrombin mutation G20210A	Results in a 2-fold risk for deep vein thrombosis or pulmonary embolism.
	Antithrombin III deficiency	(1) Can be tested with antithrombin activity and quantification. (2) Can treat with antithrombin III replacement and anticoagulation.
Medication-induced	Oral contraceptives, heparin	Hypercoagulable states can develop with the use of oral contraceptives or the development of heparin-induced thrombocytopenia.
Acquired	Malignancy	Any patient that is diagnosed with a hypercoagulable state should be evaluated for malignancy.
	Antiphospholipid antibodies	(1) The patient may present with a history of thrombosis (deep vein thrombosis, pulmonary embolism, stroke) with mild thrombocytopenia. They may also have a history of recurrent fetal loss. (2) Anticardiolipin and/or lupus anticoagulant antibodies will be present. Anticardiolipin does not change PTT. Lupus anticoagulant prolongs PTT. (3) Screen the patient for malignancy.
	Nephrotic syndrome	Will cause loss of protein C and S in the urine.
	Pregnancy	(1) Pregnancy decreases the effectiveness of the fibrinolytic system. (2) Many thrombotic events occur in the peripartum period, especially after delivery.
	Trauma or surgery	The risk depends on the nature of the surgery or injury, but circulating effector molecules following tissue injury combined with a lack of patient mobility can contribute to their hypercoagulability.
	Paroxysmal nocturnal hemoglobinuria	(1) Patients will have anemia, pain, and RBC lysis by complement (see Table 5-2). (2) Treat with prednisone and cautious iron supplementation.

occur. These thromboses may embolize or cause end-organ necrosis, depending on the location.

b. In contrast to the other causes of hypercoagulability, hyperhomocysteinemia also predisposes to arterial thrombosis. This can lead to myocardial infarction, stroke, and peripheral arterial disease, in addition to the venous thrombotic complications discussed previously.

3. Evaluation (see Table 5-4).

4. Treatment: The treatment for all hypercoagulable syndromes involves warfarin anticoagulation with a target INR of greater than 3.0. Specific additional therapies for the deficiencies are described in Table 5-4.

Arterial thrombosis will present with claudication, rest pain, a cool extremity, and absent pulses in an affected limb. Venous thrombosis will present with limb pain, edema, and limb cyanosis, but pulses may be palpable (if the edema is not so severe that it prevents evaluation).

There are several caveats to the interpretation of abnormal coagulation labs. (1) During an acute thrombotic event, levels of protein C, protein S, and antithrombin will be reduced. (2) Heparin reduces antithrombin levels. (3) Warfarin reduces protein C and protein S levels. Keep the status and medications of the patient in mind before deciding on a probable cause for the coagulopathy.

Hodgkin's disease has an incidence of 2 in 10,000 and a bimodal age distribution (predominantly affecting people between ages 15 and 25 or after age 50).

IV. Lymphoma

A. Hodgkin's Disease

1. Symptoms and signs

a. Patients have painless lymphadenopathy, usually in the neck.

b. Constitutional symptoms may include fever, sweats, and weight loss.

c. The patient may have shortness of breath (SOB) or wheezing if the airways are involved or compressed.

2. Evaluation

a. Excisional lymph node biopsy is diagnostic.

(1) Reed-Sternberg cells (large cells with multilobed nuclei) will be present in the affected lymph node (Fig. 5-3).

(2) Histologic types of Hodgkin's disease include lymphocyte predominance, nodular sclerosis, mixed cellularity, and lymphocyte depletion.

b. Bone marrow biopsy to assess for marrow involvement.

c. Splenectomy may be necessary to confirm staging before radiation therapy.

3. Staging: A staging laparotomy may be required to accurately classify the extent of disease.

a. Stage I: Restricted to a single lymph node region.

b. Stage II: Involvement of more than 2 lymph node regions on the same side of the diaphragm.

c. Stage III: Involvement of lymph node regions on both sides of the diaphragm.

d. Stage IV: Disseminated involvement of including extralymphatic organs.

4. Treatment

a. Stage I: Radiation therapy.

b. Stage II: Radiation and/or chemotherapy.

c. Stages III and IV: Chemotherapy. A commonly used combination is the ABVD regimen, which includes doxorubicin (**A**driamycin), **b**leomycin, **v**inblastine, and **d**acarbazine.

5. Prognosis: With treatment, patients with stage I or II disease have a 10-year survival of greater than 80%. Patients with stage III or IV disease have a 10-year survival of 60%.

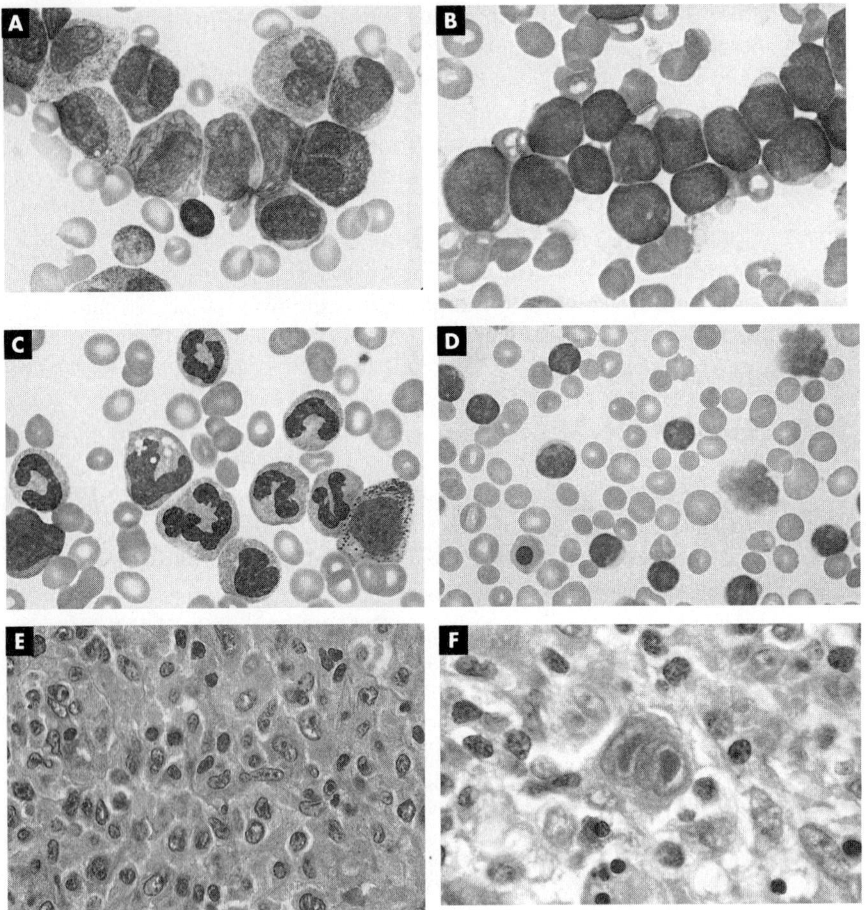

5-3: *Diagnostic features of leukemia and lymphoma, based on cell morphology. A, In acute myelogenous leukemia (AML), circulating blast cells will be present on the peripheral smear and needle-like Auer rods will be present in some cells. B, In acute lymphocytic leukemia (ALL), lymphocytosis and circulating blasts will be present, without Auer rods. C, In chronic myelogenous leukemia (CML), the peripheral smear will display a leukocytosis with varying maturation and circulating blasts. D, In chronic lymphocytic leukemia (CLL), mature-appearing lymphocytes and "smudge cells" will be present. E, Non-Hodgkin's lymphoma (NHL) will present with atypical lymphocytes in an affected organ (a lymph node, in this picture). F, Hodgkin's lymphoma may display atypical lymphocytes similar to those seen in NHL but will additionally have large, binucleate Reed-Sternberg cells.*

NHL has an incidence of 3 in 10,000. It predominantly affects patients over 50 years of age.

B. Non-Hodgkin's Lymphoma (NHL)
   1. Patients typically have nontender, diffuse lymphadenopathy. They also may have abdominal pain and bone pain.
   2. Lymph node biopsy is diagnostic (see Fig. 5-3).
      a. There are no Reed-Sternberg cells.
      b. There can be nodal and extranodal involvement.
      c. Non-Hodgkin's lymphomas are usually B-cell lymphomas.

3. Staging: Stages are the same as those for Hodgkin's lymphoma, but histologic grade is more important in NHL.
    a. Low-grade changes: Small lymphocytic, follicular pattern with small cells.
    b. Intermediate-grade changes: Follicular pattern with mostly large cells, or diffuse pattern.
    c. High-grade changes: Blastic cells, Burkitt's and non-Burkitt's lymphomas. These frequently spread to the meninges. Perform a lumbar puncture to assess for meningeal involvement.
4. Treatment: Chemotherapy with or without irradiation.
    a. Low-grade lymphoma: Use alkylating agents, fludarabine, or cladribine. Treatment often is not started until patients become symptomatic. Relapses can be treated with more chemotherapy or with rituximab (anti-CD20 antibodies).
    b. Intermediate-grade lymphoma: CHOP regimen (**c**yclophosphamide, **d**oxorubicin, vincristine (**O**ncovorin), and **p**rednisone. An anthracycline can also be used.
    c. High-grade lymphoma: High-dose chemotherapy with CNS prophylaxis (intrathecal methotrexate). Give hydration, urine alkalinization, and allopurinol to prevent tumor lysis in patients with Burkitt's lymphoma.
    d. Autologous bone marrow transplantation is another treatment option.
5. Prognosis: Patients with low-grade lymphoma have an average survival of 6 to 8 years. The prognosis for high-grade lymphoma is highly dependent on the effectiveness of chemotherapy. Chemotherapy can be curative in up to 30% of cases of high-grade lymphoma.

V. Leukemia (Table 5-5; see Fig. 5-3)

VI. Myeloproliferative Disorders
  A. Polycythemia Vera: Overproduction of erythrocytes by the bone marrow that is independent of erythropoietin levels.
    1. Symptoms and signs
      a. Patients may have a history of thrombosis (transient ischemic attack, myocardial infarction, digital pain, paresthesias, gangrene).
      b. Patients may also have symptoms of headache, visual problems, mental clouding, or pruritus after bathing.
      c. These patients are also predisposed to hemorrhage due to platelet dysfunction.
    2. Evaluation
      a. Hematocrit will be high.
      b. Erythropoietin will be low.
    3. Treatment: Patients usually die within 18 months of diagnosis if they are not treated. With treatment, the disease course is chronic and progressive.
      a. Treat with intermittent phlebotomy and low-dose chemotherapy (hydroxyurea and interferon).

TABLE 5-5
Types of Leukemia

Disorder	Symptoms and Signs	Evaluation	Treatment/Prognosis
Acute myelogenous leukemia (AML)	(1) Occurs primarily adults or children <1 year of age. The incidence is 2.5 in 100,000. (2) Most patients have a brief viral-like syndrome. Fatigue, infection, and bleeding may indicate decrease in functional blood cells. (3) If the WBC count exceeds 100,000, patients can experience headache, blurred vision, and transient ischemic attacks from leukostasis.	(1) Peripheral blood smear may show elevated WBCs with circulating blasts. (2) Bone marrow biopsy specimen is hypercellular with >30% blasts. Auer rods (eosinophilic needle-like inclusions) may also be present. (3) Tumor lysis can cause massive electrolyte abnormalities.	(1) Induction chemotherapy using a "3 + 7" regimen (3 days of idarubicin/ daunorubicin followed by 7 days of cytarabine). (2) For leukostasis, start treatment immediately with leukapheresis, hydroxyurea, and chemotherapy. (3) Bone marrow transplantation can also be attempted. (4) Complete remission can occur with therapy in up to 80% of patients.
Acute lymphocytic leukemia (ALL)	(1) This is the most common cause of childhood leukemia (usually presents between ages 3 and 7) but it also accounts for 20% of acute leukemias in adults. The incidence is 6 in 100,000. (2) Patients have fatigue, bleeding, bone pain, hepatosplenomegaly, and lymphadenopathy. Another possible complication is leukemic meningitis. (3) Risk factors include Down syndrome, radiation exposure, and a sibling with leukemia.	(1) Peripheral blood smear will show pancytopenia with circulating blasts. (2) Bone marrow biopsy specimen is hypercellular with >30% blasts. Immunostaining with TdT and CALLA will confirm the diagnosis and subtype. (3) Tumor lysis can cause massive electrolyte imbalances.	(1) Induction chemotherapy using the CHOP regimen (**c**yclophosphamide, **h**ydroxydamnomycin, vincristine [**O**ncovin], and **p**rednisone). Alternatively, vincristine and prednisone with L-asparaginase can be used. (2) CNS prophylaxis using irradiation with or without intrathecal methotrexate can be used.
Chronic myelogenous leukemia (CML)	(1) Occurs in middle-aged adults and in children. The incidence is 2 per 100,000. (2) Patients can have fevers, night sweats, fatigue, and splenomegaly. Signs of leukostasis may also be present. (3) The condition eventually evolves into acute leukemia following a blast crisis, in which blasts replace marrow cells and cause loss of other bone marrow elements.	(1) Peripheral blood smear shows leukocytosis with varying degrees of maturation and few blasts. (2) Bone marrow biopsy specimen is hypercellular with <5% blasts. Philadelphia chromosomes [t(9,22)] can be detected by polymerase chain reaction (PCR) detection of the BCR-ABL fusion.	(1) Chemotherapy with hydroxyurea and interferon alpha with or without cytarabine. (2) Bone marrow transplantation can also be attempted. (3) Average survival is 3 to 4 years with treatment.

TABLE 5-5 Types of Leukemia—cont'd

Disorder	Symptoms and Signs	Evaluation	Treatment
Chronic lymphocytic leukemia (CLL)	(1) Occurs primarily in patients over 50 years of age. The incidence is 2 in 100,000. (2) Patients have fatigue, malaise, and night sweats. (3) Lymphadenopathy, hepatosplenomegaly, or immunosuppression may also be present. (4) Other associated conditions include autoimmune hemolytic anemia and thrombocytopenia.	(1) Flow cytometry demonstrates a proliferation of a clonal population of B cells. (2) Peripheral blood smear shows lymphocytosis. (3) Bone marrow biopsy specimen has small B-cell lymphocytes with abnormal cytogenetics. (4) Lymph node biopsy specimen has small lymphocytic or diffuse small cleaved cells.	(1) Do not treat until patients are symptomatic. (2) Chemotherapy with chlorambucil and prednisone or fludarabine. (3) Splenectomy, IVIg, and/or corticosteroids for autoimmune disease. (4) Patients who are given the diagnosis in the early stages of disease can live in excess of 10 years. Patients who are given the diagnosis in the late stages of the disease often die within 2 years.

b. Treatment goals include maintenance of Hct less than 45% in men and less than 42% in women.

B. Essential Thrombocytosis
1. Symptoms and signs
a. Patients have headache, dizziness, visual changes, and burning in the hands and feet (erythromelalgia).
b. Thrombocytosis predisposes to thrombotic disease, so thrombotic symptoms may be present.
c. If present in a pregnant woman, the risk of fetal loss is high.
2. Evaluation
a. Elevated levels of platelets and WBCs (platelets >600,000 with normal RBC mass)
b. Normal iron studies
c. Bone marrow biopsy that has ruled out myelodysplasia, myelofibrosis, and Philadelphia chromosomes
3. Treatment
a. Mild symptoms: Aspirin.
b. Elderly patients or those with thrombosis history can be treated with hydroxyurea or anagrelide.
c. Pregnant patients can be treated with interferon or aspirin.

C. Myelofibrosis: Excessive marrow fibrosis leading to marrow failure.
1. Symptoms and signs
a. Patients present with fatigue and dyspnea, which progresses to early satiety and left upper quadrant abdominal pain from splenomegaly and splenic infarction. Hepatomegaly may also be present.
b. Patients may eventually develop complications of neutropenia and thrombocytopenia.

2. Evaluation
    a. CBC will display anemia with normal RBC mass.
    b. Peripheral smear will show evidence of extramedullary hematopoiesis, with teardrop erythrocytes and circulating immature blood cells.
    c. Bone marrow biopsy will display bone marrow fibrosis and an absence of Philadelphia chromosomes.
3. Treatment
    a. Hydroxyurea to decrease thrombocytosis and leukocytosis.
    b. Splenectomy for symptomatic patients, refractory thrombocytopenia, and portal hypertension.
    c. Allogenic stem cell transplantation can be tried.
    d. Ten percent of patients progress to leukemia, but the most frequent cause of death is thrombotic disease.

D. Multiple Myeloma

Multiple myeloma has an incidence of 3 in 100,000. It is predominantly found in older adults.

The presence of a monoclonal protein in the blood without Bence Jones proteinuria, hypercalcemia, or renal disease suggests a diagnosis of monoclonal gammopathy of undetermined significance (MGUS). This is a benign disorder that may progress to myeloma over the course of years. Patients may be asymptomatic, or they may have symptoms of chronic peripheral neuropathy (see Chapter 8).

1. Symptoms and signs
    a. Patients can have anemia, bone pain, and signs of hypercalcemia (kidney stones, constipation, fatigue, and altered mental status).
    b. Patients may be susceptible to recurrent infections.
    c. Overproduction of circulating antibodies and light chains can produce proteinuria, renal failure, and hyperviscosity syndromes.
2. Evaluation
    a. Serum protein electrophoresis: To identify an excess of a monoclonal antibody (M protein) in the blood.
    b. Urine protein electrophoresis: To detect light chains (Bence Jones protein) in the urine.
    c. CMP may detect a high total serum protein with a low albumin.
    d. Bone survey: To assess lytic bony lesions. These may also be noticed on a radiograph (Fig. 5-4).
    e. Beta$_2$-microglobulin: For staging.

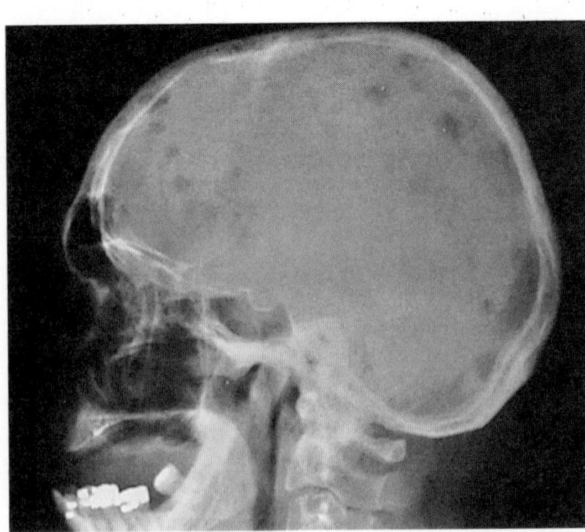

5-4: *Radiographic appearance of multiple myeloma. Skull radiograph depicting multiple lytic bone lesions, which are a common finding in multiple myeloma.*

3. Treatment
   a. Chemotherapy including melphalan + prednisone.
   b. Bisphosphonates and irradiation can decrease osteoclastic activity.
   c. Plasmapheresis for acute renal failure or hyperviscosity.
4. Prognosis: The average survival of patients with multiple myeloma is 3 years.

E. Waldenström's Macroglobulinemia: Malignancy of plasma cells that secrete large amounts of IgM.
1. Symptoms and signs
   a. Hepatomegaly, splenomegaly, and lymphadenopathy can be present, but bone involvement is rare.
   b. Patients often have symptoms of hyperviscosity, including epistaxis, retinal hemorrhages, dizziness, confusion, and cryoglobulinemia (Raynaud's phenomenon).
2. Evaluation
   a. Serum protein electrophoresis and immunofixation will detect a large amount of monoclonal IgM (>3 g/dL).
   b. Plasma cell infiltration of the bone marrow may be present on bone marrow biopsy.
3. Treatment
   a. Plasmapheresis to decrease IgM.
   b. Chemotherapy with 2-chlorodeoxyadenosine (2-CdA) and fludarabine or an alkylating agent. Prednisone can be added.

Monoclonal IgM at levels less than 3 g/dL is insufficient to cause hyperviscosity. In this case, the patient would have MGUS of the IgM type, which may be asymptomatic or associated with peripheral neuropathy.

CHAPTER 6

Infectious Disease

Children with asplenia should receive both pneumococcal and meningococcal vaccine, because the spleen is important for the clearance of encapsulated organisms. *Haemophilus influenzae* is also encapsulated, but that vaccine should be given to all children.

Otitis media can be differentiated from otitis externa because movement of the auricle causes pain in otitis externa but not in otitis media.

Viral causes of pharyngitis include rhinovirus, coronavirus, adenovirus, Epstein-Barr virus, and influenza. These infections resolve spontaneously with symptomatic treatment.

I. Immunization (Table 6-1)

II. Head and Neck Infections

A. Otitis Media (OM): Occurs most often in children 6 to 36 months of age.

1. Causes: 30% of cases are caused by viruses, 70% of cases are caused by bacteria (*Streptococcus pneumoniae, Haemophilus influenzae, Moraxella catarrhalis*). Chronic suppurative OM is more likely to be due to *Staphylococcus aureus* or *Pseudomonas aeruginosa* (often associated with spa or hot tub use).

2. Patients have ear pain, fever, and fussiness that are often preceded by cold symptoms. On otoscopic examination, the tympanic membrane looks opaque, erythematous, and immobile.

3. Treat with oral amoxicillin or ampicillin/clavulanic acid.

B. Sinusitis: Typically caused by the same organisms as OM.

1. Patients have a history of headache, fever, and chronic purulent nasal drainage. Facial pain and sinus tenderness are present on physical examination, and the infected sinus fails to transilluminate.

2. Treat with oral amoxicillin or ampicillin/clavulanic acid for 14 to 21 days. Decongestants can also be helpful.

C. Oral Candidiasis (Thrush): *Candida* infection of the mouth.

1. Can be seen in infants, immunocompromised people, and people getting broad-spectrum antibiotics.

2. Mild cases show white exudates on the buccal mucosa and pharynx. More severe cases may be painful.

3. Yeast and pseudohyphae can be seen on KOH (potassium hydroxide) treatment of exudate scrapings.

4. Treatment: The thrush may resolve after discontinuation of the antibiotics without additional treatment, or with clotrimazole. Thrush unresponsive to clotrimazole or infection of the esophagus should be treated with fluconazole or itraconazole.

D. Herpangina: Caused by enteroviruses (coxsackievirus A)

1. This occurs most commonly in spring and summer.

2. Patients initially have a high fever and very sore throat, with the development of vesicular lesions and ulcers scattered over the soft palate, tonsils, and pharynx.

3. If similar lesions are present on feet and hands, then it is called hand-foot-and-mouth disease.

4. The infection resolves without treatment in 5 to 7 days.

E. Streptococcal Pharyngitis: Caused by group A beta-hemolytic streptococci.

1. Unlike other causes of pharyngitis, streptococcal pharyngitis requires treatment because of the frequency of complications.

TABLE 6-1 Commonly Used Vaccinations and Recommended Dosing Schedules

Immunization	Diseases Covered	Time of Administration (months of age)
Hepatitis B	Hepatitis B	Birth, 1, 6 Indicated for those who are likely to be exposed to blood (including health care workers)
Hib	*Haemophilus influenzae* type b	2, 4, 6, 12
PCV	Pneumococcal	2, 4, 6, 12
IPV	Inactivated poliovirus	2, 4, 6, and then at 4 years
DTaP	Diphtheria, tetanus, pertussis	2, 4, 6, 15, and then at 4 years
Td	Tetanus	Every 10 years after 4 years of age
Varicella	Varicella zoster virus	12 months
MMR	Measles, mumps, rubella	12 months, then at 4 years
Influenza	Influenza viruses	Yearly, especially indicated for patients with lung disease All adults over 50 years of age and all patients with chronic respiratory, cardiac, or renal conditions
Hepatitis A	Hepatitis A	As needed for foreign travel
Rubella	Rubella	Also give to all women of childbearing age who do not have a record of immunization for rubella (but do not immunize if they are pregnant)
Pneumococcus	Pneumococcus	All adults over 65 years of age immunocompromised patients, diabetics, and patients with chronic respiratory, cardiac, or renal conditions.
Tetanus	Tetanus	(1) Maintenance booster should be given every 10 years (2) Give patients with dirty wounds a booster if they have not received a tetanus shot in more than 5 years

a. Suppurative complications include peritonsillar abscess and retropharyngeal abscess.
b. Nonsuppurative complications include rheumatic fever and post–streptococcal glomerulonephritis.

2. Patients are typically over the age of 3 years and have sore throat, fever, headache, and malaise. Physical examination findings include white exudate on the tonsils and tender cervical lymphadenopathy. A sandpapery rash on the trunk and extremities would give the patient a diagnosis of scarlet fever.
3. Testing includes throat culture and antigen detection testing for group A streptococci.
4. Treat with a 10-day course of penicillin to prevent the development of rheumatic heart disease (this does not prevent glomerulonephritis). Erythromycin can be used in penicillin-allergic patients.
5. Complications.
   a. Acute rheumatic fever: Occurs 3 to 4 weeks after streptococcal pharyngitis in some untreated patients. This is an inflammatory condition involving the connective tissues of the heart, joints, and CNS. Symptoms include fever, dyspnea, chest pain, cardiac murmur, and arthritis. It can cause mitral or aortic valve insufficiency or stenosis. Affected individuals should receive prophylactic penicillin treatment owing to the high rate of recurrence.
   b. Acute post–streptococcal glomerulonephritis: May follow streptococcal pharyngitis or cutaneous streptococcal infection by about 10 days. Antibiotic treatment does not prevent it. Symptoms include hematuria, edema, proteinuria, and decreased urination. Treat with penicillin, diuretics, and antihypertensives as needed.

F. Mononucleosis: Caused by Epstein-Barr Virus (EBV; 80% of cases) or cytomegalovirus (CMV; 20% of cases).
1. Patients have pharyngitis, systemic lymphadenopathy, fatigue, and atypical lymphocytosis. Exudates can be present and may lead to misdiagnosis as streptococcal pharyngitis. Hepatosplenomegaly may also be present.
2. Testing includes heterophile antibody testing, and the CBC will show lymphocytosis with up to 20% atypical cells.
3. Treat with supportive therapy, and the patient should refrain from contact sports if splenomegaly is present.
4. Complications
   a. Rash, if the patient is treated with ampicillin (which can occur if a bacterial throat infection is suspected).
   b. Neutropenia, hemolytic anemia, and thrombocytopenia (all reversible).
   c. Airway obstruction or splenic rupture rarely.

G. Epiglottitis: Caused by *H. influenzae, S. pneumoniae,* and group A streptococci.
1. Most commonly found in winter in children 2 to 7 years of age.
2. Patients have fever, sore throat, hoarseness, and stridor over 1 to 2 days. The patient will appear "toxic" and may be drooling. This condition is

life-threatening because of the tendency of the swelling to cause airway closure.

3. Soft-tissue radiograph shows a "thumbprint sign" related to epiglottic swelling.

4. Treat with intubation and empiric therapy with IV cefuroxime until the sensitivities of the causative organism are known.

III. Lower Respiratory Tract Infections

A. Croup: Most commonly caused by parainfluenza virus.

1. Croup presents in spring and fall with hoarseness, a barky cough, and inspiratory stridor.

2. Chest radiograph shows a "steeple sign" of subglottic narrowing, which differentiates croup from epiglottitis (Fig. 6-1).

3. The cough usually responds to cool air and humidity. If necessary, stridorous infants can receive nebulized epinephrine and corticosteroids.

B. Respiratory Syncytial Virus (RSV) Bronchiolitis

1. Can be life-threatening in infants (worse in infants 2 to 6 months of age, former preterm infants, or children with heart or lung disease).

2. Patients have fever, copious rhinorrhea, retraction, mouth breathing and tachypnea. Neonates may have apnea.

3. Testing includes culture or rapid antigen testing.

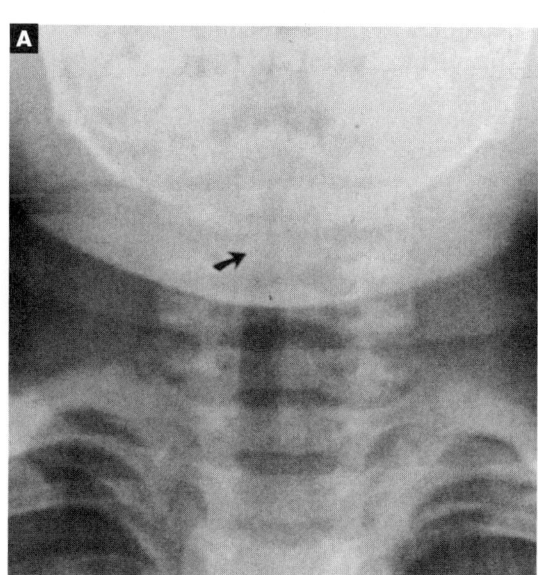

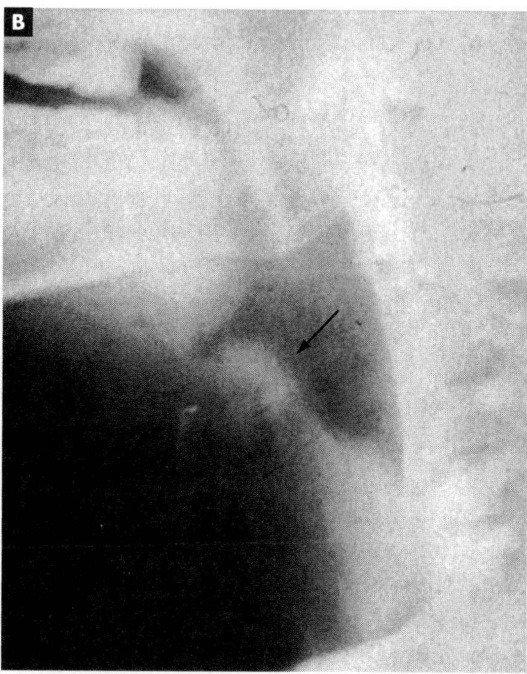

***6-1:** Use of radiography to distinguish between croup and epiglottitis. A, A steeple-shaped subglottic narrowing (arrow) can be found in croup. B, An enlarged, thumb-shaped epiglottis (arrow) can be found in epiglottitis.*

4. Treatment can include hospitalization (if the patient has an oxygen saturation of less than 95% or is in distress) and ribavirin. RespiGam (polyclonal) and Synagis (monoclonal) are trademark antibody preparations used for prophylaxis in at-risk populations.

C. Whooping Cough: Caused by *Bordetella pertussis*

1. Presentation depends on age. In adults, it causes common cold–like symptoms. In children, it presents as whooping cough with several phases of illness.
    a. Catarrhal phase: 1 to 2 weeks of low-grade fever, cough, and coryza.
    b. Paroxysmal phase: 3 to 8 weeks of paroxysms of cough followed by inspiratory stridor. Posttussive emesis may occur.
    c. Convalescent phase: Cough can persist for 3 to 12 months, but other symptoms will remit.
2. Testing includes culture or antigen testing of nasopharyngeal secretions. CBC with differential shows leukocytosis (>30,000 WBC/μL).
3. Treatment depends on severity.
    a. Hospitalization or supportive care for infants with severe disease.
    b. More mild cases can be treated with erythromycin for a 14-day course.
4. Immunization at 2, 4, 6, and 12 months and booster at 4 to 6 years can prevent severe disease, but one third of children still get mild infections.

D. Pneumonia

1. Causes
    a. Viral: RSV, adenovirus, parainfluenza, influenza, and enteroviruses.
    b. Bacterial (many cases of bacterial pneumonia also have viral disease).
        (1) *S. pneumoniae:* Most common cause of community-acquired pneumonia in otherwise healthy people.
        (2) Mycoplasmal pneumonia: Less severe, uncommon before 5 years of age. This is often called "walking pneumonia," and the chest radiograph often looks worse than the patient appears.
        (3) Chlamydial pneumonia: Found in infants at 2 to 3 months of age if their mothers had a chlamydial genitourinary infection.
        (4) Bacterial causes of pneumonia in children differ depending on the age group.
            (a) Neonatal period: Group B streptococci and *Listeria monocytogenes.*
            (b) Neonatal period to 5 years of age: *S. pneumoniae, H. influenzae* type b, *S. aureus,* and group A streptococci.
    c. "Aspiration pneumonia" can occur following the aspiration of oral or esophageal contents, which can subsequently injure the lung.
        (1) A serious situation involves the aspiration of gastric acid, which can produce cough, dyspnea, frothy sputum, and (in extreme cases) death.
        (2) Patients with aspiration injury are predisposed to the development of bacterial pneumonia, which can lead to clinical deterioration 2 to 3 days after the aspiration incident.

(3) Treat aspiration injuries by establishing an airway, suctioning the airway, and providing oxygen and supportive care to maintain high oxygen saturation measurements.

2. Symptoms and signs
   a. Patients typically have fever, chills, dyspnea, chest pain, and productive cough.
      (1) Focal findings (decreased breath sounds, dullness, asymmetric crackles) suggest a bacterial cause.
      (2) Patients with pneumonia due to mycoplasmal or viral infection may have a low-grade fever, persistent dry cough, and malaise. They will have diffuse crackles on physical examination.
   b. Presentation in children may involve more nonspecific constitutional complaints (fever, irritability, poor feeding, vomiting, lethargy).
3. Diagnostic evaluation: Chest radiographs to assess the extent of involvement and the possibility of pleural effusion. See Figure 6-2 for different abnormalities.
4. Treatment
   a. Bacterial pneumonia: Use IV cefuroxime or penicillin for inpatient cases, and amoxicillin for most outpatient bacterial cases. If *H. influenzae* or *S. aureus* is suspected cause, then amoxicillin/clavulanic acid should be used.
   b. Viral, mycoplasmal, or chlamydial pneumonia: Give supportive care as needed.
   c. Pleurocentesis can be performed for large pleural effusions if present.

E. Tuberculosis (TB): Caused by *Mycobacterium tuberculosis*
1. Patients can be asymptomatic or have productive cough, hemoptysis, weakness, weight loss, fever, and sweats. Symptoms of renal insufficiency may be present if the kidneys are infected.
2. Diagnostic evaluation (Fig. 6-3).
   a. Acid-fast stain in the sputum to detect bacilli.
   b. Chest radiograph may show enlarged, calcified lymph nodes and granulomas.
   c. Purified protein derivative (PPD) test will document exposure to TB but not infection. The PPD may be positive in patients from countries where the BCG vaccine was used, which causes seroconversion without exposure to the *M. tuberculosis* organism.
   d. Baseline liver function tests (LFTs) should be obtained before therapy is begun.
3. Treatment
   a. Respiratory isolation in a negative pressure room.
   b. Medical regimen for active TB (mnemonic—RESPI): **r**ifampin, **e**thambutol (or **s**treptomycin), **p**yrazinamide, and **i**soniazid (INH).
   c. Give vitamin B_6 (pyridoxine) to prevent INH-induced peripheral neuropathy.
   d. Young patients with no symptoms but a positive PPD test can receive INH therapy for 9 months.

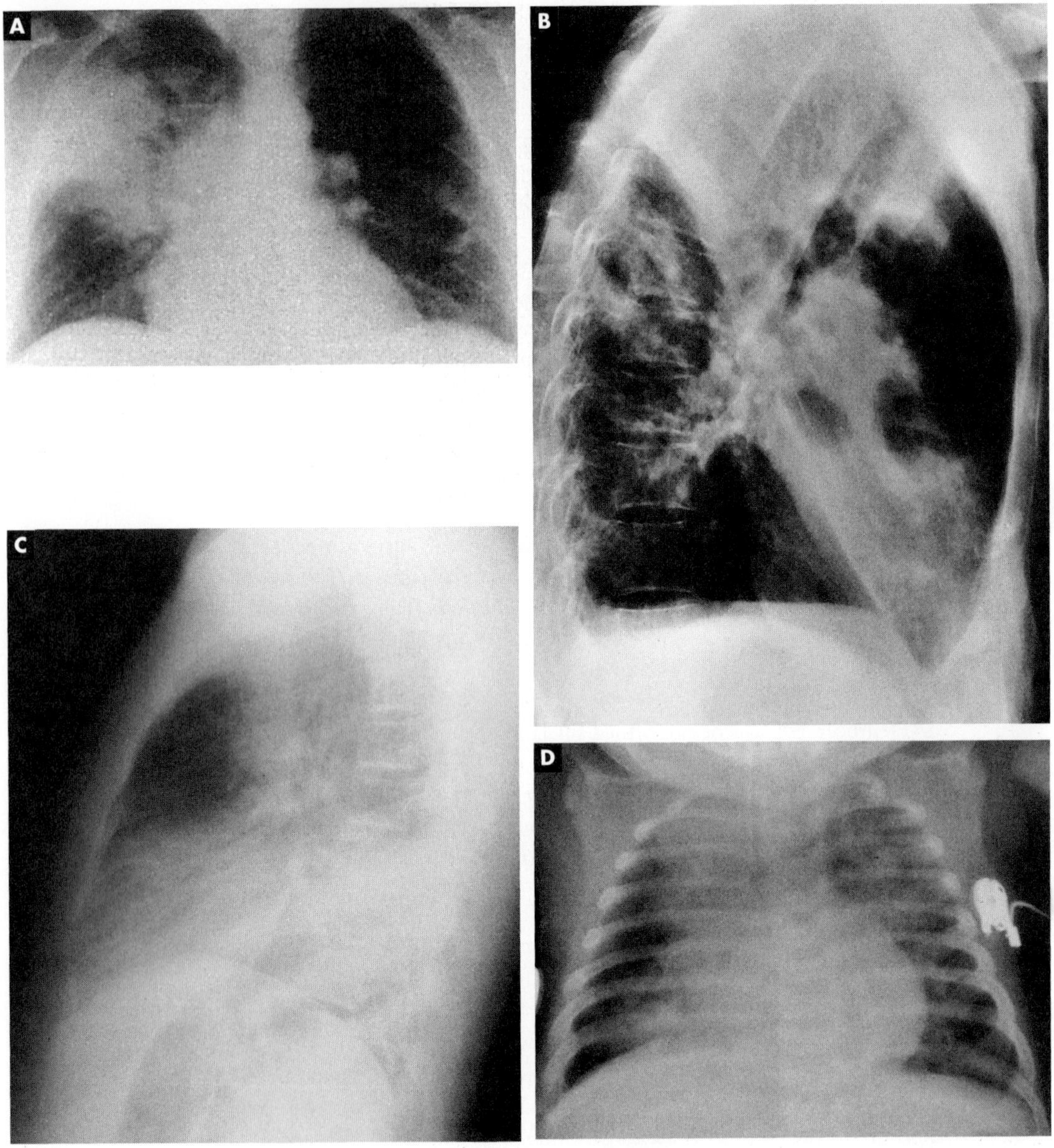

A

B

C

D

6-2: Abnormalities on chest radiograph in various types of pneumonia. Typical pneumonia often shows a pattern of lobar consolidation on radiographs. A, Lobar consolidation restricted to the right upper lobe. B, Consolidation of the right middle lobe with some involvement of the right upper lobe. C, Lobar consolidation of the right lower lobe. Note the clear diaphragmatic margin in right middle lobe consolidation, in contrast to the indistinct diaphragmatic border seen in right lower lobe consolidation. D, A diffusely infiltrative pattern is present in many cases of viral pneumonia (RSV in this case).

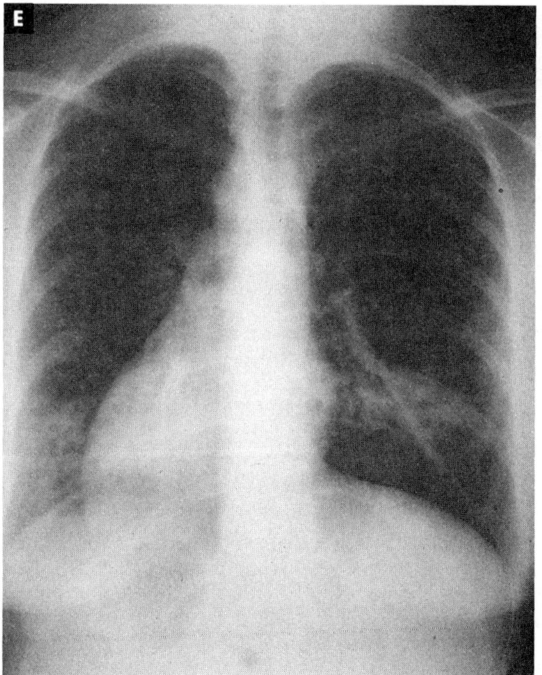

6-2, cont'd *E, A similarly diffuse pattern can be seen in atypical pneumonia caused by* Mycoplasma pneumoniae *infection.*

IV. Bacteremia and Sepsis
   A. Bacteremia: Presence of bacteria in the blood
      1. In children
         a. Transient and self-limited without obvious source of infection.
         b. Suspect bacteremia in a child 6 to 36 months of age with fever higher than 102.2°F (39°C) and leukocytosis.
         c. The majority of cases are due to *S. pneumoniae,* and they resolve within 48 hours.
      2. In adults: Identify the source of the infection (as described previously), and treat accordingly.
   B. Sepsis: Bacterial invasion of the intravascular compartment
      1. In children
         a. Uncommon in immunocompetent children older than 3 months old.
         b. Patients appear very ill and may develop shock.
         c. Evaluate with cultures (blood, urine, possibly CSF) and chest radiograph to identify the source of infection.
         d. Treat empirically with a third-generation cephalosporin and supportive care until the organism and sensitivities are known.
      2. In adults
         a. Patients can experience fever, chills, hypothermia, hypotension, mental status changes, and multisystem organ failure.

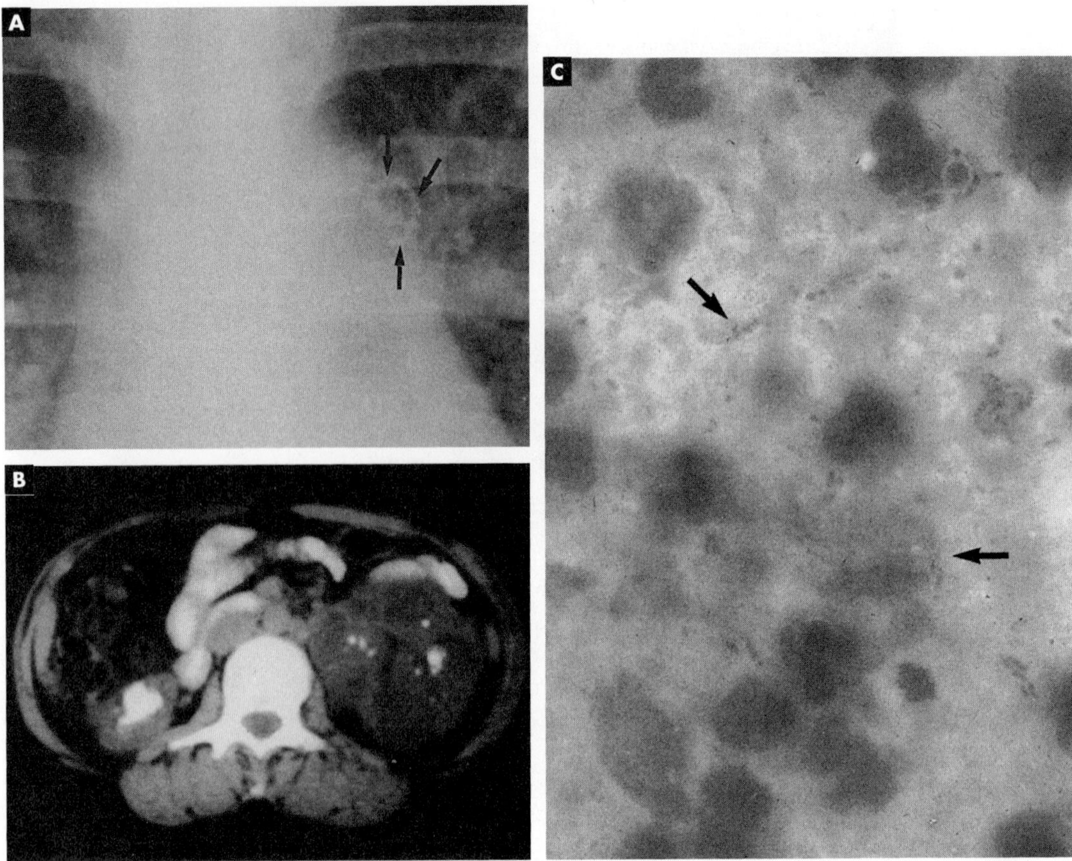

6-3: *Abnormal test results seen in tuberculosis. A, Chest radiograph depicting a calcified lung nodule* (arrows) *in a patient with tuberculosis. B, CT scan showing the appearance of the same calcified lesion. C, Acid-fast stain of a sputum sample from a patient with active tuberculosis* (arrows).

b. Evaluate with cultures (blood, urine, maybe CSF) and chest radiograph to identify the source of infection.

c. Sepsis can cause distributive shock, which in turn can cause decreased or normal pulmonary capillary wedge pressure and increased or normal cardiac output (see Chapter 2 for a comparison of the other types of shock).

d. Treat by admission to the intensive care unit and institution of therapy with fluids, oxygen, vasopressors, and empiric broad-spectrum antibiotics. Switch to a different antibiotic once the source and sensitivity are known.

V. Gastrointestinal Infections

A. Infectious Diarrhea (see Chapter 4 for a discussion of noninfectious diarrhea)

1. Causes
   a. Bacterial diarrhea: *Salmonella, Shigella, Escherichia coli, Yersinia enterocolitica* (causes severe pain in the right lower quadrant of the abdomen), *Campylobacter jejuni, Vibrio cholerae* (causes rice-water stools in patients infected during travel to Asia or Africa), and *Clostridium difficile* (if the patient has a history of antibiotic therapy or is an inpatient).
   b. Nonbacterial diarrhea: rotavirus (which occurs with upper respiratory infection symptoms between November and April) and giardiasis (which can cause frequent, foul smelling, watery stools and can be associated with camping).
2. Symptoms and signs: Patients have an increase in the frequency of bowel movements and may have some of the other characteristics described previously. The patient should be assessed for a surgical abdomen and for dehydration. Signs of liver disease or malabsorption should be evaluated to rule out noninfectious causes of diarrhea.
3. Diagnostic evaluation
   a. Evaluate electrolyte status.
   b. Stool examination and culture: Fecal leukocytes suggest a bacterial cause, and cysts may be present in giardial diarrhea. Stool culture is used for determination of antibiotic sensitivity but takes several days.
   c. Rapid antigen testing can be performed for rotavirus.
4. Treatment
   a. Electrolyte management.
   b. Antibiotic therapy: Usually only done when the infections are systemic (otherwise it prolongs the shedding period).
      (1) For most bacteria: Use trimethoprim/sulfamethoxazole (TMP-SMX).
      (2) For *C. difficile:* Use oral metronidazole.
      (3) For *Giardia:* Use furazolidone or quinacrine.
5. Complications
   a. *Salmonella* can cause meningitis, arthritis, and osteomyelitis.
   b. *Shigella* can cause neurologic signs and hemolytic uremic syndrome.
   c. *E. coli* O157:H7 can cause hemolytic uremic syndrome.
   d. *Y. enterocolitica* can cause erythema nodosum.

B. Hepatitis (see Chapter 4)

VI. Human Immunodeficiency Virus (HIV) and Acquired Immunodeficiency Syndrome (AIDS)

AIDS = HIV infection + a CD4 count less than 200 or an opportunistic infection or carcinoma (Kaposi sarcoma, non-Hodgkin's lymphoma, CNS lymphoma).

A. Modes of Transmission
1. Sexual contact (homosexual and heterosexual).
2. Parenteral exposure (to infected blood or needles).
3. Vertical transmission from mother to child: 30% of women pass HIV to their children during or after pregnancy. This risk is reduced to 8% with third-trimester AZT (zidovudine) treatment. Rate of transfer is less than 1% to 2% in patients with undetectable viral loads.

B. Symptoms and Signs

1. Adults
   a. Acute retroviral syndrome: Can occur about 4 weeks after infection and includes a salmon-colored maculopapular rash, lymphadenopathy, splenomegaly, and malaise.
   b. Symptoms associated with opportunistic infections (Table 6-2).
2. Children: Will have developmental delay and recurrent or severe opportunistic infections. AIDS-defining illnesses in children include *Pneumocystis carinii* pneumonia, lymphocytic interstitial pneumonitis, and CNS lymphoma.

C. Diagnostic Evaluation
1. For adults
   a. Enzyme-linked immunosorbent assay (ELISA) screening test: Becomes positive at 1 to 12 weeks postinfection.
   b. Western blot (confirmatory test following a positive ELISA).
   c. Polymerase chain reaction (PCR): Determines viral load and can detect HIV earlier than ELISA. It is also used to assess the efficacy of treatment regimens.
   d. CD4 lymphocyte count: Not a diagnostic test but useful for tracking progression of disease in making decisions about prophylaxis.
2. For children
   a. PCR in children less than 18 months of age.
   b. ELISA after 18 months of age to test for anti-HIV antibodies.
   c. A child is uninfected if both tests are continuously negative for the first 2 years of life.

D. Treatment
1. For adults: Regimens typically include a group A nucleoside reverse transcriptase inhibitor + a group B nucleoside reverse transcriptase inhibitor

TABLE 6-2 Opportunistic Infections in Immunocompromised Hosts

Condition/ Infection	Associated CD4 Count	Symptoms and Signs	Diagnostic Evaluation	Treatment
Kaposi's sarcoma	<500	Red or purple nodular skin lesions	Biopsy	Chemotherapy
Thrush	<500	Thick white plaques on the oral mucosa	Organisms visible on KOH treatment of exudate scrapings	Fluconazole
Tuberculosis	<500	Chronic cough, weight loss, fever, hemoptysis	Acid-fast organisms in the sputum	Pyrazinamide, isoniazid (INH), rifampin, ethambutol
Herpes simplex virus (HSV)	<500	Painful skin vesicles	Rapid antigen testing	Acyclovir
Varicella zoster virus (VZV)	<500	Pain and a cluster of vesicles in a dermatomal distribution	None	Varicella zoster immunoglobulin

TABLE 6-2 Opportunistic Infections in Immunocompromised Hosts—cont'd

Condition/ Infection	Associated CD4 Count	Symptoms and Signs	Diagnostic Evaluation	Treatment
Pneumocystis carinii pneumonia (PCP)	<200	Dry cough with dyspnea	(1) Chest radiograph shows interstitial infiltrates (2) Positive PCP sputum stain	Treat with trimethoprim-sulfamethoxazole or dapsone, and add steroids if the patient's PaO_2 is <70
Toxoplasmosis	<200	Symptoms of space-occupying intracranial lesion	Multiple ring-enhancing lesions on CT with positive toxoplasmosis serologic tests	Pyrimethamine, sulfadiazine, and folinic acid
Cryptococcosis	<200	Symptoms of meningitis (headache, neck stiffness, etc)	Positive serum or CSF *Cryptococcus* antigen	Amphotericin B for 2 weeks, then lifelong fluconazole
Histoplasmosis	<200	Meningitis or pneumonia, with exposure in the Midwest United States	Positive urinary *Histoplasma* antigen	Amphotericin B or itraconazole
Coccidiosis	<200	Meningitis or pneumonia, with exposure in the Southwest United States	DNA test	Fluconazole or amphotericin B
Cytomegalovirus (CMV)	<100	Retinitis, neuropathy, esophagitis, hepatitis	Serologic study	Treat with ganciclovir or foscarnet
Mycobacterium avium complex (MAC)	<100	Fever, lymphadenopathy, abdominal pain, pneumonia, hepatosplenomegaly	Acid-fast stain of sputum	Treat with clarithromycin + ethambutol + sometimes rifabutin
Aspergillosis	<100	Space-occupying lesion in lung, mucosa, or brain	Biopsy, imaging	Amphotericin B
CNS lymphoma (associated with Epstein-Barr virus [EBV])	<100	Headache, personality changes, focal neurologic signs	(1) CT will show single enhancing lesion (2) Positive on CSF PCR assay for EBV	Chemotherapy
Progressive multifocal leukoencephalopathy (PML)	<75	Dementia, visual problems, seizures, focal neurologic signs	(1) Multiple nonenhancing lesions on CT (2) Positive PCR for JC virus in the CSF	None

TABLE 6-3 Classes of Antiretroviral Medications and Side Effects*

Drug Class	Drug Names	Side Effects
Group A nucleoside reverse transcriptase inhibitors	Zidovudine (AZT) Stavudine	Zidovudine: Bone marrow suppression, hepatitis Stavudine: Peripheral neuropathy, pancreatitis
Group B nucleoside reverse transcriptase inhibitors	Didanosine Zalcitabine Lamivudine	Didanosine: Pancreatitis, peripheral neuropathy Zalcitabine: Peripheral neuropathy Lamivudine: Minimally toxic
Protease inhibitors	Indinavir Ritonavir Saquinavir Nelfinavir Amprenavir	Indinavir: Nephrolithiasis Ritonavir: Paresthesias Saquinavir: Headache Nelfinavir: Diarrhea Amprenavir: Rash
Nonnucleoside reverse transcriptase inhibitors	Nevirapine Delavirdine Efavirenz	Nevirapine: Rash, hepatitis Delavirdine: Rash, headache Efavirenz: CNS effects, rash, headache

*In addition to the side effects described above, most antiretrovirals also cause GI intolerance and have varying effects on the cytochrome P-450 system. Goals of antiretroviral therapy are to have a 3- to 4-fold drop in viral load within 8 weeks and to have undetectable viral load at 6 months.

+ either a protease inhibitor or a nonnucleoside reverse transcriptase inhibitor (Table 6-3).

2. Prophylaxis for opportunistic infections for adults.
   a. Tuberculosis: Give INH and vitamin B_6 for 12 months if the patient has a PPD greater than 5 mm.
   b. *P. carinii* pneumonia: Start TMP-SMX or dapsone in patients with CD4 counts less than 200 or thrush.
   c. Toxoplasmosis: Start TMP-SMX or dapsone with pyrimethamine and folic acid if the patient has a CD4 count less than 100 and positive *Toxoplasma* serologic tests.
   d. *Mycobacterium avium* complex: Start clarithromycin or azithromycin if the patient has a CD4 count less than 75.
3. For children: Give AZT and ddI (didanosine) and protease inhibitors with TMP-SMX as prophylaxis for opportunistic infections.

Severely immunocompromised patients may have no reaction to the PPD antigen (owing to their poor immune function) despite being infected with tuberculosis.

VII. Sexually Transmitted Diseases
   A. Syphilis: Caused by *Treponema pallidum.*
      1. Can be acquired in utero or sexually
      2. Symptoms and signs
         a. Congenital: Early congenital syphilis presents as hepatomegaly, splenomegaly, mucocutaneous lesions, lymphadenopathy, and snuffles. Late congenital syphilis presents as CN VIII deafness, saber shins (anterior bowing of the tibia), Hutchinson's teeth (notched), and saddle nose.

b. Acquired: Several stages of infection.

(1) Primary stage: Painless genital chancre that appears 3 weeks after infection and lasts about 3 weeks.

(2) Secondary stage: Widespread dermatologic involvement (usually an erythematous and maculopapular rash) with upper respiratory infection symptoms and condyloma latum (large, white flattened lesion) on the vulva. This appears 6 weeks to 6 months after infection.

(3) Tertiary stage: Widespread CNS, musculoskeletal, and cardiovascular involvement. Patients may develop tables dorsalis (slapping gait due to the dorsal column tract damage) and aortic aneurysms.

3. Diagnostic evaluation

a. First-line tests (screening): VDRL or RPR. These can be falsely positive in patients with some rheumatic disorders (such as systemic lupus erythematosus).

b. Second-line tests (confirmatory): FTA-ABS testing.

c. Skin scrapings can be placed under dark-field microscopy for direct visualization of the spirochetes.

4. Treatment: Parenteral penicillin G. If there is no CNS involvement, penicillin G benzathine can be used. If the CNS is involved, aqueous crystalline penicillin G can be used.

B. Herpes: Genital herpes is usually caused by herpes simplex virus (HSV) 2.

1. Patients have genital burning and itching that progress to ulcer formation. Pharyngitis may accompany primary episode. Following the resolution of symptoms, the virus can stay latent in the dorsal root ganglia and periodically reactivate.

2. Can be vertically transmitted, so any active lesions at labor are an indication for cesarean section.

3. Diagnostic evaluation

a. Rapid antigen testing.

b. Identify giant multinucleated cells with intranuclear inclusions in scrapings from the ulcer base.

4. Treatment

a. Acyclovir diminishes the length of episodes and degree of viral shedding. Lidocaine gel can be used if necessary for topical analgesia.

b. Pregnant patients who have had more than one outbreak during pregnancy and those who have had an outbreak during the last 4 to 6 weeks should be given acyclovir at 36 weeks.

C. Pelvic Inflammatory Disease (PID): Most often caused by *Chlamydia trachomatis* and *Neisseria gonorrhoeae*.

C. trachomatis is an obligate intracellular organism and is the most common cause of mucopurulent cervicitis.

1. Symptoms and signs

a. Patients have abdominal pain/tenderness, cervical motion tenderness (Chandelier sign), and adnexal tenderness.

b. Infants can be infected during passage through the birth canal. Neonatal gonorrheal infection can cause meningitis and arthritis, while neonatal chlamydial infection can cause conjunctivitis and pneumonia.

2. Diagnostic evaluation
   a. Gram's stain of endocervical smear (Fig. 6-4).
   b. ELISA tests and DNA probes are also available.
3. Treatment
   a. *N. gonorrhoeae:* Single dose of ceftriaxone or cefixime. Ciprofloxacin can also be used for a longer duration. Pregnant women who receive the diagnosis during pregnancy can be treated with ceftriaxone or penicillin and probenecid. Patients should also be treated with azithromycin or erythromycin for presumed chlamydial infection.

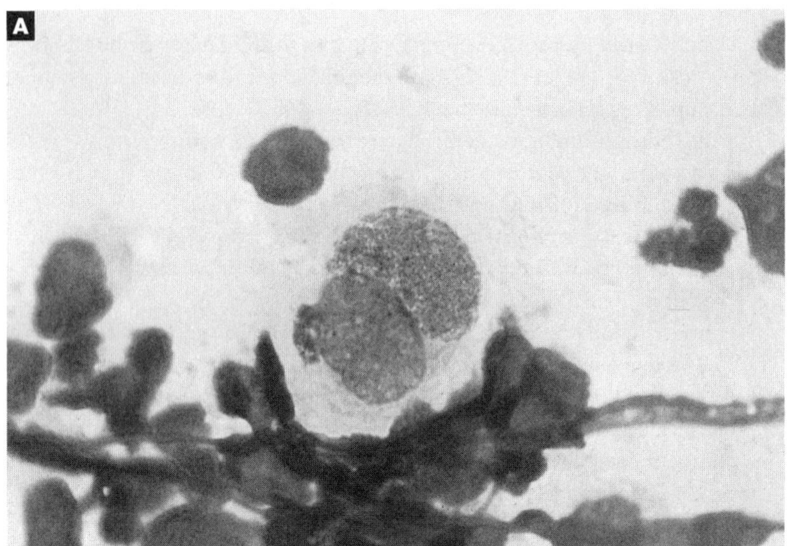

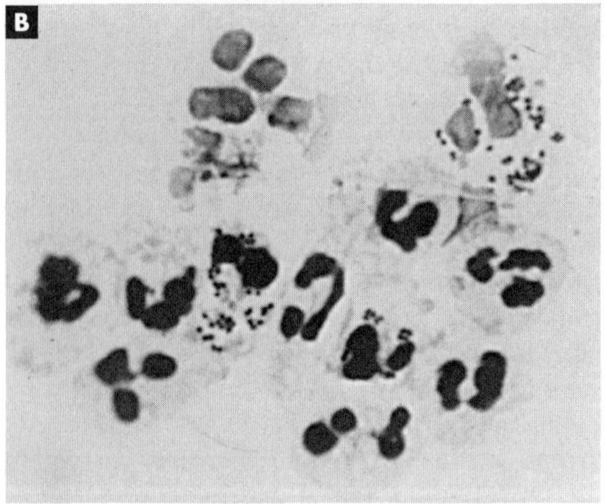

6-4: *Diagnosis of* C. trachomatis *and* N. gonorrhoeae *using histologic staining. A, This Giemsa stain shows the characteristic intracellular growth of* C. trachomatis. *B, This Gram's stain shows extracellular clusters of gram-negative cocci, indicative of* N. gonorrhoeae *infection.*

b. *C. trachomatis:* Azithromycin in one dose or doxycycline for a longer duration. Pregnant women who receive the diagnosis during pregnancy should be treated with azithromycin or erythromycin.

4. Complications

a. PID: Infertility, increased risks for ectopic pregnancy and adhesions, arthritis, and Fitz-Hugh-Curtis syndrome (perihepatitis).

b. Chlamydia: Reiter's syndrome (urethritis, conjunctivitis, arthritis).

D. Venereal Warts: Caused by human papillomavirus (HPV)

1. Patients have warts that may form clustered growths (condylomata acuminata) in the anogenital area.

2. Treat with local application of podophyllin or 5-fluorouracil. Liquid nitrogen, electrocautery, cryocautery, and laser vaporization can also be used. Relapses are common.

3. Ensure that patient has a yearly Pap smear for cervical cancer surveillance.

HPV strains 16 and 18 increase the risk for cervical cancer.

VIII. Other Genitourinary Infections

A. *Trichomonas vaginalis*

1. Symptoms and signs

a. Infection can cause a malodorous, frothy gray discharge, vaginal discomfort, and sometimes dysuria and lower abdominal pain in women.

b. Infection can cause urethritis in men.

2. Wet preparation of vaginal fluid shows neutrophils and protozoa.

3. Treat with a single dose of metronidazole.

B. Bacterial Vaginosis: Caused by *Gardnerella vaginalis, Mycoplasma hominis,* and some anaerobes

1. Patients have a foul-smelling vaginal discharge that has a fishy odor when mixed with KOH.

2. Wet preparation of vaginal fluid shows "clue cells" (epithelial cells with smudged border due to adherent bacteria).

3. Treat with a single dose of metronidazole.

C. Vaginal Candidiasis

1. Risk factors include antibiotic use, pregnancy, diabetes mellitus, immunosuppression, and oral contraceptive use.

2. Patients have thick white vaginal discharge with vaginal itching and burning.

3. Wet preparation of vaginal fluid shows yeasts and pseudohyphae.

4. Treat with over-the-counter antifungal cream or terconazole.

D. Urinary Tract Infections (UTIs): Most commonly due to *E. coli*

1. Risk factors include female sex, instrumentation, pregnancy, anatomic abnormalities of the urinary tract, and diabetes mellitus.

2. Patients typically have dysuria, urinary frequency, and urgency. UTIs can progress to cystitis and pyelonephritis. Costovertebral angle tenderness is usually present in pyelonephritis.

3. Diagnostic evaluation

a. Urine culture.

b. Urinalysis: If positive for leukocyte esterase and has increased WBCs, then the culture will most likely be positive.

c. Children may require a voiding cystourethrogram (VCUG) to evaluate for reflux and other urinary tract abnormalities.

4. Treatment can include amoxicillin, nitrofurantoin, or TMP-SMX if *E. coli* is suspected. Intravenous ampicillin and gentamycin can be used if pyelonephritis is suspected.

IX. Viral Infections that Present with Rash

A. Rocky Mountain Spotted Fever: Caused by *Rickettsia rickettsii,* a tick-borne pathogen

1. Most prevalent in summer and fall in the southeastern states and the Ohio River Valley of the United States.

2. Patients experience fever, headache, myalgias, and rash 5 to 10 days after a tick bite. The rash begins on the ankles and wrists and spreads proximally over hours.

3. Treat with tetracycline or chloramphenicol if diagnosis is made within 5 days of symptom onset.

4. Complications include multiple organ system problems, thrombocytopenia, and coagulopathy.

B. Lyme Disease: Caused by *Borrelia burgdorferi,* a tick-borne pathogen

1. Most common in the northeast, Midwest, and California-Oregon border of the United States in summer and early fall.

2. Patients have rash, fever, headache, stiff neck, malaise, and arthralgia that occur 7 to 10 days following a tick bite. The rash (erythema migrans) lasts 3 weeks, occurs at the site of inoculation, and may be followed by multiple secondary lesions.

3. Diagnostic test: ELISA with confirmation by Western blot.

4. Treatment: Children over 8 years of age should receive doxycycline for at least 14 days (or until symptoms are gone). Younger children should get amoxicillin. Severe cases can be treated with high-dose ceftriaxone.

5. Complications: After disappearance of the rash, 50% of patients develop arthritis at the large joints and neurologic problems (meningitis, cranial nerve palsies) can also occur. Other complications include myocarditis, conduction abnormalities, Guillain-Barré syndrome, and encephalitis.

C. Varicella-zoster Virus: Causes chickenpox (primary infection) and shingles (reactivation)

1. Chickenpox typically occurs in children and presents with disseminated papules that progress to vesicles, pustules, and crusted lesions. Several crops of lesions form, presenting new skin lesions at the same time as resolving ones.

2. In adults, the infection can be more serious and can progress to pneumonia. Systemic infection can be fatal in immunocompromised or pregnant hosts.

3. Following primary infection the virus is latent in dorsal root ganglia neurons. Reactivation can produce shingles (herpes zoster), which involves

the development of pain and (later) rash in the distribution of a single dermatome.

4. Treatment includes supportive care for otherwise healthy children. Infection may be prevented with vaccination. Varicella-zoster immunoglobulin (VZIG) can be given to immunocompromised, pregnant, or otherwise at-risk patients to prevent development of severe disease. Otherwise healthy patients with shingles can be treated with oral acyclovir.

X. Soft Tissue and Bone Infections

A. Cellulitis

1. Patients have localized erythema, edema, and warmth. Linear erythematous streaking indicates lymphatic spread.

2. Lower extremity cellulitis can be caused by beta-hemolytic streptococci (most commonly), but *S. aureus* and gram-negative bacilli (in immunocompromised patients) are alternative causes.

3. Treat with antibiotics with elevation of the limb.

B. Osteomyelitis

1. Patients have bone pain, fever, malaise, and night sweats.

2. Sources of infection

a. Blood: Risk factors include intravenous drug abuse (often caused by *S. aureus* or *P. aeruginosa*), IV line infections (often caused by *S. aureus, Staphylococcus epidermidis,* or *Candida*), or urinary tract infection (often caused by enterobacteria).

b. Local wound infection: Risk factors include surgery or trauma (often caused by *S. aureus* or aerobic gram-negative bacilli), bite wounds, and periodontal infections (usually caused by penicillin-sensitive anaerobes) or cutaneous ulcers (usually caused by mixed aerobes and anaerobes).

In osteomyelitis caused by stepping on a nail while wearing rubber-soled shoes, the causative organism is likely to be *P. aeruginosa.*

3. Diagnostic evaluation

a. Culture from surgical sampling or needle biopsy

b. Blood cultures

c. Radiograph or CT can show bone destruction

4. Treatment

a. Antibiotics (based on culture and sensitivity) for 4 to 6 weeks

b. Surgery if osteomyelitis remains unresponsive to therapy, infects a prosthesis, or leads to vertebral instability

C. Diabetic Foot

1. Diabetic patient has ulcer with surrounding erythema and warmth. Fever and chills may occur if the infection spreads to the blood, but tenderness may be absent owing to neuropathy. Crepitance may be present if gas-producing organisms are involved.

2. Blood cultures should be done to evaluate for sepsis; imaging should be done to rule out osteomyelitis.

3. Treatment

a. Bedrest

b. Antibiotics

(1) Mild cases: First-generation cephalosporin

(2) Limb-threatening cases: Fluoroquinolone with clindamycin or ampicillin/sulbactam

(3) Life-threatening cases: Imipenem or vancomycin with aztreonam and metronidazole

D. Necrotizing Fasciitis

1. Patients have cellulitic skin with poorly defined margins that spread rapidly with systemic signs and bullae formation. The skin may darken to bluish gray.

2. Diagnostic evaluation

a. Aspiration of the necrotic center for gram staining and culture

b. Radiograph or CT may demonstrate gas in the soft tissue

3. Treatment

a. Surgical débridement and fasciotomy

b. Broad spectrum antibiotics: Clindamycin with penicillin and an aminoglycoside

c. Hyperbaric oxygen

E. Clostridial Myonecrosis (Gas Gangrene): Caused by *Clostridium perfringens*

1. Patients have an acute onset of pain that increases rapidly with systemic signs. There is also bronze discoloration of the skin with bullae containing dark fluid, and crepitus may be present.

2. Diagnostic evaluation

a. Gram's stain of discharge will show large, gram-positive bacilli with blunt ends.

b. Radiograph may show gas in soft tissues.

3. Treatment

a. Surgical exploration and débridement

b. Antibiotic treatment with penicillin G and clindamycin

c. Hyperbaric O_2

CHAPTER 7

Nephrology and Electrolyte Disturbances

I. Azotemia and Uremia
   A. Azotemia
      1. An increase in blood urea nitrogen (BUN) and creatinine, usually due to a decreased glomerular filtration rate (GFR).
      2. Can be caused by prerenal (hypoperfusion), renal, or postrenal (urinary obstruction) factors.
   B. Uremia
      1. Azotemia combined with a variety of symptoms and signs, including anorexia, vomiting, confusion, or coma. It can also cause pericarditis, serositis, hyperkalemia, metabolic acidosis, and anemia.
      2. Treat emergently with dialysis.

II. Nephrotic Syndrome
   A. Cause: Noninflammatory processes involving the glomerulus. Fatty casts may be seen on microscopic analysis of the urine.
   B. Patients have proteinuria (>3.5 g/day), hypoalbuminemia, hyperlipidemia, and edema.
   C. Types
      1. Minimal change disease
         a. This is the most common cause of nephrotic syndrome in children, but it can also occur in adults. In children (<7 years of age) with nephrotic syndrome, prednisone therapy can be attempted without performing a renal biopsy. Corticosteroid-responsive cases are given the diagnosis of minimal change disease, and nonresponsive cases necessitate a biopsy.
         b. Adults with nephrotic syndrome require a renal biopsy. Minimal change disease is diagnosed if there are no morphologic abnormalities on light microscopy and immunofluorescence. Electron microscopy will show podocyte foot process effacement as the sole abnormality.
         c. Treatment for adults and children is prednisone. Cyclophosphamide can be attempted for cases that are unresponsive to prednisone.
      2. Focal segmental glomerulosclerosis (FSGS)
         a. FSGS refers to the presence of sclerotic lesions that are present focally throughout the renal cortex and segmentally within a portion of the glomerulus.
         b. FSGS can be due to a primary idiopathic process or secondary to focal glomerular damage in a variety of conditions (e.g., HIV, sickle cell disease, IgA nephropathy).

c. Symptoms will not be initially responsive to prednisone therapy. However, prolonged treatment with prednisone (for 6 to 12 months) or cyclosporine (for 4 to 6 months) can cause remission and stop progression to end-stage renal disease (ESRD) in some patients.

3. Membranous glomerulonephropathy
   a. The most common cause of nephrotic syndrome in adults.
   b. It can be associated with the use of certain medications (penicillamine, gold, captopril, or NSAIDs) or as a finding in other medical conditions (systemic lupus erythematosus [SLE], hepatitis B or C, syphilis, schistosomiasis, malaria, diabetes mellitus, or thyroiditis).
   c. Glomerular damage is due to an antibody-mediated autoimmune process.
   d. Diagnosis can be made by observing antibody binding to the glomerulus by immunofluorescence of renal biopsy specimens.
   e. Corticosteroids or chlorambucil may be beneficial, but the relapsing/remitting course of the disease makes it difficult to determine their therapeutic efficacy.

III. Nephritic Syndromes
- A. Caused by inflammatory lesions in the glomerulus.
- B. Presents with hematuria (tea colored), azotemia (increased BUN and creatinine), oliguria, edema, and hypertension.
- C. Types
  1. Poststreptococcal glomerulonephritis (PSGN)
     a. Associated with streptococcal throat or skin infections. Nephritic symptoms follow the streptococcal infection by 8 to 12 days.
     b. High IgG antistreptococcal antibodies and depressed complement levels are found in the blood. IgG and complement deposition are found in the kidney (glomerular humps), but renal biopsy usually is not performed if the diagnosis is suspected clinically.
     c. Most cases resolve spontaneously within weeks.
  2. IgA nephropathy
     a. Most common cause of nephritic syndrome in adults worldwide. Typically occurs in children and young adults.
     b. Patients have relapsing/remitting episodes of hematuria without significant proteinuria.
     c. Diagnosis can be made by observing IgA deposits on the glomerular mesangial cells upon immunofluorescence of renal biopsy specimens.
     d. No treatment is currently available. Corticosteroid and cytotoxic agent therapy can be attempted when IgA nephropathy is severe enough to cause rapidly progressive glomerulonephritis.
  3. Membranoproliferative glomerulonephropathy (MPGN)
     a. Most cases occur between the ages of 5 and 30 years. Patients have nephrotic syndrome, asymptomatic proteinuria, or nephritic syndrome.
     b. Patients will have concurrent hematuria and proteinuria on urinalysis.

c. Renal biopsy displays immunocomplex and complement deposition. Subtypes of MPGN are defined by features demonstrated by electron microscopy.

d. This is a progressive disease that puts 30% of patients in chronic renal failure 10 years after diagnosis. Treat with renal transplant. Type 1 MPGN has a 25% recurrence rate, and type 2 MPGN has a 100% recurrence rate.

4. Alport's syndrome
   a. Progressive inherited nephritis in which the glomerular basement membrane is weak and tends to rupture and scar.
   b. Usually found along with bilateral hearing loss.
5. Rapidly progressive glomerulonephritis (RPGN)
   a. Rapid deterioration of renal function that can lead to death from renal failure in weeks to months.
   b. Can be caused by Goodpasture's syndrome (with anti–glomerular basement membrane [GBM] antibodies), by pauci-immune RPGN (associated with antineutrophil cytoplasmic antibodies [ANCAs]), or by severe cases of other forms of glomerulonephritis.
   c. Pulmonary hemorrhage can occur in RPGN associated with Goodpasture's syndrome or with ANCA antibodies.
   d. Serologic tests are available for anti-GBM antibodies and ANCA. The characteristic finding of RPGN on renal biopsy is the formation of cellular crescents within the glomeruli.
   e. Treatment
      (1) Corticosteroid therapy and cytotoxic agents with or without plasmapheresis if anti-GBM antibodies are present. Typically, corticosteroid therapy will prevent pulmonary hemorrhage but will not stop the progression of renal disease.
      (2) For ANCA-associated disease, cyclophosphamide and corticosteroids can be highly effective.

ANCA antibodies are associated with a variety of vasculitic syndromes, including Wegener's granulomatosis, microscopic polyangiitis, and polyarteritis nodosa (see Chapter 14).

IV. Diabetic Nephropathy
   A. Microalbuminuria is the first indication, and patients reach end-stage renal disease in 7 to 10 years after proteinuria starts.
   B. Diagnostic Evaluation
      1. Diabetes causes persistent albuminuria (>300 mg/24 hr), persistently declining GFR, and raised arterial blood pressure.
      2. Further diagnostic testing is required if the patient has no proteinuria, has no retinopathy, or has red blood cell casts.
      3. Biopsy tissue may show Kimmelstiel-Wilson nodular glomerulosclerosis or diffuse glomerulosclerosis with increased hyaline material in the mesangial areas.
   C. Treatment
      1. Control blood glucose (see Chapter 3).
      2. Control hypertension. ACE inhibitors are the most protective for the kidneys in diabetic nephropathy.
      3. Low protein diet.

V. Adult Polycystic Kidney Disease
   A. Inherited disease with an autosomal dominant inheritance.
   B. Patients typically are 30 to 50 years old and have slowly progressive azotemia or uremia, with abdominal masses and (rarely) abdominal or flank pain.
   C. Cysts are present in the kidneys, liver, and pancreas. Cerebral berry aneurysms (which can cause death from rupture and subarachnoid hemorrhage) and mitral valve prolapse are also frequently found in these patients.
   D. Patients can be treated with dialysis or transplantation, and the disease will not recur in the transplanted kidney.

Renal insufficiency is defined as a GFR of 20% to 50% of normal. Renal failure is defined as a GFR of 20% to 25% of normal. End-stage renal disease (ESRD) is defined as a GFR of less than 5% of normal.

VI. Acute Renal Failure
   A. Causes: Can be separated into prerenal, renal (intrinsic), and postrenal. Prerenal causes involve insufficient blood flow to the kidney, renal causes involve damage to the kidney itself, and postrenal causes involve an obstruction of the urinary tract (Table 7-1).
   B. Symptoms and Signs
      1. Prerenal renal failure causes symptoms of dehydration or congestive heart failure.
      2. Intrinsic causes of renal failure produce symptoms of venous congestion, muscle pain, and obtundation.
      3. Postrenal causes of renal failure produce urinary retention and mass-related symptoms depending on the type of obstruction (e.g., enlarged prostate, flank pain due to renal stones).
   C. Diagnostic Evaluation
      1. A distinction between prerenal and renal causes of acute renal failure can be made on the basis of urinalysis and the basic metabolic profile (Table 7-2).
      2. Urine sediment analysis: The type of casts present in a urine sample can indicate the cause of renal failure.
         a. Hyaline casts: Prerenal
         b. Red blood cells (RBCs) or RBC casts: Glomerulonephritis
         c. White blood cells (WBCs) or WBC casts: Allergic tubulointerstitial nephritis
         d. Granular casts or renal tubular cells: Acute tubular necrosis
      3. Renal ultrasound and prostate-specific antigen (PSA) can be used to investigate possible postrenal urinary tract obstructions. Ultrasound can detect many physical obstructions, as well as any hydronephrosis that has developed due to renal damage. The PSA level can be elevated when benign prostatic hypertrophy or prostatic cancer is causing an obstruction.

Urinalysis can also detect proteinuria and hematuria. In rhabdomyolysis, 4+ blood is detected on the dipstick test, with only 2 to 5 RBCs seen on microscopic examination. This result occurs because the myoglobin in the urine registers as blood on the dipstick examination.

   D. Treatment
      1. First-line therapy includes loop diuretics (furosemide), IV hydration, and alkalinization of the urine with sodium bicarbonate.
      2. If patients do not improve, consider hemodialysis.
      3. Indications for emergent dialysis (mnemonic—AEIOU)
         a. **A**cidemia
         b. **E**lectrolyte disorder (hyperkalemia)
         c. **I**ntoxication (methanol, polyethylene glycol)

When potassium is greater than 7 mg/dL, dialysis should be started immediately.

TABLE 7-1
Causes of Acute Renal Failure

Condition	Symptoms and Signs	Evaluation	Treatment
Renal artery stenosis (prerenal)	(1) Causes decreased juxtaglomerular perfusion and subsequent release of renin, which results in fluid retention. (2) Two thirds of stenoses are due to atherosclerosis, one third due to fibromuscular dysplasia. (3) Suspect renal artery stenosis in a young woman with hypertension. Headache is another common complaint. (4) Physical signs include diastolic hypertension, flank bruits, and decreased renal function.	(1) Arteriogram is the gold standard test. (2) Intravenous pyelography can demonstrate delayed filling of contrast in kidneys. (3) Renal vein renin ratio is abnormal (one renal vein contains >1.5 times the renin of the other vein). (4) A captopril provocation test causes a drop in blood pressure.	(1) Do not treat these patients with angiotensin converting enzyme inhibitors (ACE-Is), because they will cause renal insufficiency. (2) Percutaneous renal transluminal angioplasty (PRTA) is especially good for stenosis caused by fibromuscular dysplasia. (3) Other surgical techniques include resection, bypass, vein/graft interposition, and endarterectomy.
Hypoperfusion (prerenal)	Inadequate arterial volume (due to hypovolemia or poor delivery) will shunt blood away from the kidneys. Symptoms of hypovolemia, liver failure, CHF, sepsis, or anaphylaxis may be present.	Urinalysis may display hyaline casts.	Volume resuscitation and maintenance of blood pressure.
Glomerulonephritis (renal)	(1) Hematuria, oliguria, and hypertension several weeks following an infection (usually streptococcal). (2) See Chapter 11.	(1) RBCs and RBC casts are present on urinalysis. (2) Renal biopsy may show antibody deposition.	Supportive.
Nephrotoxic drugs (renal)	Can be caused by NSAIDs, aminoglycosides, cisplatin, ACE-Is, and polyethylene glycol.	Hematuria may be present.	Discontinue exposure to nephrotoxic agents.
Endogenous nephrotoxins (renal)	(1) Myoglobin in rhabdomyolysis. (2) Uric acid in gout. (3) Azotemia in hepatorenal syndrome.	(1) In rhabdomyolysis, urine dipstick examination will display 4+ blood, but urine microscopic examination will show few RBCs. (2) Direct tests for uric acid and myoglobin are available.	Dialysis may be necessary to remove toxins.
Acute tubular necrosis (renal)	Can be due to ischemia, pigment deposition, or drugs (contrast dye, aminoglycosides, amphotericin, cisplatin).	Urinalysis can display coarsely granular casts and possibly tubular cells.	Discontinue exposure to nephrotoxic agents, and provide supportive therapy.

continued

TABLE 7-1 Causes of Acute Renal Failure—cont'd

Disorder	Symptoms and Signs	Evaluation	Treatment
Acute interstitial nephritis (renal)	Can be due to drug allergy, infection, or autoimmune disease.	Neutrophils and eosinophils will be present in the urine.	Treat or discontinue exposure to causative agent.
Urinary tract obstruction (postrenal)	Patients may have renal stones, tumors, adhesions, or prostatic enlargement.	CT imaging and intravenous pyelography may reveal the site of obstruction.	Surgical correction to remove or bypass the obstruction.

d. **O**verload of volume

e. **U**remia

4. Calcium chloride, glucose, albuterol, furosemide, and sodium polystyrene sulfonate (Kayexalate) also can be used if hyperkalemia develops.

5. For acute tubular necrosis (ATN), provide adequate protein calories, treat hyperkalemia, and perform dialysis if necessary.

VII. Chronic Renal Failure

A. Occurs in cases of long-standing renal disease, usually in the context of renal function that progressively declines over the course of years.

B. Chronic renal insufficiency occurs when the patient has consistently elevated creatinine levels (between 1.5 and 3.0) for long periods. The cause of the renal failure should be investigated, and measures should be taken to treat the underlying cause.

Dialysis is equivalent to 10% to 15% of renal function, so it should not be considered an option until the patient's GFR has dropped below that level.

C. Renal replacement therapy, which consists of either dialysis or renal transplantation, should be attempted when the serum creatinine reaches 4 to 6 mg/dL in women or 6 to 8 mg/dL in men.

D. Dietary protein should be restricted to minimize urea production and subsequent complications of uremia.

VIII. Urinary Tract Infection (UTI)

A. Symptoms

1. Patients typically have dysuria, urinary urgency, and increased urinary frequency.

TABLE 7-2 Distinctions Between Prerenal and Renal Types of Acute Renal Failure

Test	Type of Acute Renal Failure: Prerenal	Renal
BUN/creatinine	>20	10–20
Urine Na^+	<20 mEq/L	>40 mEq/L
Fractional excretion of Na^+ (FENa)	<1%	>1%
Urine osmolality	>500 mOsm/kg	<350 mOsm/kg
Urine specific gravity	>1.04	~1.01

2. Other symptoms may suggest the location of the infection within the urinary tract.
   a. Urethral discharge may be present in urethritis.
   b. Outlet obstruction may be present in prostatitis.
   c. Shaking, chills, and back pain may be present in pyelonephritis.
   d. Symptoms may persist following antibiotic therapy in renal abscess.

B. Diagnostic Evaluation
1. Urinalysis
   a. Findings can include pyuria (WBCs in urine), bacteriuria, and possibly hematuria. WBC casts can be present in pyelonephritis.
   b. Sterile pyuria may indicate urethritis, tuberculosis, or urinary obstruction.
2. Urine gram staining and culture: Cystitis is most commonly caused by *Escherichia coli* or *Staphylococcus saprophyticus.*
3. Rapid assays are available for *Chlamydia* and *Neisseria gonorrhoeae.*
4. Abdominal CT if renal abscess is suspected.

C. Treatment
1. For cystitis, use metronidazole or a fluoroquinolone for 10 to 14 days.
2. For urethritis, treatment depends on the cause (ceftriaxone or ofloxacin for gonorrhea, doxycycline or azithromycin for *Chlamydia*). However, patients with gonorrhea should be treated presumptively for *Chlamydia* because coinfection is common and *Chlamydia* is less symptomatic.
3. For prostatitis, use metronidazole or a fluoroquinolone.
4. For pyelonephritis, use a fluoroquinolone, ampicillin/clavulanic acid, or ampicillin with IV gentamycin (for inpatients).
5. For renal abscess, treat with drainage and either a fluoroquinolone or ampicillin/clavulanic acid or ampicillin with IV gentamycin.

IX. Nephrolithiasis (Renal Stones)

A. Patients can have hematuria, flank pain, urinary tract infection, or signs of postrenal acute renal failure.

B. Diagnostic Evaluation
1. Proof of stones can be obtained using several imaging studies (radiography, intravenous pyelography, or positron emission tomography [PET]).
2. Urinalysis and basic metabolic profile to assess for renal failure.
3. Urine culture and sensitivity to evaluate for UTI.
4. Uric acid levels to evaluate for urate stones and gout.
5. 24-hour urine test and dietary evaluation for recurrent stones.

C. Treatment
1. Acute treatment
   a. Analgesia with aggressive hydration.
   b. Antibiotics if a UTI is present.
   c. Lithotripsy, cystoscopic stenting, percutaneous nephrostomy, or stone removal by a urologist, if necessary. This is usually indicated if the stones are greater than 8 mm, are located in the upper ureter or renal pelvis, or produce increasing hydronephrosis, infection, or intractable pain.

2. Chronic treatment (for recurrent stones)
   a. Increase fluid intake.
   b. Calcium stones: Give thiazide diuretics, and decrease the patient's meat and sodium intake.
   c. Uric acid stones: Urine alkalinization and allopurinol.
   d. Citrate stones: Potassium citrate replacement.
   e. Magnesium phosphate (struvite) stones: These usually are the result of recurrent UTIs due to urease-producing organisms (*Proteus*). Treat the infections, and evaluate for urinary tract obstruction.
   f. Cystine stones: Treat with penicillamine or tiopronin. If this is unsuccessful, use ultrasonic lithotripsy, *not* extracorporeal shock wave lithotripsy.

X. Acid/Base Disturbances
   A. Determination of Abnormalities (Figs. 7-1 and 7-2)
      1. The predominant abnormality will be indicated by the deviation of the overall pH: pH less than 7.35 indicates acidosis, and pH greater than 7.45 indicates alkalosis.

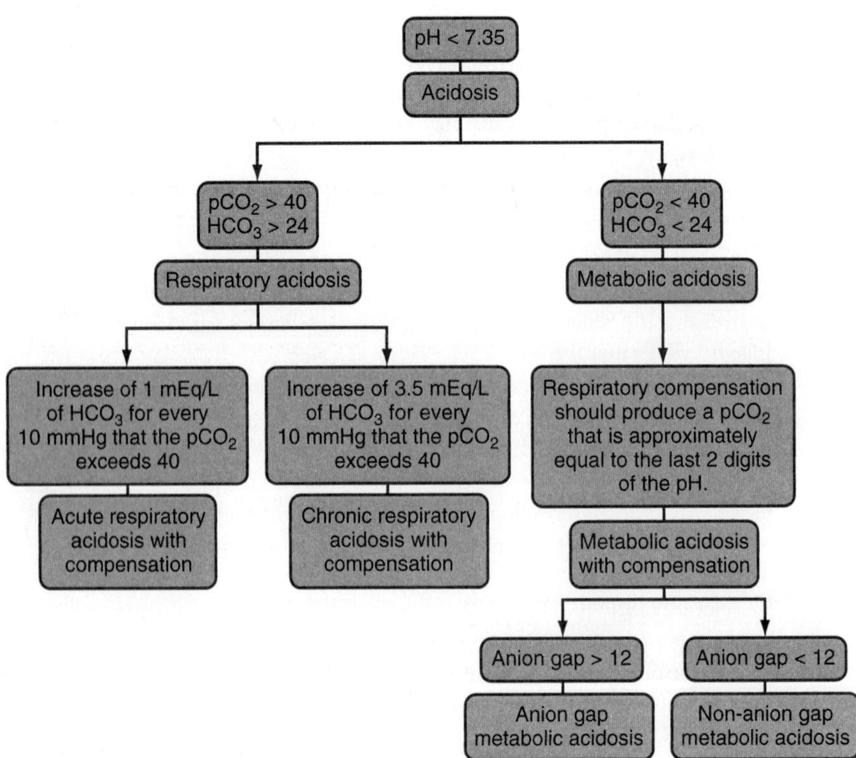

7-1: *Algorithm for the characterization of acidosis.*

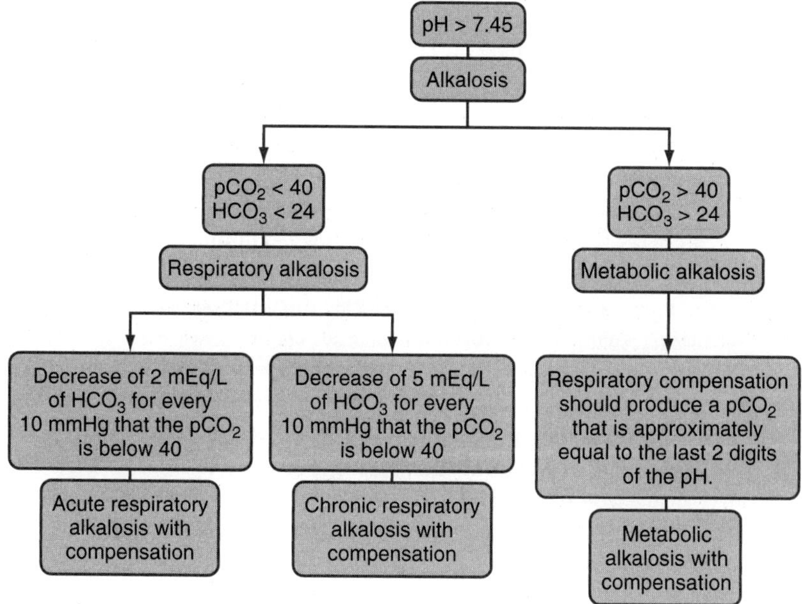

7-2: *Algorithm for the characterization of alkalosis.*

2. Determine whether the deviation is due to respiratory or metabolic causes.
3. Determine whether compensation has occurred.
4. Calculation of anion gaps may assist in determining the cause of the abnormality.

B. Respiratory Acidosis/Alkalosis: In respiratory acidosis, the patient will have a pH of less than 7.35 with a pCO_2 of greater than 40. In respiratory alkalosis, the patient will have a pH of greater than 7.45 with a pCO_2 of less than 40.
1. Normal CO_2 is 40. In acute respiratory acidosis, the expected compensation would involve an increase of 1 mEq/L of HCO_3 for every 10 mm Hg of CO_2 above 40 measured. For example, a patient with a pH of 7.30 and a pCO_2 of 50 would be expected to have an HCO_3 of 25 as a result of metabolic compensation.
2. In chronic respiratory acidosis, the expected compensation would involve an increase of 3.5 mEq/L of HCO_3 for every 10 mm Hg of CO_2 above 40 measured. For example, a patient with a pH of 7.30 and a pCO_2 of 50 would be expected to have an HCO_3 of 27 to 28 as a result of metabolic compensation.
3. In acute respiratory alkalosis, the expected compensation would involve a decrease of 2 mEq/L of HCO_3 for every 10 mm Hg of CO_2 below 40 measured. For example, a patient with a pH of 7.50 and a pCO_2 of 30 would be expected to have an HCO_3 of 22 as a result of metabolic compensation.
4. In chronic respiratory alkalosis, the expected compensation would involve a decrease of 5 mEq/L of HCO_3 for every 10 mm Hg of CO_2 below 40

measured. For example, a patient with a pH of 7.50 and a pCO_2 of 30 would be expected to have an HCO_3 of 19 as a result of metabolic compensation.

5. Situations in which the expected metabolic compensation do not occur may be caused by the presence of multiple acid-base disturbances in the same patient.

C. Metabolic Acidosis/Alkalosis: In metabolic acidosis, the patient will have a pH of less than 7.35 with an HCO_3 of less than 24. In metabolic alkalosis, the patient will have a pH of greater than 7.45 with an HCO_3 of greater than 24.

1. Compensation for metabolic acid/base disturbances occurs through ventilatory changes, as indicated by the pCO_2 in the arterial blood gas (ABG). You can estimate the pCO_2 expected in compensation for a metabolic acid-base change by using the last 2 digits of the pH measurement. For instance, in a patient with metabolic acidosis who has a pH of 7.30, the predicted respiratory compensation would result in an arterial pCO_2 of 30 mm Hg. Conversely, a patient with metabolic alkalosis and a pH of 7.50 would be expected to have a pCO_2 of 50 mm Hg.

2. The cause of a metabolic acidosis can be further evaluated using the anion gap values:

$$\text{anion gap} = \text{Na} - (\text{Cl} + \text{HCO}_3).$$

a. Anion gaps of greater than 12 can be due to the presence of other anions.

b. Causes of anion gap acidosis (mnemonic—MULEPAK).

(1) **M**ethanol
(2) **U**remia
(3) **L**actic acidosis
(4) **E**thylene glycol
(5) **P**araldehyde
(6) **A**spirin
(7) **K**etoacidosis

D. Treatment

1. Respiratory acidosis: Usually due to hypoventilation, so increasing ventilation (through bronchodilation, mechanical ventilation, etc.) can alleviate the acid-base abnormality.

2. Respiratory alkalosis: Caused by hyperventilation, so alleviation of the stimulus causing the hyperventilation will allow recovery of normal acid-base status. If the patient is on a ventilator, this can be done by turning down the respiratory rate.

3. Metabolic acidosis: Treatment is dependent on cause. In cases of lactic acidosis or ketoacidosis, the underlying causes should be treated. In cases of acidosis due to ingestion, hemodialysis may be required. In particularly severe cases ($pH < 7.0$), sodium bicarbonate can be used to normalize the pH.

4. Metabolic alkalosis: Often due to loss of HCl following periods of vomiting. Dehydration also can occur, and IV fluid resuscitation is a treatment of choice.

XI. Electrolyte Disturbances (Table 7-3)

In diabetes insipidus (DI) either antidiuretic hormone (ADH) is not present (central/neurogenic) or the kidney is unresponsive to ADH (nephrogenic). Central DI can be caused by CNS trauma or disease. Nephrogenic DI can be caused by rheumatic kidney disease, sickle cell disease, electrolyte imbalance (hypercalcemia, hypokalemia), or medications (lithium, amphotericin, demeclocycline).

Causes of hyperkalemia include renal failure, hypoaldosteronism, hyporeninemia, type IV renal tubular acidosis (RTA), adrenal disease (Addison's disease, congenital adrenal hyperplasia), myeloma, amyloidosis, SLE, and medications (NSAIDs, heparin, potassium-sparing diuretics, and cyclosporine).

TABLE 7-3 Common Electrolyte Abnormalities

Condition	Presentation	Evaluation	Treatment
Hyponatremia	(1) Usually occurs as a result of increased antidiuretic hormone (ADH). (2) The patient may have signs of low blood volume. (3) Brain swelling may cause mental status changes or coma.	(1) Measure serum osmolality to determine whether the hyponatremia is hypertonic (usually due to hyperglycemia) or hypotonic. Normal serum osmolality is 275–295 mOsm/kg. (2) Hypotonic hyponatremia can be further assessed by assessing volume status, urine Na^+, and urine osmolality. (a) Hypovolemia with a urine Na^+ of >20 mEq/L indicates a renal sodium loss (from diuretics, hypoaldosteronism, or salt-wasting nephropathy). (b) Hypovolemia with a urine Na^+ of <10 mEq/L indicates an extrarenal sodium loss (from GI loss, third spacing, or insensible losses). (c) Euvolemia with a urine osmolality of >100 units indicates the syndrome of inappropriate antidiuretic hormone (SIADH) secretion. SIADH may be caused by hypothyroidism, adrenal insufficiency, malignancy, drugs (antipsychotics, antidepressants, thiazides), and pulmonary or intracranial pathology. (d) Euvolemia with a urine osmolality of <100 units indicates ADH suppression by polydipsia. Investigate these patients for psychiatric problems. (e) Hypervolemia indicates renal failure if the urinary Na^+ is >20 mEq/L. (f) Hypervolemia indicates CHF, cirrhosis, or nephritic syndrome if the urinary Na^+ is <10 mEq/L.	(1) Hypovolemic hyponatremia can be treated with Na^+ replacement. The rate of replacement should not exceed 0.5 mEq/L/hr in order prevent neurologic complications. Brain edema can cause seizures, and central pontine myelinolysis can cause a locked-in syndrome. (2) Hypervolemic hyponatremia can be treated with restriction of sodium and water. (3) SIADH can be treated with free water restriction. Demeclocycline can be given in chronic cases. (4) In emergencies, hypertonic fluid replacement and loop diuresis can be used.
Hypernatremia	(1) Patients may display signs of fluid overload. (2) Frequently caused by an inability to concentrate urine.	(1) Hypovolemic hypernatremia should be further evaluated with urine osmolality measurement. (a) Urine osmolality <300 units indicates diabetes insipidus. Central and	(1) Correction of hypernatremia must happen at a rate of less than 0.5 mEq/L/hr in order to prevent neurologic complications (see above).

continued

TABLE 7-3 Common Electrolyte Abnormalities—cont'd

Condition	Presentation	Evaluation	Treatment
		nephrogenic diabetes insipidus (DI) can be distinguished using vasopressin. Vasopressin administration will correct central DI, but not nephrogenic DI. (b) Urine osmolality 300–600 units indicates DI or renal disease. (c) Urine osmolality >600 units indicates extrarenal water losses. (2) Hypervolemic hypernatremia is caused by Na^+ retention due to infusion or mineralocorticoid excess.	(2) Hypovolemic hypernatremia can be treated by volume replacement with hypotonic saline. (3) Hypervolemic hypernatremia can be treated with loop diuretics and IV fluids. (4) Central DI can be treated with desmopressin (DDAVP). (5) Nephrogenic DI can be treated by treating the underlying cause, Na^+ restriction, and thiazide diuresis.
Hypokalemia	Patients have weakness, nausea, vomiting, muscle cramps, paralysis, and confusion.	(1) Urinary potassium >30 mEq/L indicates renal losses. (2) Hypertensive hypokalemia suggests hyperaldosteronism or pseudohyperaldosteronism (occurs with Cushing's syndrome and licorice ingestion). (3) Normotensive hypokalemia requires acid/base evaluation. (a) Acidemia indicates diabetic ketoacidosis or renal tubular acidosis. (b) Alkalemia indicates diuretics or vomiting as a cause. (c) Magnesium deficiency can cause either acidemia or alkalemia. (4) Electrocardiography can show U waves, atrioventricular block, and ventricular ectopy.	(1) Potassium repletion. In cases of hypomagnesemia with hyperkalemia, correct the magnesium first and the potassium may spontaneously correct. (2) Treat underlying cause.
Hyperkalemia	(1) Patients have weakness, cardiac arrest, and small bowel ulcers. (2) Associated with some medications (beta-blockers, digoxin) and metabolic conditions (insulin deficiency, acidosis).	(1) Calculate the glomerular filtration rate (GFR) based on the patient's creatinine clearance: $C_{cr} = U_{cr}V/P_{cr}$. (a) Low GFR indicates renal failure as the cause. (b) Normal GFR indicates hypoaldosteronism. (2) Electrocardiogram shows peaked T waves, increased PR interval, and increased QRS width progressing to sine wave pattern.	(1) Acute treatment with calcium gluconate, insulin, and bicarbonate. (2) Long-term treatment with Kayexalate, diuresis, and hemodialysis, if necessary.

TABLE 7-3 Common Electrolyte Abnormalities—cont'd

Condition	Presentation	Evaluation	Treatment
Hypocalcemia	(1) Patients have alopecia, cataracts, hypotension, and steatorrhea. (2) Physical signs include Chvostek's sign (contraction of the facial muscles after the cheek is tapped) and Trousseau's sign (carpal spasm following inflation of blood pressure cuff).	(1) Check calcium, magnesium, and phosphate. Hypomagnesemia can cause hypocalcemia by causing parathyroid resistance or deficiency. Low phosphate may indicate vitamin D abnormalities. (2) ECG displays prolongation of the QT interval.	(1) Slow infusion of IV calcium gluconate with calcitriol. (2) Replace magnesium as needed.
Hypercalcemia	(1) Symptoms include bone fractures, kidney stones, constipation, fatigue, and altered mental status. (2) Associated with medications (vitamin D, estrogen, thiazides, theophylline, and lithium), cancer, and hyperparathyroidism.	(1) ECG shows shortening of the QT interval. (2) Evaluate endocrine function with parathyroid hormone, thyroid-stimulating hormone, vitamin D, and phosphate measurements.	(1) Volume expansion with saline. (2) Loop diuretics can be used to facilitate Ca^{++} excretion after volume status is normal. (3) Bisphosphonate. (4) Surgery as needed for hyperparathyroidism.

CHAPTER 8

Neurology

I. Basic Neuroanatomy

A. Upper versus Lower Motor Neuron Lesions (Box 8-1)

1. Signs of upper motor neuron lesions
   a. Hyperactive reflexes
   b. Spastic tone
   c. Fasciculations with atrophy of muscle groups rather than of individual muscles
   d. Normal findings on electromyography (EMG)
2. Signs of lower motor neuron lesions
   a. Decreased or absent reflexes
   b. Flaccid tone
   c. Fasciculations and focal atrophy
   d. Abnormal findings on EMG and fibrillation

B. Neuroanatomy Review: Focal lesions (e.g., ischemic strokes) can produce discrete neurologic deficits that allow physicians to localize the site of the infarction. Table 8-1 and Figure 8-1 correlate the sites of infarction with the associated symptoms.

C. Symptoms Affecting Executive Functions

1. Aphasia: Loss of previously acquired language ability
   a. Injury to different regions of the brain results in various deficits affecting the use and understanding of language (Table 8-2).
   b. A common cause is an ischemic stroke in the distribution of the middle cerebral artery.
   c. Affects the ability to use both written and spoken language.
   d. Aphasia vs dysarthria: Dysarthria involves impaired speech due to weakness or poor coordination of the muscles involved in speaking. The ability of a dysarthric patient to communicate through written language would not be impaired.

Aphasia = loss of language; apraxia = loss of motor skills.

Dysarthria - impaired speech due to weakness or poor coordination of muscles *written language NOT impaired

2. Apraxia: Loss of the ability to perform learned motor tasks
   a. Can involve activities such as dressing, combing hair, and eating.
   b. Significant alteration in the patient's daily behavior is usually an indication of bilateral damage to the parietal association cortices. This can occur in some neurodegenerative disorders, including Alzheimer's disease.

II. Cerebrovascular Disease (Stroke)

A. Risk Factors for Stroke

1. Hypertension
2. Smoking cigarettes
3. Consumption of alcohol
4. Diabetes

BOX 8-1

SIGNS OF INJURY:
UPPER MOTOR NEURONS VERSUS LOWER MOTOR NEURONS

The CNS acts to calibrate the tone and reflexes of the peripheral neuromuscular system, allowing appropriate reflexes to sensory stimuli. Injury to the brain, brainstem, or spinal cord tracts (upper motor neurons) can interrupt these control mechanisms and produce spasticity with hyperactive reflexes. In contrast, lesions of the motor system at the level of the peripheral nerve or anterior horn cells (lower motor neurons) are associated with hypotonia and areflexia due to the interruption of reflex pathways or the innervation of the muscle itself. Clinical signs that are helpful in determining the location of a lesion when a pure upper or lower motor neuron injury occurs are discussed throughout this chapter. In addition, injuries involving the vertebral column and spinal cord, or degenerative diseases such as amyotrophic lateral sclerosis or subacute combined degeneration, may involve the loss of both upper and lower motor neurons.

TABLE 8-1
Focal Lesions

Location	Symptoms
Motor cortex	Contralateral weakness (-paresis) or paralysis (-plegia) with sparing of legs (in cases of middle cerebral artery occlusion) or with sparing of upper body (in cases of anterior cerebral artery occlusion)
Sensory cortex	Contralateral loss of all sensory modalities Sensory cortical lesions are also likely to involve neighboring motor cortex, causing additional symptoms of weakness
Broca's area	Expressive aphasia (see text, section IC1)
Wernicke's area	Receptive aphasia (see text, section IC1)
Frontal lobe	Disinhibition, poor judgment, apathy, and amotivation Patient may also display a return of infantile reflexes (suck, snout, rooting, grasp)
Parietal lobe	Dominant lesions cause visual and/or tactile agnosias (resulting in defective recognition of objects by sight and touch, respectively) Nondominant lesions can cause anosognosia (neglect of contralateral side of body)
Occipital lobe	Cortical blindness or visual agnosias, depending on location

continued

TABLE 8-1
Focal Lesions—cont'd

Location	Symptoms
Temporal lobe	Hippocampal lesions cause global impairment of declarative memory functions (impaired recall of factual information without impairment of learned motor skills) Lesions of amygdala can cause Klüver-Bucy syndrome (hypersexuality, hyperorality, loss of anxiety, depressed aggression) Lesions in other areas may cause seizures
Internal capsule	Damage results in paralysis of contralateral face, arms, and legs to an equivalent degree
Thalamus	Sensory loss of all modalities on contralateral side of body; motor function may be completely spared
Midbrain	Cranial nerve palsies with fixed, midposition pupils
Pons	Cranial nerve palsies with pinpoint pupils Severe lesions may cause a locked-in syndrome that interrupts efferent tracts but spares afferent ones; affected patients can sense stimuli, but they are only able to respond through eye-blinking
Cerebellum	Ipsilateral ataxia with intact motor strength; nystagmus and vertigo may also occur
Medulla	Occlusion of vertebral artery or posterior inferior cerebellar artery (PICA) can cause lateral medullary syndrome (Wallenberg's syndrome) Patients have numbness on ipsilateral face and contralateral body, ipsilateral limb ataxia, vertigo, and ipsilateral Horner's syndrome, but motor function is spared
Spinal cord	Occlusion of posterior spinal artery causes bilateral infarction of posterior column tracts and loss of vibration and proprioception below spinal level Occlusion of anterior spinal artery causes loss of motor function and pain sensation below spinal level with sparing of proprioception (see margin notes for other spinal cord injury patterns)

TABLE 8-2
Types of Aphasia

Type	Structures Involved	Signs and Symptoms
Broca's (expressive)	Posterior inferior frontal lobe adjacent to motor cortex	Able to understand what is heard but unable to communicate fluently. Contralateral hemiparesis may be present if adjacent motor cortex is affected.
Wernicke's (receptive)	Posterior superior temporal lobe	Able to speak fluently but unable to comprehend what is being said or written.
Conductive	Arcuate fasciculus connecting Broca's and Wernicke's areas	Fluent speech and good comprehension but unable to repeat what is said.
Global	Broca's area, Wernicke's area, and arcuate fasciculus	Unable to comprehend or use language.

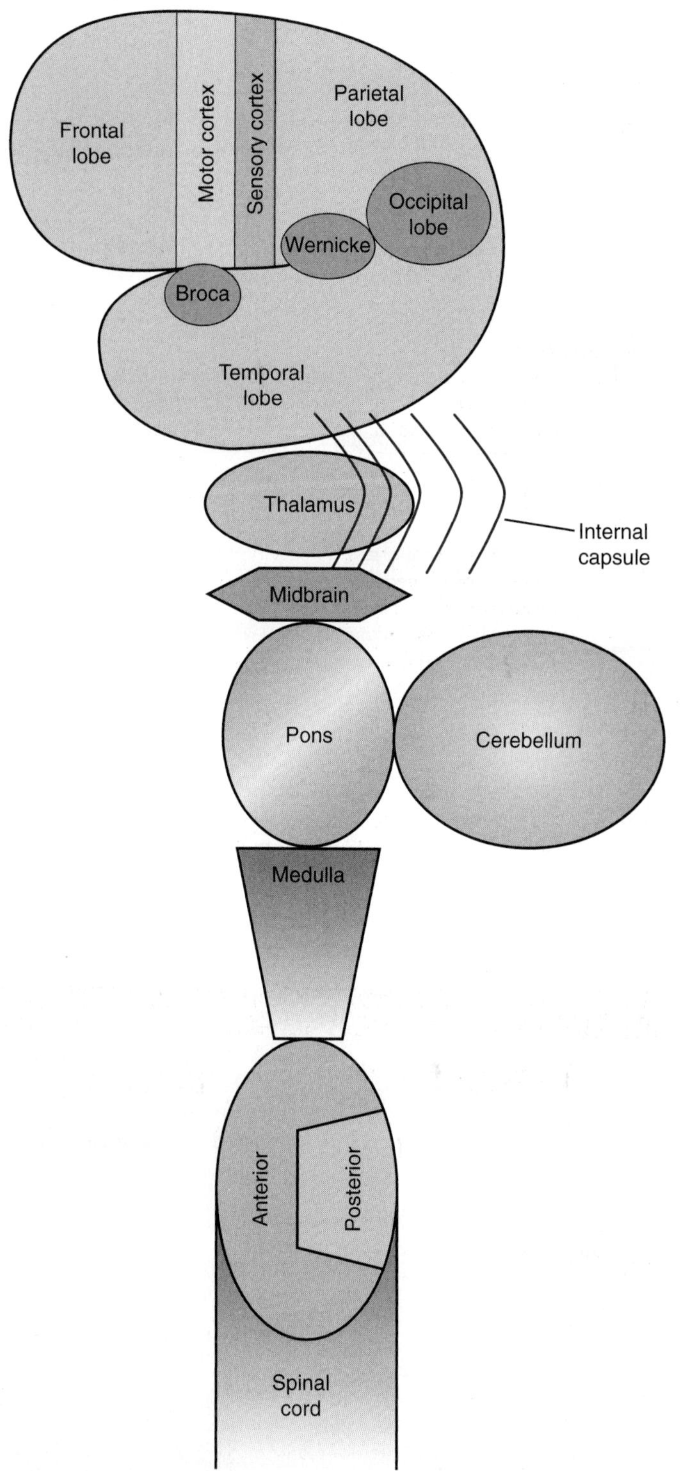

***8-1:** Simplified schematic depicting the pertinent locations for most focal neurologic deficits.*

5. Heart disease
6. Carotid artery stenosis
7. History of transient ischemic attacks (TIAs)

B. TIAs: Focal, temporary deficits produced by occlusion of the cerebral vasculature by emboli. The embolus dissolves before permanent ischemic damage can occur.
1. Signs and symptoms
   a. Transient focal neurologic deficits (e.g., motor deficits, aphasia).
   b. Amaurosis fugax: Temporary blindness of one visual field with onset similar to the pulling down of a shade.
2. Evaluation
   a. CT scan to assess for hemorrhage. If the scan shows no hemorrhage, a follow-up MRI scan can be performed to assess the extent of damage.
   b. Carotid duplex ultrasound and echocardiography.
   c. Angiography, if necessary.
3. Treatment
   a. Prophylaxis: Anticoagulation and control of risk factors (e.g., smoking cessation, control blood glucose in diabetic patients).
   b. Carotid endarterectomy: Indicated especially for patients with 70% of greater occlusion of the carotid arteries or symptomatic patients.

C. Ischemic Stroke: Ischemia producing permanent neurologic deficits.
1. Signs and symptoms
   a. Focal neurologic deficits: Depend on the site of the infarct (Figs. 8-1 and 8-2A).
   b. Strokes of the major cerebral arteries can produce typical symptom complexes.
      (1) Anterior cerebral artery (see Fig. 8-2B): Contralateral hemiparesis with relative sparing of the upper limb and face.
      (2) Middle cerebral artery (see Fig. 8-2C): Contralateral hemiparesis with relative sparing of the lower limb. Aphasias can also occur.
      (3) Posterior cerebral artery (see Fig. 8-2D): Homonymous hemianopsia of the contralateral visual field.
   c. Symptoms may be dependent on cause.
      (1) Thrombotic strokes typically occur during sleep and may progress to maximal deficit over hours.
      (2) Embolic strokes may be associated with cardiac disease and frequently occur while awake. The progression to maximal deficit occurs over minutes.
2. Evaluation
   a. CT scan can confirm the location of the infarct (but often not until hours or days postinfarction).
   b. CT scan is useful for excluding hematomas, arteriovenous malformations (AVMs), mass lesions, and hemorrhagic strokes as the cause of focal neurologic deficits.
3. Treatment
   a. During a stroke: To avoid decreasing cerebral perfusion, do *not* treat patients with moderate hypertension. Intra-arterial thrombotic agents

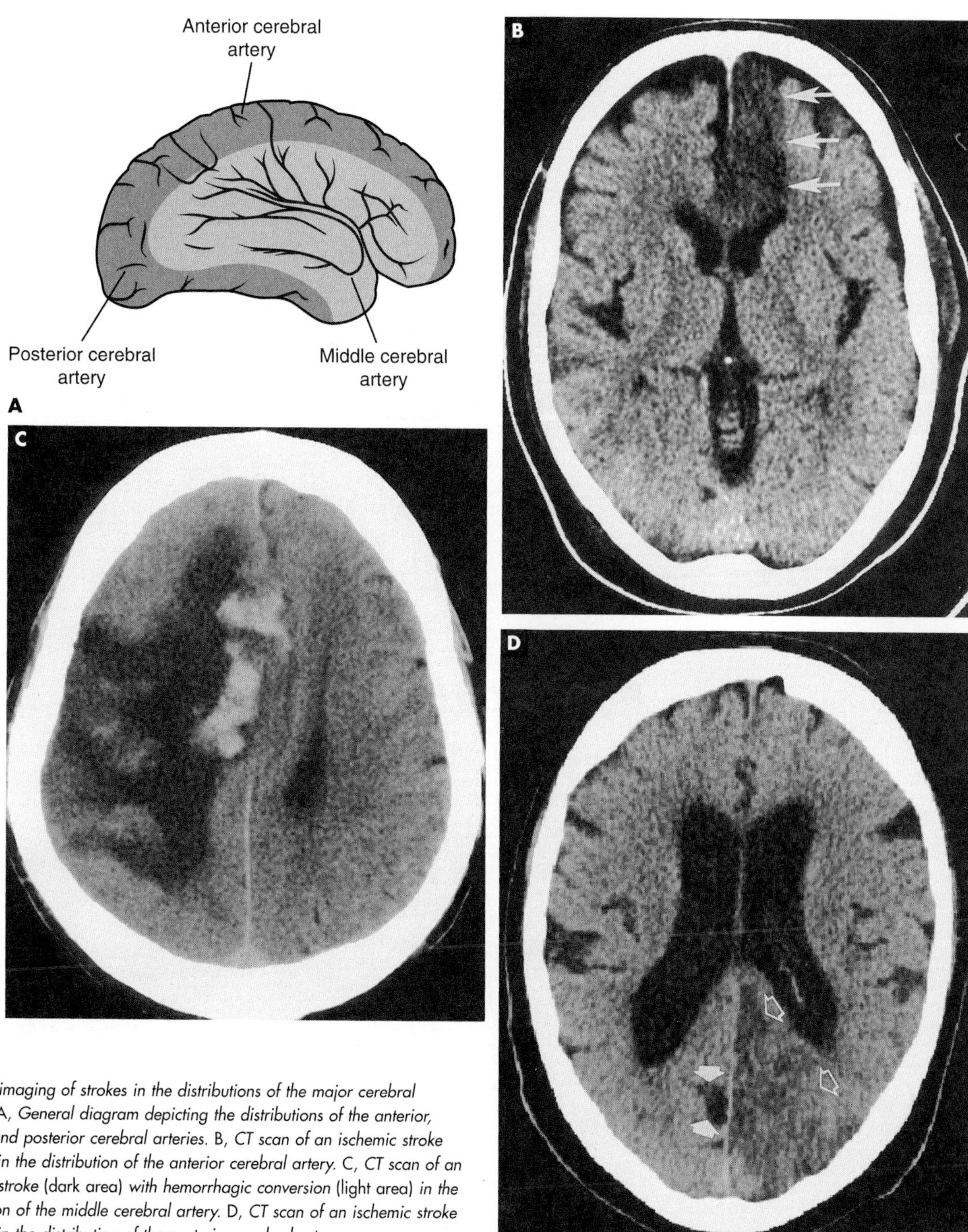

8-2: *CT imaging of strokes in the distributions of the major cerebral arteries.* A, *General diagram depicting the distributions of the anterior, middle, and posterior cerebral arteries.* B, *CT scan of an ischemic stroke* (arrows) *in the distribution of the anterior cerebral artery.* C, *CT scan of an ischemic stroke* (dark area) *with hemorrhagic conversion* (light area) *in the distribution of the middle cerebral artery.* D, *CT scan of an ischemic stroke* (arrows) *in the distribution of the posterior cerebral artery.*

may be used if the stroke began less than 6 hours earlier, but these agents increase the risk of conversion to hemorrhagic stroke.

b. Thrombolysis
   (1) Indications
      (a) Presence of an ischemic stroke diagnosed using clinical and imaging criteria.
      (b) Ability to administer the agent within 3 hours of symptom onset.
   (2) Contraindications
      (a) Evidence of hemorrhage
      (b) Evidence of recent major infarction (mass effect or edema)
      (c) Patient currently receiving anticoagulant therapy (heparin or warfarin)
      (d) Onset of symptoms more than 3 hours before therapy can be initiated
c. Stroke prevention
   (1) Decrease risk factors (e.g., quit smoking; control hypertension, cholesterol, and blood glucose).
   (2) Anticoagulation therapy with warfarin or heparin.
   (3) Antiplatelet drugs (acetylsalicylic acid, clopidogrel, dipyridamole).
   (4) Carotid endarterectomy: For patients with symptomatic carotid artery stenosis of 70% or greater.

D. Hemorrhagic Stroke
   1. Types (Table 8-3)
      a. Subarachnoid hemorrhage: Bleeding into the subarachnoid space.
      b. Parenchymal hemorrhage: Hemorrhage within the substance of the brain.
   2. Causes
      a. Hypertension: Most common cause of parenchymal hemorrhage.
      b. Vascular malformation
         (1) AVM
         (2) Aneurysm: Congenital berry aneurysm, located in the anterior circle of Willis, is a common cause of subarachnoid hemorrhage.

Berry aneurysm is associated with adult polycystic kidney disease.

      c. Reperfusion injury: Occurs when perfusion is restored after the endothelial cells of the blood vessels are damaged during an ischemic stroke. The vessel may no longer be able to support the blood pressure, and the ischemic stroke undergoes a conversion to a hemorrhagic stroke.
      d. Trauma
      e. Use of illicit substances
   3. Signs and symptoms, evaluation, and treatment (see Table 8-3)

III. Headache
   A. Types of Headache (Table 8-4)
      1. Migraine: Common in females under 30 years of age
      2. Cluster headache: Common in males
      3. Tension headache

TABLE 8-3 Types of Hemorrhagic Stroke

Type	Signs and Symptoms	Evaluation	Treatment
Subarachnoid hemorrhage	"The worst headache of my life." Hemorrhage occurs while patient is awake and active; deficits progress over ~30 minutes. Elevated ICP: headache, impaired consciousness. Focal neurologic deficits due to impingements or mass effects (posterior communicating artery can compress CN III and cause oculomotor palsy). Sentinel bleeding may cause mild headache in weeks preceding aneurysm rupture as well as meningeal signs (Kernig's and Brudzinski's signs, nuchal igidity) owing to meningeal irritation by blood.	CT scan without contrast to show recent or current hemorrhage. Angiography for visualization of AV malformation or aneurysm. Lumbar puncture to diagnose hemorrhage too small to be seen on CT scan if ICP is normal.	Surgical removal; success depends on timing of surgery and location of hemorrhage. Aneurysm repair using clipping or coiling procedures. Nimodipine (Ca^{++} channel blocker) and hemodilution can reduce postoperative complications. Phenytoin for postoperative seizure prophylaxis.
Parenchymal hemorrhage	Lethargy, headache, and other signs of increased ICP.	Same as above.	Treat bleeding and elevated ICP same as for subarachnoid hemorrhage.

AV, arteriovenous; ICP, intracranial pressure.

4. Traction (postlumbar puncture): Occurs owing to a drop in cerebrospinal fluid (CSF) pressure after lumbar puncture
5. Pseudotumor cerebri
   a. Occurs owing to elevated intracranial pressure in the absence of a mass lesion, most likely as a result of impaired CSF circulation
   b. Commonly associated with obesity
6. Temporal arteritis
   a. Inflammatory condition causing vasculitis and increased sedimentation rate
   b. Common in the elderly

B. Important Features of Patient History
   1. Distribution and timing of the pain
   2. Any precipitants
   3. Any accompanying symptoms

Precipitants of migraine headache: emotional stress, various foods, menstrual cycle.

TABLE 8-4
Types of Headache

Type	Signs and Symptoms	Treatment
Migraine	Visual disturbances (usually shimmering arc of light in visual field that may spread or migrate over minutes) preceding onset of incapacitating unilateral headache. Light and sound intolerance. Nausea and vomiting.	Avoidance of precipitants. Symptomatic relief with analgesics and antiemetics (metoclopramide). Prevention: beta-blockers, Ca^{++} channel blockers, methysergide, tricyclic antidepressants, valproic acid. Migraines in progress: ergot alkaloids, triptans. Incapacitating headaches: intravenous dihydroergotamine.
Cluster	Episodic, daily headache for at least 3 consecutive weeks (often several per day); can recur within several years. Unilateral periorbital pain with an ipsilateral red, watery eye. Nasal discharge, nasal congestion, and ipsilateral Horner's syndrome may be present.	Acute therapy with 100% oxygen, ergot alkaloids, or sumatriptan. 3-Week course of corticosteroids. Prophylaxis: ergot alkaloids, Ca^{++} channel blockers, prednisone, lithium, valproate, and topiramate.
Tension	Pressure or bandlike bilateral pain often not as severe or incapacitating as migraine that may persist for days, weeks, or years.	Mild analgesics or muscle relaxants (which usually relieve symptoms).
Traction (postlumbar puncture)	Symptoms are exacerbated by sitting or standing and relieved when lying flat.	Epidural blood patch administered at site of lumbar puncture.
Pseudotumor cerebri	Symptoms of elevated ICP (headache, nausea, mental status changes).	Acetazolamide or CSF shunt procedure.
Temporal arteritis	Severe headache and jaw claudication (worsening when chewing); can be associated with muscle pain (polymyalgia rheumatica).	Prompt treatment with corticosteroids to prevent possibility of permanent blindness.

CSF, cerebrospinal fluid; ICP, intracranial pressure.

C. Evaluation
  1. Noncontrast CT scan to evaluate for intracranial bleeding
  2. Temporal arteritis: Definitive diagnosis requires temporal artery biopsy.
D. Treatment (see Table 8-4)

Petit mal seizures are the most common type in children and can be induced by hyperventilation or photic stimulation.

IV. Seizures
  A. Types of Seizure (Table 8-5)
  B. Causes of Seizure

TABLE 8-5
Types of Seizures

Type	Signs, Symptoms, and Specific Treatments
Simple partial	Focal jerking (motor) or isolated sensory disturbance without loss of consciousness.
Complex partial	Begins with aura (usually sensory disturbance with dreamy alteration of consciousness) that lasts up to 15 seconds, followed by loss of consciousness while body continues to perform behaviors. Patients usually regain consciousness within several minutes with no recollection of actual seizure.
Nonconvulsive generalized (absence or petit mal)	Typically involves altered consciousness with 3-Hz bilateral discharges on EEG. Treat petit mal seizures with ethosuximide or, alternatively, valproic acid.
Convulsive generalized (tonic-clonic and myoclonic)	Tonic-clonic (grand mal): Sustained extension sometimes accompanied by loud cry. Loss of bladder continence, followed by progression to myoclonic jerks lasting ~2 minutes. Postictal phase (15–30 min) can involve sleepiness, confusion, and altered consciousness; EEG shows 10- to 12-Hz spikes. Myoclonic seizures with muscle jerks occur in toxic or metabolic disorders.
Status epilepticus	Persistent or repeated seizure for at least a 30-minute period; can also be recurrence of seizure prior to recovery from postictal state. Prolonged seizure activity can cause irreversible neurologic damage owing to excitotoxicity. Treat immediately with rapid-acting benzodiazepines followed by longer-acting anticonvulsants.
Anoxic	Typical presentation: patient faints owing to anoxia but does not fall to a horizontal position, preventing return of blood flow to brain.
Febrile	Commonly occurs in children <5 years of age as fever is rising during illness, and lasts <5 minutes. Lumbar puncture is indicated if the seizure lasts >10 minutes, if recurrent, or if meningitis is suspected. Anticonvulsants should be avoided, if possible. Antipyretics can be used to treat fever. In patients with high risk for later seizure disorder, phenobarbital or diazepam per rectum can be used at first sign of fever.
Juvenile myoclonic epilepsy	Commonly occurs in teenagers in the form of morning myoclonic jerks that generalize into convulsions. EEG shows 4- to 6-Hz spikes. Treat with valproate.

EEG, electroencephalogram.

1. Brain injury (trauma, anoxia)
2. Metabolic derangement
    a. Substance use (cocaine)
    b. Drug withdrawal (alcohol, benzodiazepines)
    c. Toxins (tetanus)
    d. Electrolyte disturbances (hypoglycemia, hyponatremia)
3. Congenital brain malformation
4. Tumor
5. Infection

C. Seizure Phases
1. Tonic phase
    a. Contraction of muscles leading to stiffness
    b. Possible loss of consciousness
2. Clonic phase
    a. Synchronous twitching of limbs, jaw, and face that may lead to tongue trauma
    b. Excessive salivation
3. Postictal phase
    a. Rapid breathing
    b. Fatigue and confusion that can last more than 30 minutes
    c. Incontinence
    d. Lack of memory of the seizure event

D. Simple versus Complex Seizures
1. Simple
    a. Jerking or twitching of a body part without loss of consciousness
    b. Focal (no generalization to other brain regions)
    c. No postictal state
2. Complex
    a. Impaired consciousness.
    b. Automatisms (repeated performance of complex coordinated tasks) may be present.
    c. Most commonly associated with origin in the temporal lobe.
    d. Postictal confusion.

E. Evaluation
1. CT or MRI scan to evaluate structural causes and stroke.
2. Electroencephalogram
    a. During a seizure: Should show a spike-wave pattern.
    b. Quiescent seizure foci can show focal slowing of brain wave activity.
3. Perform a lumbar puncture if infection is suspected.
4. Telemetry may be required to differentiate seizures from pseudoseizures.

Only 50% of patients who have had a single seizure will ever have another one.

F. Treatment
1. Initial management
    a. Implement seizure safety precautions (prevent falls and aspiration, roll the patient on his or her side).
    b. Treat life-threatening potential causes (hypoglycemia, infection, hyponatremia).
2. Specific therapies (see Table 8-5)

3. Seizure prophylaxis
   a. Carbamazepine, phenytoin, valproate
   b. Benzodiazepines or phenobarbital
4. Surgery: If the seizure focus is accessible and small, with minimal postoperative risks of persistent deficits

V. Neoplasms
  A. Primary
    1. Origin: Arise from cells within the central nervous system (CNS), usually as a single lesion.
    2. Most common: Medulloblastomas and astrocytomas in children; meningiomas in adults.
    3. Types and description (Tables 8-6 and 8-7).

Patients with neurofibromas are at increased risk of developing other types of cancers.

TABLE 8-6 Primary Benign Neoplasms of the Nervous System

Type	Description	Treatment
Meningioma	Slow-growing tumor of the dura.	Surgical removal if location is accessible
Pituitary adenoma	Local mass effect can cause bitemporal hemianopsia through compression of the optic chiasm. Can cause hormone excess or insufficiency, depending on whether tumor is functional.	Surgical removal through transsphenoidal approach
Schwannoma	Commonly found at cerebellopontine angle, arising from nerve sheath of vestibular nerve (the term *acoustic neuroma* is a misnomer).	Surgical removal, which may damage CN VII (facial nerve) and/or CN VIII (vestibulocochlear nerve)
Neurofibroma (NF)	Associated with formation of neural tumors (neurofibromas) that occur throughout peripheral nerves and subcutaneous tissue. Other features: numerous hyperpigmented areas (café-au-lait spots), nodules on iris (Lisch nodules), optic gliomas, vestibular schwannomas (acoustic neuromas), axillary freckling, and learning disabilities. Subtypes NF type 1: Due to mutation in neurofibromin on chromosome 17. NF type 2: Due to mutation on chromosome 22; in addition to typical signs of neurofibromatosis, these patients commonly have bilateral acoustic neuromas and may have meningiomas.	Surgery to remove neurofibromas for cosmetic reasons or if mass is in danger of compressing important structures

TABLE 8-7 Primary Malignant Neoplasms of the Nervous System

Type	Description	Treatment
Astrocytoma	Most progress slowly; exception is glioblastoma multiforme (grade IV astrocytoma). May cause paralysis of CN V (trigeminal nerve), VI (abducens nerve), VII (facial nerve), and X (vagus nerve).	High-grade astrocytomas: radiation therapy with or without chemotherapy
Ependymoma	Most often located in the posterior fossa (which may impinge on the fourth ventricle) in children or the filum terminale in adults.	Debulking surgery followed by radiation therapy
Medulloblastoma	Can lead to increased ICP owing to compression of fourth ventricle. Can lead to seeding of subarachnoid space with malignant cells.	Debulking surgery if tumor is accessible Combination therapy with irradiation and chemotherapy
Oligodendroglioma	Slow-growing tumor most commonly located in frontal lobe.	Removal of low-grade lesions Removal of high-grade lesions and chemotherapy
Lymphoma	More common in patients with AIDS. Can be metastatic.	Chemotherapy

ICP, intracranial pressure.

B. Metastases
1. Origin: Arise from the metastatic spread of tumors located elsewhere in the body.
2. Most common: Melanoma and lung, breast, kidney, and colon cancer.
3. Diagnostic features
   a. Metastatic tumors are typically found at the gray-white junction and can be multifocal.
   b. Focal deficits are dependent on the location of the mass (see Fig. 8-1 for symptoms of focal CNS damage).
   c. Spread of tumor cells throughout the CSF can lead to meningeal carcinomatosis (widespread seeding of the meninges and nerve roots), producing signs of neuropathy and elevated intracranial pressure.
4. Prognosis: Usually fatal within 18 months of presentation

C. Signs and Symptoms
1. Slowly developing focal deficits
   a. Motor or sensory deficits
   b. Seizures
2. Signs of increased intracranial pressure
   a. Headache

b. Papilledema
c. Oculomotor (CN III) palsy
3. Nerve compression caused by mass effects from the tumor.
4. Cognitive deficits

D. Treatment
1. Primary tumors: Specific therapies as described in Tables 8-6 and 8-7.
2. Metastases
a. Surgical removal with subsequent irradiation to treat a single accessible lesion.
b. Dexamethasone to decrease cerebral edema.
c. Chemotherapeutic agents often cannot cross the blood-brain barrier but can be used to treat a primary lesion elsewhere in the body.

VI. Trauma

A. Skull Fracture
1. Signs and symptoms
a. Rhinorrhea (due to leakage of CSF)
b. Cranial nerve damage (Table 8-8).
c. Focal deficits due to trauma and possible hemorrhage of underlying brain tissue
2. Evaluation
a. Radiograph may depict linear or depressed fractures.
b. CT scan will show any underlying hemorrhage or mass effects.
3. Treatment: Removal of irreversibly damaged tissue and mending of meningeal tears to prevent CSF leakage.

B. Brain Contusion
1. Bruising of the brain that occurs from contact between brain tissue and the skull during a traumatic head injury.
2. Classification: Depends on the surface with which the brain collides.
a. Coup: Occurs at the site of impact.
b. Contrecoup: Occurs on the side opposite to the site of impact.
3. Injury to the ventral aspect of the frontal lobes and the anterior temporal lobe can occur from contact with the rough surfaces of the calvaria of the skull.

C. Cerebral Edema
1. Cause: Can be a response to any type of brain injury, including traumatic.
2. Signs and symptoms
a. Increased intracranial pressure.
b. Cushing's reflex: Elevated systemic blood pressure with lowered pulse.
c. Brain ischemia due to restriction of cerebral blood flow by elevated intracranial pressure.
d. Herniation of the uncus of the temporal lobe can lead to compression of CN III (oculomotor nerve), causing an ipsilateral fixed and dilated pupil with the paralysis of all extraocular movements except abduction (controlled by CN VI, abducens nerve).

TABLE 8-8 Symptoms of Cranial Nerve Injury

Nerve	Signs and Symptoms	Comments
Olfactory (CN I)	Anosmia: absence or loss of sense of smell. Rhinorrhea may occur if head trauma causes shearing of olfactory nerves and subsequent CSF leak.	
Optic (CN II)	Relative afferent pupillary defect: swinging light test shows dilation of eyes when light is shined into one eye, owing to incomplete transmission of light information through damaged optic nerve. Visual field defects: can localize where a lesion has occurred in optic nerve or tract (see Figs. 8-4 and 8-5). Optic neuritis: sudden visual loss in one eye accompanied by pain; may be associated with multiple sclerosis.	
Oculomotor (CN III), trochlear (CN IV), and abducens (CN VI)	Diplopia due to paralysis of the extraocular muscles. Inability to abduct the eye (medial rectus muscle paralysis) can occur in CN III lesion. While the inability to adduct the eye (lateral rectus muscle paralysis) can occur in CN VI paralysis, superior oblique paralysis from trochlear nerve (CN IV) injury is not usually noticeable by the patient.	
Trigeminal (CN V)	Injury May cause loss of sensation from lower jaw (mandibular division), upper jaw (maxillary division), or forehead (ophthalmic division). Jaw deviation to side of injury due to paralysis of ipsilateral muscles of mastication; this does *not* occur with unilateral upper motor neuron lesions. Trigeminal neuralgia (tic douloureux) Episodic severe stabbing or "electric" pain in distribution of trigeminal nerve that may be triggered by touching target area. No weakness or numbness in facial nerve distribution.	Usually caused by compression of CN V by tortuous superior cerebellar artery near the pons. Treatment: carbamazepine, surgical repositioning of blood vessels near CN V or CN V branch destruction.

TABLE 8-8 Symptoms of Cranial Nerve Injury—cont'd

Nerve	Signs and Symptoms	Comments
Facial (CN VII)	Facial nerve palsy: paralysis of the muscles of facial expression, which may be associated with changes in auditory and gestatory function (see Fig. 8-6).	
	Bell's palsy: sudden onset of CN VII palsy with no associated trauma.	Caused by inflammation of CN VII and impingement within the petrous bone. Treatment: corticosteroids. Patients usually recover function.
Vestibulocochlear (CN VIII)	Sensorineural hearing loss: Rinne and Weber tests (placing vibrating tuning fork on mastoid process and top of head, respectively) show that bone conduction is no better than air conduction.	
	Nystagmus: eyes drift to one side and jerk rapidly toward other side; direction of nystagmus is named after fast component, which is usually contralateral to vestibular lesion.	Caused by damage to vestibular nerve or semicircular canals.
	Dizziness: general complaint that can be further narrowed to vertigo (conscious feeling of spinning), syncope (blacking out), unsteadiness, or lightheadedness (dizziness in the absence of cardiovascular problems).	Often associated with CN VIII lesions, inadequate CNS circulation, weakness, sensory deficits, anxiety, and side effects of medications.
	Benign paroxysmal positional vertigo: triggered by changes in head position when there is a blockage of the semicircular canals.	Evaluation: seated patient is asked to lie backward rapidly so that one ear is lower than the table; symptoms of nystagmus and vertigo should appear when affected side is lowered below table. Treatment: positional maneuvers that promote clearance of the clogging debris.
	Ménière's disease: Damage to membranous labyrinth causes periodic vertigo, tinnitus, and deafness. Vertigo disappears between episodes, but the deafness (low frequency) is progressive.	Treatment: anticholinergics (e.g., meclizine or scopolamine patch) and head and neck exercises to preserve reflexes; may also include low-salt diet and acetazolamide.

continued

TABLE 8-8 Symptoms of Cranial Nerve Injury—cont'd

Nerve	Signs and Symptoms	Comments
Glossopharyngeal (CN IX)	Dysphagia or choking, ipsilateral droop of the palate, decreased gag reflex, and deviation of uvula to unaffected side.	Usually associated with CN X lesion.
Vagus (CN X)		Usually occurs with CN IX injury. In addition to symptoms of CN IX injury, hoarseness may be present due to innervation of the larynx through the recurrent laryngeal nerve.
Accessory (CN XI)	Weakness of sternocleidomastoid and trapezius muscles.	
Hypoglossal (CN XII)	Upper motor neuron lesions do *not* show symptoms, because of bilateral cortical control of the tongue. Lower motor neuron lesions cause deviation of tongue to side of lesion when patient protrudes tongue; atrophy and fasciculations may also be present on ipsilateral tongue.	

e. Herniation of the medulla through the foramen magnum can cause compression of the medullary respiratory centers, resulting in ataxic breathing followed by respiratory arrest.

D. Subdural Hematoma (Figs. 8-3A and 8-3B)
1. Cause: Damage of the subdural bridging veins
2. Signs and symptoms
   a. Typical presentation: Focal deficit and altered mental status following a fall in an elderly person.
   b. May be slowly progressive.
2. Evaluation
   a. CT scan shows a localized collection of blood causing compression of nearby brain tissue.
   b. Bleeding pattern: Less convex and more diffuse than that occurring in epidural hematoma.
3. Treatment
   a. Acute hemorrhage can be drained through a burr hole in the skull.
   b. Chronic hemorrhage (with clots) can be removed surgically following a local craniotomy.

E. Epidural Hematoma (see Fig. 8-3C)
1. Most common: Laceration of the middle meningeal artery caused by a fracture of the temporal bone.

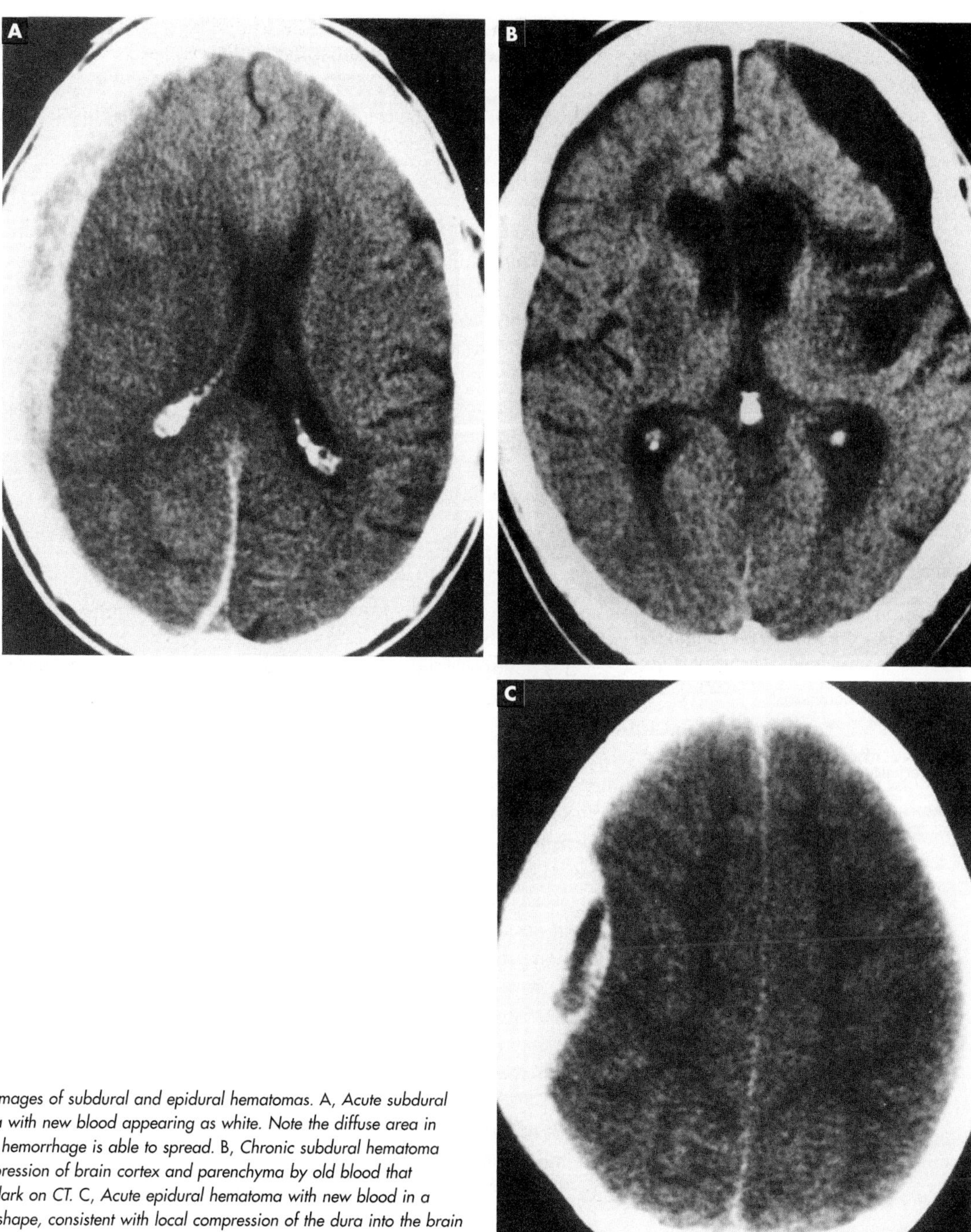

8-3: *CT images of subdural and epidural hematomas. A, Acute subdural hematoma with new blood appearing as white. Note the diffuse area in which the hemorrhage is able to spread. B, Chronic subdural hematoma with compression of brain cortex and parenchyma by old blood that appears dark on CT. C, Acute epidural hematoma with new blood in a biconvex shape, consistent with local compression of the dura into the brain parenchyma.*

2. Typical presentation: Traumatic injury followed by a lucid interval with subsequent rapid neurologic deterioration.
3. Evaluation
   a. CT scan can show skull fracture and significant diffuse bleeding with compression of the underlying brain tissue.
   b. Bleeding pattern: Convex in shape.
4. Treatment
   a. Management of intracranial pressure: Hyperventilation and diuretics; if that fails, induction of coma through barbiturate therapy.
   b. Craniectomy to allow decompression.

F. Spinal Cord Trauma
1. Signs and symptoms
   a. Spinal shock
      (1) Absence of upper motor neuron signs despite obvious damage to the spinal cord.
      (2) Can last for days to weeks after the initial injury.
   b. High cervical cord lesion (above C3)
      (1) Paralysis of the diaphragm.
      (2) Sympathetic lesion: bradycardia.
   c. Brown-Séquard lesion (spinal cord hemisection)
      (1) Ipsilateral side: Loss of position sense, vibration sense, and motor control.
      (2) Contralateral side: Loss of pain and temperature sensation.
   d. Intramedullary spinal cord lesions
      (1) Originate near the center of the spinal cord and extend outward.
      (2) Loss of pain and temperature sensation below the level of the lesion, with sparing in the sacral dermatomes.

Syringomyelia (cavitary lesion) is the most common type of intramedullary lesion.

2. Evaluation: CT or MRI scan
3. Treatment
   a. Stabilization of the spine.
   b. Within 8 hours of injury: Methylprednisolone to prevent edema.
   c. Surgical decompression if symptoms continue to worsen.
   d. Long-term physical therapy to promote recovery.

VII. Confusional States

A. Dementia
1. Cognitive impairment that is gradual in onset with a slowly progressive course.
2. Types of dementia
   a. Most common: Alzheimer's disease, vascular dementia (multi-infarct).
   b. Table 8-9 lists types of dementia and diagnostic features.
3. Evaluation
   a. Mini-mental status examination: Documents cognitive decline.
   b. Imaging can often show cortical atrophy or vascular etiologies of dementia.
   c. Blood studies and neuropsychiatric testing can be done to exclude other causes of dementia.

TABLE 8-9
Types of Dementia

Type	Description	Diagnostic Features
Alzheimer's disease	Age of onset: Usually >65 years; incidence increases dramatically with age. Familial types (10% of cases) may manifest before age 50 and may have accelerated disease course. Chronic progressive memory loss that can develop into poor judgment and personality changes (common as disease progresses). Incontinence, inability to care for self; may progress to terminal vegetative state.	Postmortem examination shows diffuse cortical atrophy. Presence of β-amyloid plaques and neurofibrillary tangles composed of tau protein found throughout brain, but especially in hippocampus, amygdala, and sensory association cortices.
Lewy body dementia	Clinically indistinguishable from Alzheimer's disease.	Presence throughout cortex of Lewy bodies made of α-synuclein.
Frontal lobe dementia	Personality changes occur before memory deficits. Apathy or disinhibition may also be present.	CT or MRI may show frontal lobe atrophy.
Pick's disease	Progressive dementia that may manifest as personality changes and/or progressive aphasia. Often symptomatically indistinguishable from other dementias.	Cortical atrophy of anterior temporal lobes and fibrillary inclusions in neurons of frontal and temporal lobes.
Subcortical dementia	Can be found in association with progressive supranuclear palsy, Parkinson's disease, Huntington's disease, or subcortical strokes. Slow thought processes, dysarthria, depression, and forgetfulness, combined with progressive dementia.	See text for discussion of specific diseases.
Vascular dementia	Multi-infarct dementia: due to destruction of brain by many small strokes, often with rapid onset, stepwise progression, and focal neurologic signs. Lacunar state: small subcortical infarcts, causing language difficulty and pseudobulbar palsy (slow dysarthric speech with emotional incontinence). Binswanger's disease: destruction of white matter due to multiple infarcts of deep penetrating vessels.	CT, MRI, and postmortem examination may show infarction and ischemia.

continued

TABLE 8-9 Types of Dementia—cont'd

Type	Description	Diagnostic Features
Prion disease	Rapidly progressive dementia that can include ataxia, myoclonus, and pyramidal and extrapyramidal motor dysfunction. Death usually occurs within 6 months of diagnosis, but some patients survive up to 2 years after diagnosis.	CSF test for protein kinase inhibitor 14-3-3 is an indicator of neuronal loss. Postmortem examination shows spongiform change and may show inclusion bodies.

d. Postmortem examination: Assesses pathologic changes, including atrophy, ischemia, and the presence of pathognomonic inclusions throughout the brain.

4. Treatment
   a. Acetylcholinesterase inhibitors (tacrine, donepezil, rivastigmine).
   b. Supportive care.
   c. Management of symptoms of depression and agitation.
   d. Myoclonus (seen in prion diseases) can be treated with benzodiazepines.

B. Delirium

1. Cognitive impairment that is reversible, rapid in onset, and fluctuating in course.
2. Conditions predisposing to delirium: Sensory deprivation, orthopedic surgery (predisposes to fat emboli), nondominant parietal strokes, increased levels of γ-aminobutyric acid (GABA).
3. Major mechanism: General decrease in acetylcholine and cerebral metabolism.
4. Major causes: Mnemonic—HIDE
   a. **H**ypoxia
   b. **I**nfection
   c. **D**rugs
   d. **E**lectrolyte disturbances
5. Drugs that can cause delirium: Mnemonic—4 BLT P
   a. **B**enadryl (diphenhydramine)
   b. **B**eta-blockers
   c. **B**arbiturates
   d. **B**enzodiazepines
   e. **L**ithium
   f. **T**ricyclic antidepressants
   g. **P**henytoin
6. Distinguishing feature: visual-spatial disturbances
7. Treatment
   a. Atypical psychotropics (risperidone).
   b. Haloperidol, droperidol, and benzodiazepines to combat agitation (Caution: the side effects of these drugs can also contribute to delirium).

Most patients with dementia can draw a clock, but those who are delirious cannot.

VIII. Movement Disorders

A. Coordinated Movement: Produced as a result of a balance between circuits that facilitate movement and those that inhibit movement. In patients with parkinsonism, the circuit facilitating movement is impaired, leading to an overwhelming inhibition of movement by the subthalamic nucleus and the globus pallidus.

B. Parkinson's Disease

1. Signs and symptoms

a. Typical presentation: Mnemonic—TRAP

(1) **T**remor (pill rolling at rest)

(2) **R**igidity (cogwheel)

(3) **A**kinesia

(4) **P**ostural changes (stooped posture, shuffling gait, wide-based turning, frequent falls)

b. Depression

c. Shy-Drager syndrome (autonomic dysfunction causing postural hypotension)

2. Evaluation

a. Rule out potentially treatable causes: Manganese poisoning, carbon monoxide poisoning, or excessive dopamine antagonist use (haloperidol).

b. Postmortem examination

(1) Gross examination shows pallor of the substantia nigra, locus ceruleus, and dorsal motor nucleus of the vagus.

(2) Microscopic examination shows Lewy body inclusions.

3. Treatment

a. Levodopa/carbidopa

(1) Levodopa is a dopamine precursor; carbidopa is a decarboxylase inhibitor that extends the half-life of levodopa.

(2) Provides symptomatic relief in Parkinson's disease but is *not* effective in treating other forms of parkinsonism (progressive supranuclear palsy, striatonigral degeneration, Shy-Drager syndrome).

(3) Serious side effects: Psychosis, chorea, and dystonia.

(4) Regimen becomes less effective over time as neurodegeneration progresses.

b. Amantadine: Can enhance dopamine release.

c. Dopamine agonists (bromocriptine, pergolide).

d. Monoamine oxidase B inhibitors (selegiline).

e. Surgery: Goal is to decrease the activity of the pathway inhibiting movement through ablation or electrical suppression of the globus pallidus or the subthalamic nucleus (sometimes called *deep brain stimulation*).

C. Progressive Supranuclear Palsy

1. Signs and symptoms

a. Bradykinesia, axial rigidity, dystonia, and dysarthria

b. Difficulty with vertical gaze

2. Degenerated regions contain neurofibrillary tangles, not Lewy bodies.

3. Unresponsive to levodopa therapy.

D. Spinal Muscular Atrophy (SMA): A type of multiple system atrophy
   1. Cause: Disease in the anterior horn cells of the spinal cord
   2. Types of SMA
      a. Werdnig-Hoffman: Infantile SMA
         (1) Fatal.
         (2) Lower motor neuron lesions in the spinal cord lead to flaccid paralysis.
      b. Kugelberg-Welander: Adolescent or adult SMA
   3. Signs and symptoms
      a. Atrophy, weakness, and fasciculation.
      b. Loss of reflexes.
      c. Symptoms of parkinsonism that are unresponsive to levodopa therapy.

E. Huntington's Disease
   1. Signs and symptoms
      a. Choreoathetosis: Irregular involuntary movements thought to be due to the loss of inhibitory (GABA) innervation to the lateral globus pallidus.
      b. Mood disorder: Depression, emotional lability, suicide. These can often be the presenting symptoms and are often misdiagnosed as schizophrenia.
      c. Dementia
      d. Family history (autosomal dominant) with onset between 35 and 40 years of age.
   2. Evaluation
      a. Positive result on blood testing for multiple trinucleotide repeats in the huntingtin gene on chromosome 4. Healthy individuals have fewer than 32 repeats; symptomatic patients typically have more than 40 repeats.
      b. CT or MRI scans show selective atrophy of the caudate nucleus.
   3. Treatment
      a. Dopamine antagonist drugs (haloperidol or thioridazine) to decrease choreoathetosis and counteract some of the mood problems.
      b. Buspirone for anxiety.
      c. Nortriptyline or fluoxetine for depression.
      d. Carbamazepine or valproate for bipolar symptoms.

F. Hemiballismus
   1. Wild flailing of an arm due to a stroke in the subthalamic nucleus
   2. Treatment: High doses of haloperidol

IX. Other Neurodegenerative Disorders

A. Amyotrophic Lateral Sclerosis (ALS): Lou Gehrig disease
   1. Signs and symptoms
      a. Weakness and atrophy of a limb that progressively spreads to other areas of the body.
      b. Both upper and lower motor neuron signs are present due to the concomitant injury to both the anterior horn and the corticospinal and corticobulbar tracts.
      c. All muscle groups can be impaired *except* the extraocular muscles and those controlling the bladder.
      d. Sensation is intact.

Difficulty swallowing is a common early symptom of ALS.

2. Evaluation
   a. Rule out autoimmunity or mercury poisoning as a potential cause.
   b. EMG and muscle biopsy show motor denervation and reinnervation.
   c. Use imaging to exclude spinal cord injury.
   d. Postmortem examination shows degeneration of the corticospinal, corticobulbar, and anterior horn cells.
3. Treatment
   a. Riluzole (glutamate antagonist) can decrease excitotoxic damage and prolong life by several months.
   b. Symptomatic therapies
      (1) Baclofen or diazepam for severe spasticity
      (2) Quinine for severe muscle cramps

B. Multiple sclerosis (MS)
1. Signs and symptoms
   a. Pattern of multiple neurologic lesions that are disseminated in time and space; most often diagnosed in women during early adulthood.
   b. Most common symptoms on presentation: Optic neuritis and sensory or motor deficits in the lower limbs.
   c. Other common symptoms: Trigeminal neuralgia and internuclear ophthalmoplegia (see Table 8-8).
2. Evaluation
   a. MRI scan can show multiple white matter lesions that may be due to active demyelination or chronic myelin loss.
   b. Visual evoked potentials assess afferent conduction in the optic nerve and tract.
   c. Somatosensory evoked potentials assess afferent conduction of the sensory systems.
   d. CSF analysis: oligoclonal IgG bands are found in 90% of patients with MS.
3. Disease progression: Can correspond to one of several patterns, but most patients have a relapsing remitting course.
4. Treatment
   a. Interferons
   b. Copolymer (glatiramer acetate)
   c. Intravenous corticosteroids for severe exacerbations
   d. Physical therapy and symptomatic relief

X. Cranial Nerve Dysfunction and Special Senses
   A. Symptoms of Cranial Nerve Injury (see Table 8-8)
   B. Lesions Affecting Visual Fields and Conjugate Gaze Pathways (Figs. 8-4 and 8-5)
   C. Lesions Affecting Facial Nerve, CN VII (Fig. 8-6)

XI. Cerebellar Syndromes
   A. Signs and Symptoms
   1. Kinetic tremor: Present only during movement; actions such as eating or drinking may be impossible.

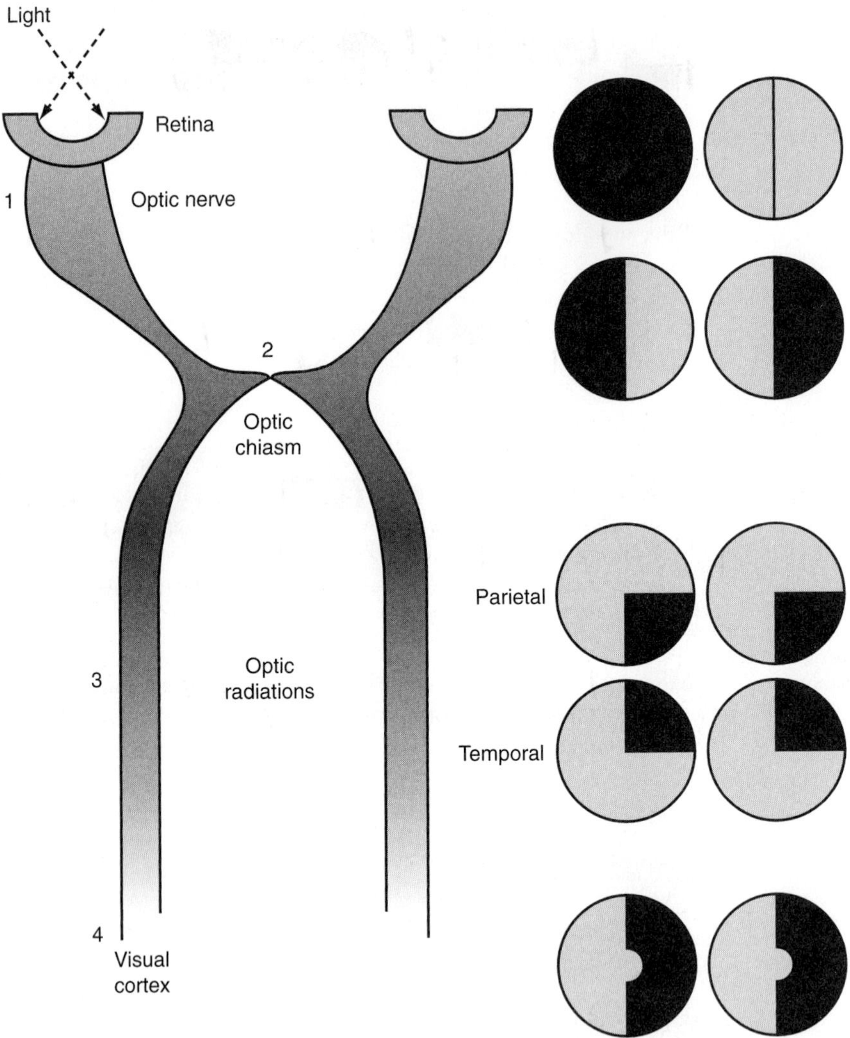

8-4: *Visual field defects arising from lesions of the optic pathways. There are several key locations at which unique visual field deficits can arise. Lesions at site 1, which could involve damage to either the retina or the optic nerve distal to the optic chiasm, can result in monocular blindness. Lesions at site 2, which typically involve compression of the optic chiasm by pituitary tumors, can result in bitemporal hemianopsia. Lesions at site 3, which involve damage to the optic radiations in either the parietal or temporal lobes, result in inferior or superior homonymous quadrantanopsia, respectively. Lesions at site 4, which involve damage to the primary visual cortex, result in a contralateral homonymous hemianopsia with macular sparing. When predicting these patterns, do not forget to take into account the pathway that the light takes into the eye.*

2. Dysmetria: Inaccuracy in finger-to-nose or heel-to-shin maneuvers.
3. Decomposition of movement: Nonfluent movements that are normally smooth.
4. Dysdiadochocinesia: Difficulty performing rapid alternating movements with the hands.

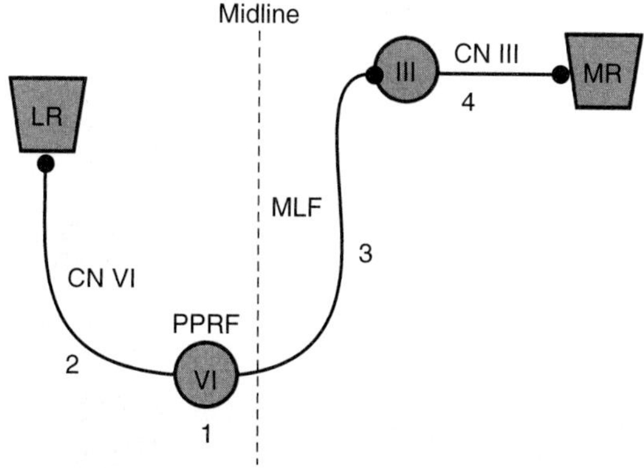

8-5: *Simplified schematic of the conjugate gaze pathways. Questions involving conjugate gaze dysfunction can be isolated to four basic types of lesion. Lesions at site 1 will involve the abducens nucleus and the paramedian pontine reticular formation (PPRF). These lesions result in conjugate gaze paralysis that manifests as the inability to voluntarily move either eye to the side of the lesion. In addition, ipsilateral facial paralysis may be found due to the course of the facial nerve through this region as it exits the brainstem. Lesions at site 2 (abducens nerve itself) result in an inability to look laterally with no dysfunction of the contralateral medial rectus. Lesions at site 3 (medial longitudinal fasciculus; MLF) cause internuclear ophthalmoplegia, which results in an interruption of conduction between the PPRF and the oculomotor nucleus. These patients have intact gaze laterally without any ability to conjugately move the other eye medially. Intact oculomotor function, however, is evidenced by the lack of other extraocular muscle paralyses, as well as intact pupillary constriction reflexes. Lesions at site 4 (oculomotor nucleus or nerve) result in the impairment of all of the muscles innervated by the oculomotor nerve, as well as the inability for that eye to pupilloconstrict directly or consensually. LR, lateral rectus muscle; MR, medial rectus muscle.*

B. Friedreich's Ataxia: Autosomal recessive inheritance
   1. Onset: Between 8 and 15 years of age.
   2. Produces lesions of the following tracts
      a. Spinocerebellar: Dysmetria, ataxia, and dysarthria
      b. Corticospinal: Weakness, upper motor neuron signs
      c. Posterior column lesions: Loss of proprioception and vibration
   3. Patients also have skeletal deformities (scoliosis) and cardiac problems (hypertrophy and arrhythmia).
   4. Confirmable through a blood test used to detect excessive trinucleotide repeats on chromosome 9.

XII. Peripheral Neuropathies
   A. Methods of Classification
      1. Axonal versus demyelinating
         a. Axonal damage
            (1) Produces decreased amplitude of the conducted impulse.
            (2) Conduction velocities are normal.
         b. Demyelination
            (1) Produces slowing of conduction but may *not* decrease the amplitude of the impulse.
            (2) Block of conduction may occur if large areas are demyelinated or if secondary axonal damage occurs as a result of the demyelinating process.

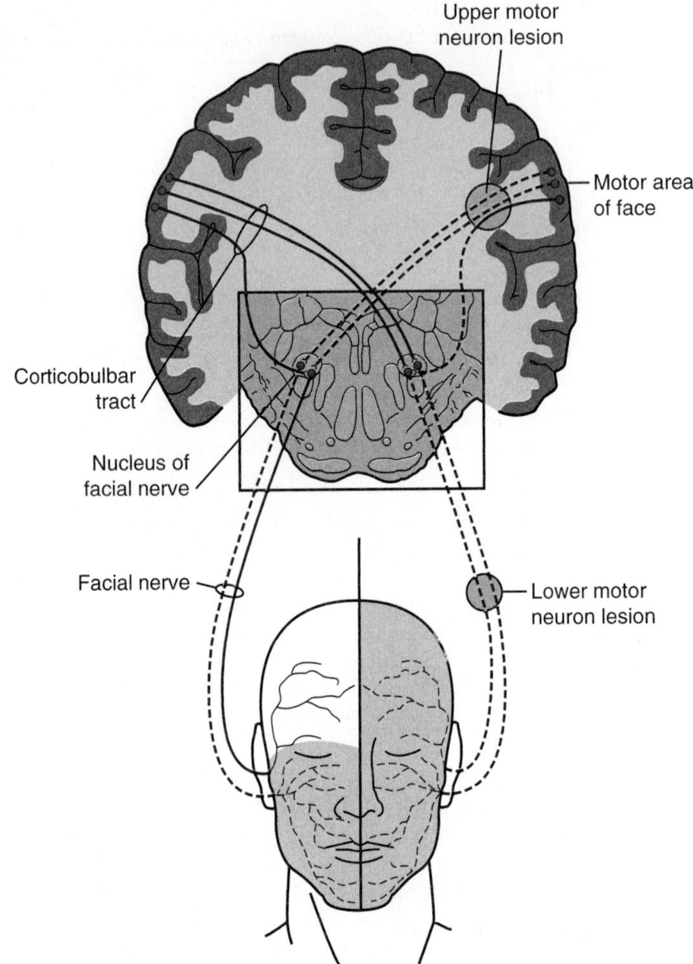

8-6: *Lesions associated with facial weakness. The muscles of facial expression are innervated by the facial nerve, which is, in turn, controlled by the motor cortices. Neurons of the motor cortex project bilaterally to the facial nuclei in the pons, providing innervation to the entire contralateral face and partial innervation to the ipsilateral forehead through the corticobulbar tract. Because of the bilateral innervation of the forehead, lesions of the corticobulbar tract cause paralysis only of the contralateral lower face. In contrast, lesions of the facial nucleus or of the facial nerve itself cause paralysis of the entire ipsilateral face. If a facial nerve lesion is located proximal to the stylomastoid foramen, then taste sensation to the anterior two thirds of the tongue (chorda tympani) and/or hyperacusis (branch to the stapedius) may also be impaired due to damage to fibers traveling with the facial nerve.*

2. Sensory versus motor
   a. Sensory polyneuropathy
      (1) Paresthesias: Tingling sensation.
      (2) Dysesthesias: Pain in response to stimuli that are normally non-noxious.
      (3) Reflexes may be impaired as a result of loss of the afferent limb.

b. Motor neuropathy
(1) Weakness: Distal muscle groups are usually affected before proximal muscle groups.
(2) Reflexes may be impaired as a result of loss of the efferent limb of the pathway.
(3) Atrophy and fasciculations of the target muscles.
3. Distribution
a. Mononeuropathy: Dysfunction of a single nerve due to compression or trauma.
b. Polyneuropathy: Loss of sensory function in several peripheral nerves simultaneously.
(1) Stocking-and-glove pattern polyneuropathy typically involves loss of sensation in the most distal portions of the hands and feet.
(2) This pattern is a common early symptom in diseases caused by circulating neurotoxic factors (autoantibodies or toxins) such as Guillain-Barré syndrome, because the longest peripheral nerves (those extending to the distal extremities) are most likely to encounter a circulating toxic factor.

B. Exogenous Causes
1. Drugs (vincristine, cisplatin, nitrofurantoin)
2. Metals (arsenic, lead, thallium)
3. Organic compounds (hexane, acrylamide, organophosphates)

C. Evaluation
1. Electrophysiology
a. EMG and/or compound muscle action potential (CMAP) recordings can assess the distribution and severity of neuropathy.
b. Nerve biopsy studies may be useful when more definitive diagnoses are needed.
2. Diagnostic studies
a. Complete blood count.
b. Serum protein electrophoresis (SPEP) to detect serum monoclonal antibodies (in paraproteinemic neuropathy).
c. Screening for metabolic causes, including blood glucose, antibody, electrolyte, and liver function tests, and erythrocyte sedimentation rate.
3. Lumbar puncture may indicate infectious etiologies (syphilis, Lyme disease, cytomegalovirus).

D. Types of Peripheral Neuropathy
1. Radiculopathies
a. Causes: Typically occur due to compression of the nerves as they exit the vertebral column.
b. Signs and symptoms: Cervical and lumbar root syndromes (Table 8-10).
c. Evaluation: MRI scans may show nerve compression but should be reserved for use in patients with possible spinal cord compression or permanent neurologic damage.
d. Treatment

TABLE 8-10 Cervical and Lumbar Radiculopathies

Root	Signs and Symptoms
C3, C4	Sensory impairment in shoulder Weakness of diaphragm
C5	Sensory impairment in deltoid area Weakness of deltoid and biceps Impaired biceps reflex
C6	Sensory impairment of thumb Weakness of biceps and brachioradialis Impaired biceps reflex
C7	Sensory impairment of second, third, and fourth digits Weakness of triceps and fingers Impaired triceps reflex
C8	Sensory impairment of fifth digit Weakness of hand Impaired triceps reflex
L3	Sensory impairment of lateral thigh Weakness of quadriceps Impaired patellar reflex
L4	Sensory impairment of medial leg Weakness of quadriceps and anterior tibial muscles Impaired patellar reflex
L5	Sensory impairment of anterior lower leg and great toe Weakness of toe extensors
S1	Sensory impairment of posterior leg and little toe Weakness on eversion of foot Impaired ankle reflex

(1) Trial of anti-inflammatory therapy for nonemergent cases.
(2) Imaging and surgical decompression for patients whose dysfunction is refractory to medical therapy and in whom the compression can be corrected.

2. Autonomic neuropathies
    a. Horner's syndrome
        (1) Most often due to a lesion in the superior cervical ganglion
        (2) Presents with a triad of ptosis, miosis, and facial anhidrosis
    b. Orthostatic hypotension
    c. Urinary incontinence: Due to parasympathetic sacral nerve damage
    d. Male impotence
        (1) Can occur due to autonomic damage; manifests as loss of an ability to have erections with no loss in libido.
        (2) Testosterone or local injection of vasoactive drugs (papaverine, prostaglandin E_1) may be helpful.
3. Entrapment syndromes (Table 8-11).

TABLE 8-11 Nerve Entrapment Syndromes

Type	Cause	Signs and Symptoms	Treatment
Carpal tunnel syndrome	Median nerve compression at wrist Associated with late pregnancy, diabetes mellitus	Pain and tingling at night in hand, radiating to forearm. Tinel's sign: tingling in first and second digits is produced by percussing carpal tunnel. Phalen's sign: tingling in the hand when both hands are hypoflexed against each other.	Wrist splints, anti-inflammatory drugs, surgery
Ulnar nerve entrapment	Fracture, repeated trauma, or arthritis	Numbness, weakness, and eventually clawlike deformity of fourth and fifth digits.	Behavioral modification, rest, surgery
Meralgia paresthetica	Entrapment of lateral cutaneous nerve of thigh by the inguinal ligament	Burning sensation over anterolateral part of thigh. Symptoms become worse with standing but improve with walking.	Weight loss and avoidance of constrictive clothing
Peroneal palsy	Entrapment of peroneal nerve between the fibula and peroneus longus muscle	Footdrop and weakness of eversion of foot and extension of great toe.	Allow nerve to recover while correcting footdrop with supports

4. Diabetic neuropathy
   a. Polyneuropathy: Loss of sensation in the feet, burning dysesthesias, and weakness of the foot on dorsiflexion.
   b. Mononeuritis multiplex: Multiple isolated lesions of single nerves producing cranial nerve abnormalities or asymmetric neurologic deficits.
5. Hereditary neuropathies
   a. Charcot-Marie-Tooth disease
      (1) Group of disorders involving defects of Schwann cell myelin proteins
      (2) Signs and symptoms
         (a) Gradual wasting of the foot and calf muscles, with formation of a clubfoot and high arches.
         (b) Disability may not manifest until adulthood.
      (3) Evaluation: DNA tests can provide more specific diagnosis.
   b. Familial amyloid polyneuropathy
      (1) Sensory and autonomic neuropathy producing loss of temperature sensation in the feet, orthostatic hypotension, and incontinence.

(2) Nerve biopsy specimens show amyloid deposits.

(3) Some forms are due to transthyretin deficiency. These patients may benefit from liver transplantation.

6. Immune-mediated neuropathy: Often occur due to an autoimmune attack on peripheral nerve myelin antigens (Table 8-12).

7. HIV neuropathy

a. Usually presents as a slowly progressive, distal, symmetric sensory neuropathy with pain.

TABLE 8-12 Autoimmune Peripheral Neuropathies

Type	Signs and Symptoms	Evaluation	Treatment
Acute inflammatory demyelinating polyneuropathy (Guillain-Barré syndrome)	Weakness ascending from legs to upper limbs and muscles of respiration that gradually worsens over days or weeks. Often associated with antecedent viral illness, immunization, or diarrhea due to *Campylobacter jejuni* infection that preceded symptoms by ~4 weeks. Symptoms usually peak ~4 weeks after onset.	EMG: demyelination of multiple nerves CSF analysis: ↑ protein	Severe disease may necessitate use of respirator and ICU treatment. Plasmapheresis: beneficial in patients with antibody-mediated disease. IVIg: beneficial if treatment is started early in disease course.
Chronic inflammatory demyelinating polyneuropathy (CIDP)	Polyneuropathy in adults >40 years of age with both weakness and painless sensory deficits.	EMG: conduction slowing	Long-term treatment with corticosteroids, IVIg, or plasmapheresis.
Multifocal motor neuropathy	Progressive, symmetric weakness of distal muscles with areflexia. Sensation is spared.	EMG: conduction block of motor nerves	Short term: IVIg. Long term: cyclophosphamide.
Paraproteinemic neuropathies	Polyneuropathy associated with monoclonal gammopathy; usually multiple myeloma or monoclonal gammopathy of undetermined significance (MGUS). IgM autoantibodies that bind myelin-associated glycoprotein in patients, with destruction of nerves caused by monoclonal autoantibodies against neural antigens.	EMG: consistent with polyneuropathy Serum protein electrophoresis (SPEP): to detect monoclonal antibodies in patient's serum	Plasmapheresis and/or IVIg.

CSF, cerebrospinal fluid; EMG, electromyogram; ICU, intensive care unit; IVIg, intravenous immunoglobulin.

b. EMG shows axonal degeneration.
c. Other causes of neuropathy in HIV-infected patients include
(1) Nucleoside analog antiretroviral therapy (didanosine, zalcitabine, and stavudine): Manifests with similar symptoms (sensory neuropathy with pain), but course is more acute. Stopping the offending agent eventually leads to improvement.
(2) Cytomegalovirus infection: Rapid, painful paraparesis of the lumbosacral plexus. Treatment consists of intravenous ganciclovir.
(3) Syphilis: Degeneration of the dorsal column tracts in tertiary syphilis causes loss of vibration and proprioception. The classic presentation is a patient with intact pinprick sensation who walks with a slapping gait.
(4) Herpes zoster reactivation: Patients have with burning pain in the distribution of a single dermatome.
d. Treatment (highly variable, depending on the cause): Nonsteroidal anti-inflammatory drugs (NSAIDs), topical capsaicin, or corticosteroids.

XIII. Myopathies and Muscular Dystrophy
A. Myopathy versus Neuropathy
1. Myopathies typically have proximal muscle weakness as a presenting sign. Most neuropathies show distal weakness at presentation.
2. Reflexes are intact in most myopathies, but they are impaired in neuropathies.
3. Creatine kinase is elevated in most myopathies, but is usually normal in neuropathies.
B. Duchenne Muscular Dystrophy
1. Cause: Deficiency of dystrophin (<5% of normal) related to a structural problem on the X chromosome.
2. Signs and symptoms
a. Pseudohypertrophy of the calves with proximal weakness.
b. Lumbar lordosis with a waddling gait.
c. Cardiac involvement.
d. Gower maneuver: Proximal muscle weakness prevents patients from rising from a chair in the usual manner. To rise from a seated position, these patients must push the arms against the thighs and progressively "climb" to a standing position.
3. Evaluation
a. Can be detected at birth due to elevated level of creatine phosphokinase (CPK) in muscle.
b. EMG shows characteristic myopathic changes.
c. Western blot technique shows deficiency of dystrophin and can distinguish between Duchenne and Becker types.
d. Muscle biopsy specimen shows degenerative changes and an increase in fat and connective tissue (the cause of the pseudohypertrophy).
4. Prognosis
a. Patients lose the ability to walk between the ages of 9 and 12 years.
b. Often fatal by age 30 duc to respiratory muscle weakness.

5. Treatment
   a. Physical therapy to minimize contractures.
   b. Splints and braces, which can extend the ability to walk for months to years.
   c. Surgery to correct scoliosis.

C. Becker Muscular Dystrophy
   1. Dystrophin deficiency is less severe (10% to 30% of normal) than in Duchenne muscular dystrophy.
   2. Clinical course is less severe. Patients retain the ability to walk much longer and have a greater overall life span than those with Duchenne muscular dystrophy.

D. Myotonic Dystrophy
   1. Due to an autosomal dominant abnormality on chromosome 19.
   2. Signs and symptoms
      a. "Hatchet face" due to wasting of the facial muscles, with marked ptosis.
      b. Distal weakness of the hands and feet.
      c. Myotonia: Inability to relax the muscles after contraction.
      d. Can also be associated with cataracts, frontal baldness, testicular atrophy, low IQ, and cardiac arrhythmias.
   3. Treatment
      a. Splints for extremity weakness
      b. Phenytoin for myotonia
      c. Pacemaker, if necessary, for cardiac conduction problems
      d. Surgery if cataracts develop

E. Mitochondrial Myopathies: Accumulations of abnormal mitochondria typically give the muscle fibers a "ragged red fiber" appearance in muscle biopsy specimens.
   1. Kearns-Sayre syndrome
      a. Progressive external ophthalmoplegia, pigmentary retinal degeneration, heart block, ataxia, and elevated CSF protein levels.
      b. May also be associated with hearing loss, diabetes, and hyperparathyroidism.
      c. Patients usually die of cardiac arrest before age 40.
   2. MELAS (**m**itochondrial **e**ncephalopathy, **l**actic acidosis, and **s**troke-like episodes)
      a. Manifests in childhood with migraine-like headaches.
      b. Lactic acidosis can occur at rest.
      c. Stroke-like episodes, most often in the parietal or occipital cortices.
   3. MERRF (**m**yoclonic **e**pilepsy with **r**agged **r**ed **f**ibers): Patients have myoclonus, myopathy, cerebellar ataxia, optic atrophy, hearing loss, and dementia.

F. Inflammatory Myopathies
   1. Polymyositis and dermatomyositis
      a. Signs and symptoms
         (1) Polymyositis: Proximal muscle inflammation and weakness; can include head droop and/or difficulty swallowing.

(2) Dermatomyositis: Polymyositis with skin involvement (erythematous rash on sun-exposed areas)
(a) Butterfly (red) and heliotrope (purple) rashes on the face and eyelids
(b) Scaling and cracking of the skin on the hands
(c) Vasculitis and Raynaud's phenomenon

b. Evaluation
(1) Elevated levels of CPK, lactate dehydrogenase, and aspartate aminotransferase (AST).
(2) Presence of anti-Jo, anti-Mi, and antinuclear antibodies.
(3) EMG and muscle biopsy: Abnormal findings document muscle involvement.

c. Treatment: High-dose corticosteroids and cytotoxic therapy (azathioprine, cyclophosphamide, methotrexate).

2. Inclusion body myositis
a. Causes progressive muscle weakness in patients greater than 50 years of age.
b. Muscle biopsy specimen shows characteristic vacuoles containing membranous material.
c. Corticosteroids are *not* useful.

3. Corticosteroid myopathy
a. Long-term treatment with high-dose corticosteroids causes proximal muscle weakness.
b. Muscle biopsy specimen shows atrophy of type II muscle fibers.
c. CPK level usually is normal. This measurement can help differentiate corticosteroid myopathy from an exacerbation of the underlying inflammatory myopathy (in which CPK level is usually elevated).

Myopathy: normal CPK = corticosteroid induced; elevated CPK = inflammatory.

G. Disorders of the Neuromuscular Junction

1. Myasthenia gravis: Autoimmune disorder in which autoantibodies attack the acetylcholine receptors (AChR) in the neuromuscular junction.

a. Signs and symptoms
(1) Typically starts as ptosis and weakness of the extraocular muscles, followed by general weakness throughout the body
(a) Extraocular paralysis may be intermittent and will not correspond to any specific brainstem syndrome.
(b) Pupils are not affected.
(c) Limb weakness is more marked proximally than distally.
(2) Sensation and reflexes are preserved.
(3) Myasthenic crisis: Concurrent infection may cause dramatic worsening of the patient's weakness and can cause respiratory failure.
(4) May be associated with thymomas.

b. Evaluation
(1) Tensilon test: Tensilon (edrophonium chloride) is an acetylcholinesterase inhibitor that increases the amount of acetylcholine in the neuromuscular junction by preventing its degradation. Intravenous administration of edrophonium

Cholinergic crisis causes severe weakness and respiratory failure that can be difficult to distinguish from myasthenic crisis.

chloride decreases symptoms of weakness in patients with myasthenia gravis.
(2) EMG shows impaired neuromuscular transmission.
(3) Supramaximal repetitive stimulation shows initially normal neuromuscular responses that decrease with successive stimuli.
(4) Elevated levels of serum antibodies against AChR.

c. Treatment
(1) Anticholinesterase drugs (pyridostigmine, neostigmine) decrease the patient's symptoms of weakness, but high doses of these drugs can result in cholinergic crises.
(2) Thymectomy
(3) Immunosuppressant drugs (prednisone, azathioprine)
(4) Plasmapheresis or intravenous immunoglobulin

2. Lambert-Eaton myasthenic syndrome
a. Autoimmune disorder in which presynaptic calcium channels are destroyed, thus impairing acetylcholine release.
b. Often related to an underlying cancer (small cell lung carcinoma is the most frequent association). The cancer cells are thought to express antigens similar to the presynaptic calcium channels.
c. Signs and symptoms: Proximal limb weakness and autonomic symptoms.
d. Evaluation: EMG
(1) Circulating anti–calcium channel antibodies may be present.
(2) Supramaximal stimulation does not show a decrease in response with successive stimuli. The calcium blockade is overcome by tetanic stimulation, and the response may improve.
e. Treatment
(1) Treat the cancer, if present.
(2) Enhancement of acetylcholine release
(a) Anticholinesterase medications
(b) Guanidine; 3,4-diaminopyridine
(c) Immunosuppression
(d) Plasmapheresis

XIV. Sleep Disorders

A. Insomnia
1. Inadequate quality and quantity of sleep.
2. Common causes: Pain, poor sleep habits, alcohol or substance use, jet lag.

B. Obstructive Sleep Apnea
1. Intermittent upper airway obstruction that causes snoring and apneic episodes throughout the night.
2. Patients experience decreased rapid eye movement (REM) sleep and wake up tired.
3. Evaluation: Overnight sleep study using polysomnography.
4. Treatment: Continuous positive airway pressure mask, weight reduction in obese persons, surgery.

C. Narcolepsy
1. Signs and symptoms
a. Inappropriate sleep attacks.
b. Cataplexy: Episodic loss of muscle tone caused by emotional stimuli.
c. Hypnagogic hallucinations with the onset of sleep.
d. Transient paralysis while waking from sleep.
e. Family history of narcolepsy.
2. Evaluation: Sleep latency tests using polysomnography show early onset of REM sleep.
3. Treatment
a. Planned sleep
b. Stimulants (methylphenidate) to prevent narcoleptic attacks
c. Tricyclic antidepressants (clomipramine) to relieve cataplexy

XV. Coma and Brain Death
A. Coma
1. Signs and symptoms
a. Unarousable, unresponsive state.
b. Presence of brainstem reflexes but no demonstrable cortical function.
c. Long-term coma may develop into a persistent vegetative state, characterized by return of pain responsiveness and eye movements without any meaningful return in cortical function.
d. Abnormal breathing patterns
(1) Cheyne-Stokes respirations: Crescendo-decrescendo hyperpnea followed by apnea. This pattern may be caused by metabolic encephalopathy or bilateral cortical structural lesions.
(2) Hyperventilation: May result from a lesion of the low midbrain or upper pons. The coma in this case may be due to the disruption of the reticular formation.
(3) Ataxic respiration: Completely irregular. Caused by injury in the medulla or compression of the medulla from elevated intracranial pressure. Patients are in danger of respiratory arrest due to injury of the medullary respiratory centers.
e. Pupillary findings
(1) Large, fixed pupils: Midbrain lesion involving the parasympathetic fibers.
(2) Small, fixed pupils: Pontine lesion involving the sympathetic fibers; can also be a side effect of cholinergic eyedrops used to treat glaucoma.
(3) Single enlarged pupil
(a) Compression of CN III due to uncal herniation; increased intracranial pressure.
(b) Immediate action is required to prevent respiratory arrest from medullary compression.
f. Eye movements in coma
(1) Oculocephalic (doll's eyes) reflex: Turning the patient's head causes the eyes to move in the opposite direction in a comatose patient with intact brainstem function.

Cervical spine stability must be assessed before testing eye movements in a comatose patient.

(2) Oculovestibular (cold caloric) reflex: Irrigation of the ear with cold water ipsilaterally inhibits the vestibular input, causing the eyes to move toward the irrigated ear in a comatose patient with intact brainstem function. Demonstrate ear canal patency and ensure that the tympanic membrane is intact before testing this reflex.

g. Posturing
   (1) Decorticate posturing: Flexion of the upper arms and extension of the lower limbs due to a cortical or hemispheric lesion.
   (2) Decerebrate posturing: Extension of upper and lower limbs due to a lesion below the red nucleus in the midbrain.

2. Evaluation: To determine the cause of the coma, if possible.
   a. Blood studies to assess for electrolyte or toxic dysfunction.
   b. Blood and CSF cultures to identify infection.
   c. CT or MRI scan to assess for mass lesions or strokes.
3. Treatment: Directed at the underlying cause, if possible.
   a. Dialysis, replenishment, or antidote for electrolyte or toxic causes.
   b. Diuresis or shunt for brain edema.
   c. Surgery, if indicated.

B. Brain Death: Medical requirements
   1. Known cause for the patient's symptoms that has been adequately treated without improvement.
   2. Absence of drug intoxication, shock, or hypothermia.
   3. Absence of brainstem and cerebral activity for more than 6 hours.
      a. Absent bedside reflexes for brainstem function.
      b. No responsiveness to pain or spontaneous respirations.
      c. Absence of activity on electroencephalogram or on cerebral blood flow scans.

"You're not dead until you're warm and dead."

XVI. Neurotoxicology
A. Tetanus: Produced by *Clostridium tetani*
   1. Toxin prevents release of an inhibitory neurotransmitter (GABA) onto motor neurons. This leads to the disinhibition of these motor neurons and causes a spastic paralysis.
   2. History of soil-contaminated wounds or use of dirty needles.
   3. Signs and symptoms
      a. Painful muscle spasms of the jaw (trismus), back (opisthotonus), and face (risus sardonicus)
      b. Seizures
   4. Treatment
      a. Supportive care in an intensive care unit
      b. Sedation with neuromuscular blockade
      c. Antibiotics
      d. Human tetanus immunoglobulin
B. Botulism: Produced by *Clostridium botulinum*
   1. Toxin prevents the release of acetylcholine at the neuromuscular junction and autonomic nerve terminals and causes a flaccid paralysis.

2. History of ingestion of improperly canned or stored food or wound infections. Also may occur in infants who are fed contaminated honey.
3. Signs and symptoms
    a. Early symptoms: Ocular weakness (ptosis, diplopia)
    b. Progression to generalized weakness of the face, limbs, and respiratory muscles
4. Treatment
    a. Equine antitoxin (20% risk of allergic reaction)
    b. Supportive care in an intensive care unit
    c. Guanidine: Facilitates release of acetylcholine

C. Carbon Monoxide Poisoning
1. History of exposure to poorly ventilated areas or malfunctioning heaters, stoves, or car exhaust
2. Signs and symptoms
    a. Early: Headache and nausea, with cherry-red discoloration of the skin and any blood that is drawn.
    b. Late: Coma, seizures, and death
3. Treatment: 100% oxygen. Survivors may develop cognitive deficits or parkinsonism due to CNS ischemia.

D. Alcohol Toxicity
1. Signs and symptoms of chronic alcohol use
    a. Peripheral neuropathy
    b. Traumatic lesions
    c. Wernicke's encephalopathy: Nystagmus, ataxia, confusion, and ophthalmoplegia
        (1) Caused by thiamine deficiency
        (2) Reversible with thiamine administration
    d. Korsakoff's psychosis: Amnesia and confabulation due to the destruction of the mammillary bodies and fornix.
2. Signs and symptoms of alcohol withdrawal
    a. Anxiety, tachycardia, diaphoresis
    b. Hallucinations and confusion
    c. Seizures: May occur up to 5 days after discontinuation of alcohol
    d. Delirium tremens (DTs)
        (1) Severe seizures associated with hyperthermia and hallucinations
        (2) Can be fatal
3. Treatment of alcohol withdrawal involves a tapering regimen of benzodiazepine therapy (usually chlordiazepoxide) to prevent seizures and minimize withdrawal symptoms (see Chapter 12).

XVII. Infections of the Nervous System

A. Meningitis
1. Cause: Viral or bacterial
2. Signs and symptoms
    a. Fever, headache, and malaise
    b. Confusion or drowsiness

c. Nuchal rigidity
d. Signs of meningeal irritation
(1) Kernig's sign: Patient or examiner cannot fully extend the patient's knee when the hip is flexed to 90 degrees.
(2) Brudzinski's sign: Flexion of the hips and knees occurs when the neck is flexed.
3. Evaluation: CSF analysis
a. Low glucose level and high WBC count (>500 mg/dL, predominantly neutrophils) indicates a bacterial cause.
b. Normal glucose level and normal WBC count (<500 mg/dL) indicates a viral cause.
c. Low glucose level and low WBC count (<500 mg/dL) indicates tuberculosis, fungi, or syphilis as cause.
4. Treatment
a. Viral meningitis usually is nonfatal and resolves spontaneously without treatment.
b. Bacterial meningitis is a serious infection. When suspected, empiric antibiotic treatment is started even before lumbar puncture is performed (Table 8-13).

B. Encephalitis
1. Cause: Usually viral; history may include a recent insect, tick, or animal bite
2. Signs and symptoms
a. May manifest as fevers, headaches, impaired consciousness, confusion.
b. Presence of seizures and/or focal deficits distinguishes encephalitis from meningitis.
3. Types
a. Herpes encephalitis
(1) Associated with herpes simplex virus 1 (oral herpes) infection.
(2) Can cause aphasia, memory impairment, and behavioral changes due to damage to the frontal and temporal lobes.

TABLE 8-13 Causes and Treatments of Bacterial Meningitis

Patient Characteristics	Causative Organism	Treatment
Neonate (<1 month old)	Group B streptococcus, *Escherichia coli*	Ceftriaxone with ampicillin
Children (<15 years old)	Meningococcus, *Streptococcus pneumoniae*	Ceftriaxone with vancomycin
Adults (>15 years old)	*S. pneumoniae*, meningococcus, *E. coli*	Ceftriaxone with vancomycin
Immunosuppressed	All of the above, plus tuberculosis, fungi, syphilis	Dependent on etiology

(3) Mortality rate is as high as 70% without treatment. With acyclovir therapy, the rate decreases to 20%.

b. Insect- or tick-borne encephalitis
   (1) California group (LaCrosse)
      (a) Viral prodrome can progress to fever, somnolence, obtundation, and seizures.
      (b) Most severe in children 4 to 11 years of age.
   (2) St. Louis encephalitis
      (a) Viral prodrome progresses to confusion, disorientation, stupor, tremors, and convulsions.
      (b) Severity increases with age.
   (3) West Nile virus infection
      (a) Viral prodrome can progress to a maculopapular rash, diarrhea, and encephalitic symptoms.
      (b) Distinguishing feature: May cause axonal neuropathy, resulting in a presentation similar to Guillain-Barré syndrome.
   (4) Colorado tick fever: Viral prodrome progresses to a fever that recurs every 2 to 3 days along with other symptoms of encephalitis and aseptic meningitis.

C. Poliomyelitis: Weakness due to infection of motor neurons in the brain and spinal cord.

D. Prion Diseases
   1. Occur in several species, including cows (bovine spongiform encephalopathy), sheep (scrapie), deer (chronic wasting disease), and humans (Creutzfeldt-Jakob disease, Gerstmann-Straüssler-Scheinker disease, fatal familial insomnia, and kuru).
   2. Transmission appears to be by infectious proteinaceous particles that differ from normal protein in terms of solubility, proteinase resistance, and infectivity but not primary structure. A post-translational mechanism is thus indicated in the modification.
   3. Evaluation: Workup is similar to that for dementia.

E. Intracranial Abscess
   1. Signs and symptoms
      a. Systemic infection
      b. Elevated intracranial pressure
      c. Focal neurologic deficits produced by mass effects
      d. Seizures
   2. Treatment
      a. Antibiotic treatment
      b. Surgical excision

F. HIV-associated complications
   1. Primary CNS lymphoma
   2. Progressive multifocal leukoencephalopathy
      a. Cause: Papovavirus infection (JC virus).
      b. Signs and symptoms: Patchy demyelination of CNS white matter with a symptom pattern similar to that of MS.

c. Evaluation: Imaging and brain biopsy.
d. Treatment: None is currently available.

3. Opportunistic brain infections
   a. Toxoplasmosis
   b. Cryptococcosis
   c. Cytomegalovirus infection
   d. Fungal or other bacterial infections

CHAPTER 9

Obstetrics and Gynecology

OBSTETRICS

I. Examination of the Pregnant Patient

A. Perform the complete physical examination, with several additional necessary steps.

1. Determine fetal lie using the Leopold maneuver: Palpate the abdomen to determine whether the fetus lies horizontally or vertically.
2. Check for rupture of membranes. Do a sterile speculum examination, and perform the following tests.
   a. Pool test: Look for a collection of fluid in the vagina.
   b. Nitrazine paper test: A pH-sensitive swab will turn blue in the presence of alkaline amniotic fluid.
   c. Fern test: The crystallization pattern of the fluid under a light microscope will look like a fern.
   d. Ultrasound: Can show oligohydramnios where the fluid level had previously been normal.
3. Examine the cervix for assessment of labor. Components of the score include the following:
   a. Degree of cervical dilation: Fully dilated = 10 cm.
   b. Cervical effacement: Measurement of the thinness of the cervix.
   c. Station: Relation of the fetal head to the ischial spines. Station is 0 at the level of the spines, +1 to +3 if the head is below the spines, and −1 to −3 if the head is above the spines.
   d. Cervical consistency: Firmness or softness of the cervix.
   e. Cervical position: posterior/mid/anterior.

B. Monitor the Fetus

1. External monitors measure both fetal heart rate and uterine contractions.
   a. Fetal heart tones should be assessed with respect to their range, long-term variability, and the presence of accelerations, decelerations, and reactivity of the fetus (Fig. 9-1).
   b. Tocometers measure uterine contractions. These are useful for determining the frequency and timing of contractions, but not the strength of contraction.
2. Fetal scalp electrodes are useful in cases of repetitive decelerations or in infants difficult to trace with Doppler imaging. Contraindications include maternal hepatitis or HIV or fetal thrombocytopenia.
3. Intrauterine pressure catheters (IUPCs) are useful when the strength of contraction needs to be determined or when external tocometers cannot detect contractions (obesity).

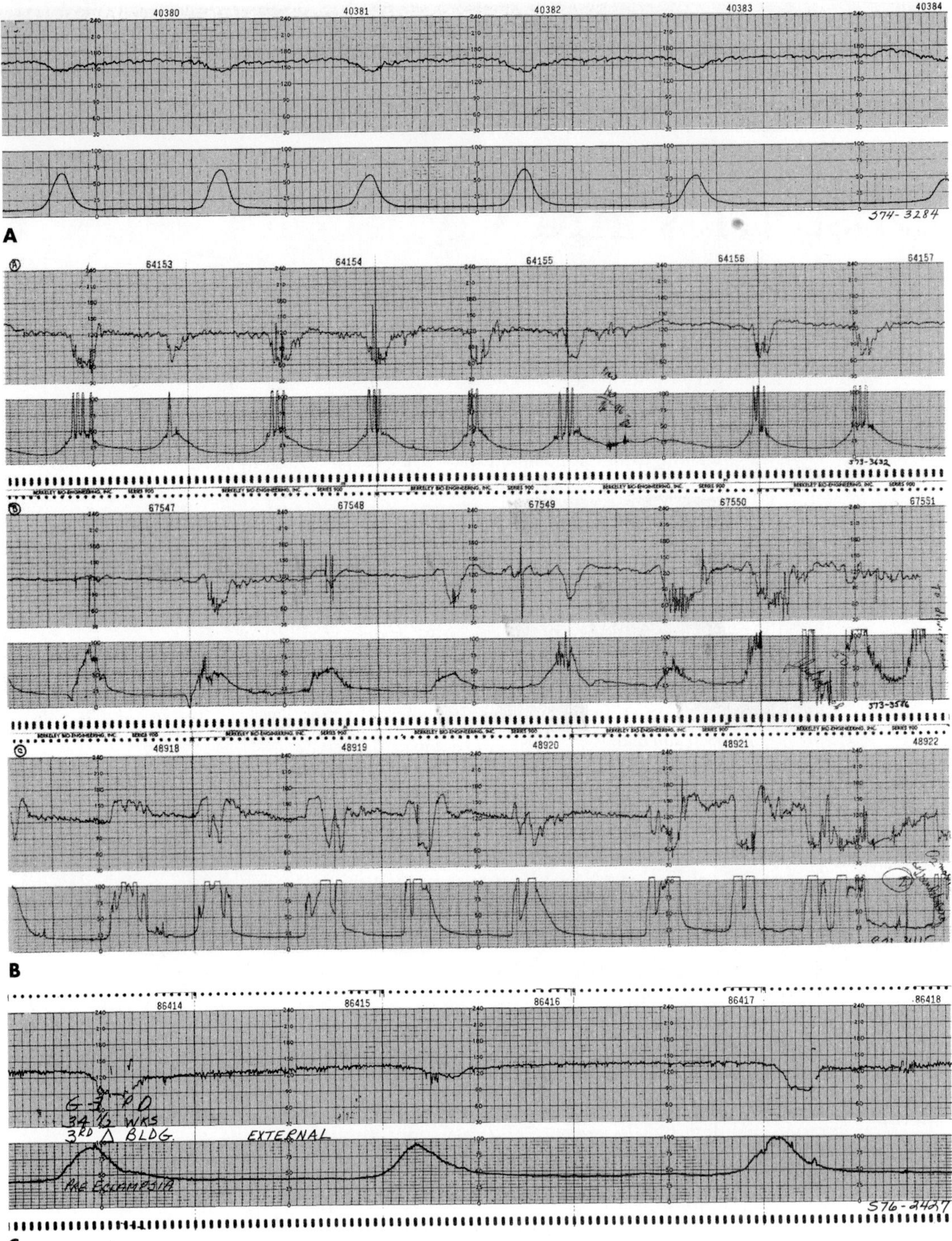

9-1: *Abnormalities found on fetal heart monitors. Decelerations of the fetal heart rate from baseline should be assessed with respect to the timing of the contractions. A, Early decelerations start and end with uterine contractions and are usually due to compression of the fetal head. B, Variable decelerations have a variable onset with a quick resolution and are usually due to compression of the umbilical cord. C, Late decelerations start after the beginning of the contraction and finish after the end of the contraction and are usually due to fetal hypoxia.*

4. Fetal scalp pH measurements can directly assesses fetal hypoxia. Measurements greater than 7.25 are reassuring, while measurements less than 7.20 are nonreassuring.

II. Medical Complications of Pregnancy
   A. Hypertension in Pregnancy
      1. Hypertension occurs in up to 20% of all pregnancies.
      2. Risk factors include age at first pregnancy (<20 years old), high blood pressure before pregnancy, large body size, family history, multiple pregnancy, diabetes, and vascular or connective tissue disease.
      3. Types of hypertension in pregnancy are described in Table 9-1.
   B. Diabetes Mellitus in Pregnancy
      1. Types of diabetes include insulin-dependent diabetes (type 1), non-insulin-dependent diabetes (type 2), and gestational diabetes (type 3).
      2. Risk factors for gestational diabetes include
         a. Age older than 25 years
         b. Obesity
         c. Family history of diabetes
         d. History of a macrosomic (>4 kg), stillborn, or deformed infant in a previous pregnancy
         e. History of polyhydramnios, recurrent spontaneous abortions, or gestational diabetes in a previous pregnancy
      3. Gestational diabetes is classified according to the White system (Table 9-2).
      4. Screening
         a. Patients with risk factors should be screened at the first prenatal visit. Other patients should be screened between weeks 24 and 28 of gestational age (GA).
         b. Paradigm for glucose tolerance testing is shown in Figure 9-2.
         c. Hemoglobin A_{1c} (HbA_{1c}) can be used to monitor the patient's glucose control over the past 6 to 8 weeks.
      5. Treatment
         a. American Diabetes Association diet of at least 1800 calories per day. If the patient's fasting blood glucose levels are less than 105 mg/dL and her 2-hour postprandial blood glucose level is less than 120 mg/dL after starting the diet, she can be controlled by diet alone.
         b. Oral hypoglycemic agents are usually not used because they cross the placenta.
         c. Insulin does not cross the placenta, so it can be used. Target glucose is generally between 60 and 105 units (see Chapter 3 for insulin dosing).
         d. Encourage activity, and change insulin dose if degree of activity changes.
         e. Start antenatal testing of the fetus at weeks 30 to 32 GA to assess any fetal changes. This includes the use of serial ultrasounds (every 4 to 6 weeks), nonstress tests, biophysical profiles, and daily kick counts.

TABLE 9-1 Hypertensive States in Pregnant Patients

Disorder	Description	Treatment	Complications
Preeclampsia/ eclampsia	(1) Preeclampsia causes edema, hypertension, and proteinuria in pregnant women after 20 weeks of gestational age. (2) Hypertension before 20 weeks should arouse suspicion of a hydatidiform mole, drug use or withdrawal, fetal chromosomal abnormalities, or undiagnosed chronic hypertension. (3) Mild cases have a third-trimester systolic BP > 140 or diastolic BP > 90 with proteinuria (>300 mg/24 hr) and edema. (4) Severe cases have a third-trimester systolic BP > 160 or a diastolic BP > 110 with more severe proteinuria (>5 g/24 hr) and edema. Other symptoms may include altered consciousness, visual changes, headache, abdominal pain, impaired liver function, oliguria, pulmonary edema, cyanosis, and thrombocytopenia. (5) Eclampsia is diagnosed when grand mal seizures occur in the preeclamptic patient that are not attributable to other causes. 25% of seizures occur before delivery, 50% during labor, and 25% within 10 days after delivery (most within the first 48 hrs).	(1) Mild preeclampsia: induce labor with NSVD for term pregnancies or unstable preterm pregnancies. Stable preterm patients can be treated with bed rest and observation. $MgSO_4$ can be used for seizure prophylaxis. Control BP with hydralazine. (2) Severe preeclampsia or eclampsia: patients should receive $MgSO_4$ for seizure prophylaxis and delivery via NSVD should be done as soon as possible. Control BP with hydralazine. (3) Mg^{++} overdose is indicated by loss of deep tendon reflexes. Treat with $CaCl_2$ or calcium gluconate.	(1) Fetal complications include prematurity, acute uteroplacental insufficiency (abruption, intrapartum fetal distress, stillbirth), chronic uteroplacental insufficiency (intrauterine growth retardation), and oligohydramnios. (2) Maternal complications include ischemia or infarction affecting a variety of organs, which can cause seizures, pulmonary edema, renal failure, disseminated intravascular coagulation, or hepatic failure. A higher complication rate is associated with delivery. (3) HELLP syndrome: syndrome including *h*emolytic anemia, *e*levated *l*iver enzymes, and *l*ow *p*latelets. These patients are often multiparous and <36 weeks of gestational age at time of presentation. Results in a high rate of stillbirth and fetal death, DIC, and multisystem organ failure.
Chronic hypertension	Hypertension that is present before conception, before 20 weeks of gestational age, or persisting for >6 weeks postpartum.	Safest agents during pregnancy include methyldopa and hydralazine.	IUGR, preeclampsia, premature delivery, abruption, and others.
Chronic hypertension with superimposed preeclampsia	(1) Worsening hypertension, increases of 30 mm Hg systolic BP or 15 mm Hg diastolic BP above the patient's average values, or worsening proteinuria in the third trimester. (2) Most often due to a hypertensive disorder of renal origin that is aggravated by pregnancy.	Same as treatment for preeclampsia.	Abruption, DIC, acute tubular necrosis, premature delivery, IUGR, and others.

TABLE 9-1 Hypertensive States in Pregnant Patients—cont'd

Disorder	Description	Treatment	Complications
Transient hypertension	New onset of hypertension that develops between mid pregnancy and the first 48 hr after delivery and occurs without the other signs of preeclampsia. Diagnosis can be made only in retrospect, when it is established postpartum that no preeclamptic changes occurred during pregnancy.	Same as treatment for preeclampsia, since the diagnosis is retrospective.	Fewer medical complications than other types, but it is likely to recur in subsequent pregnancies.

BP, blood pressure; DIC, disseminated intravascular coagulation; IUGR, intrauterine growth retardation; NSVD, normal spontaneous vaginal delivery.

f. Labor should be induced at 38 to 40 weeks if lung maturity is present. Waiting longer is a risk. Induce earlier if acidosis, hypertension, worsening diabetes, or fetal compromise indicates need for delivery.

g. Cesarean section is indicated for obstetric indications or if the fetus is more than 4500 g.

h. Following labor, most gestational diabetic patients will not require insulin. Others will require a decrease in insulin dose. Give a glucose tolerance test at 6 weeks postpartum.

6. Complications of diabetes

a. Obstetric complications include polyhydramnios, preeclampsia, miscarriage, infection, postpartum hemorrhage, and increased incidence of cesarean section.

b. Diabetic emergencies include hypoglycemia, ketoacidosis, and diabetic coma.

TABLE 9-2 White Classification System for Gestational and Other Types of Diabetes

Type	Description
A1	Gestational diabetes, diet controlled
A2	Gestational diabetes, insulin controlled
B	Diabetes with onset at >20 years old or duration of <10 years
C	Diabetes with onset at 10–19 years old or duration of 10–19 years
D	Diabetes with onset before 10 years old or duration of >20 years
F	Diabetes with diabetic nephropathy
R	Diabetes with proliferative retinopathy
RF	Diabetes with both retinopathy and nephropathy
H	Diabetes with ischemic heart disease
T	Diabetes with prior renal transplantation

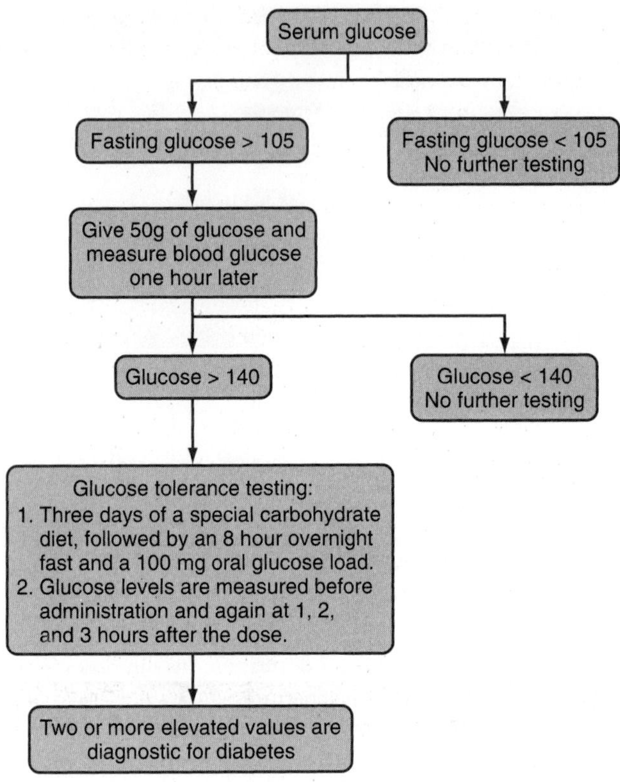

***9-2:** Algorithm for glucose tolerance testing in gestational diabetes.*

c. Vascular disease, cardiac disease, neuropathy, and gastroparesis can occur.

d. Gestational diabetes is a significant risk factor for the development of type 2 diabetes later in life.

e. Fetal complications of gestational diabetes include perinatal death, macrosomia, delayed organ maturity, congenital abnormalities, and intrauterine growth restriction.

C. Hyperemesis Gravidarum

1. Nausea and vomiting that results in dehydration and possible electrolyte abnormalities.

2. Treatment includes rehydration, antiemetic medications (prochlorperazine, promethazine, trimethobenzamide, metoclopramide, ondansetron) and maintenance of adequate nutrition.

D. Coagulation Disorders

1. Pregnancy is a hypercoagulable state.

2. Patients may have superficial vein thromboses, deep vein thromboses, or pulmonary embolism.

3. Superficial thromboses can be treated with symptomatic care. Treat deep vein thromboses and pulmonary emboli with intravenous or subcutaneous heparin for the remainder of the pregnancy.

E. Substance Abuse in Pregnancy (Table 9-3)

III. Induction and Augmentation of Labor

A. Induction is starting contractions when none are present, whereas augmentation is increasing the strength and frequency of contractions that have already begun.

B. Indications for induction or augmentation include post-term pregnancy, preeclampsia, premature rupture of membranes, nonreassuring fetal testing, and intrauterine growth retardation (IUGR).

C. Agents Used to Induce or Augment Labor

1. Prostaglandins

a. Soften the cervix. PGE_2 pessary (dinoprostone) or PGE_{1M} (misoprostol) are often used.

b. Contraindications include asthma, glaucoma, previous cesarean section, and nonreassuring fetal testing.

c. Possible side effects include uterine hyperstimulation or tetany.

TABLE 9-3 Effects of Substance Abuse during Pregnancy

Substance	Description
Alcohol	(1) Can produce fetal alcohol syndrome (FAS) when pregnant women drink 2–5 drinks per day. (2) Symptoms include growth retardation, mental retardation, abnormal facies, and sometimes cardiac abnormalities (3) Treat by counseling the mother to quit drinking, and use barbiturates for withdrawal symptoms (do not use benzodiazepines in pregnant women because of teratogenicity)
Caffeine	There is a higher risk of first- and second-trimester miscarriages if maternal caffeine intake exceeds 150 mg/day (1 cup of coffee)
Nicotine	(1) Has been correlated with increased risk of spontaneous abortions, preterm births, abruptions, and decreased birth weight (2) Children are also at higher risk for sudden infant death syndrome (SIDS) and respiratory illnesses after delivery
Cocaine	(1) Associated with abruption, fetal distress, growth restricted infants, and an increased risk of preterm labor and delivery (2) Can also cause congenital anomalies (cardiac defects, skull abnormalities, genitourinary malformations), intracranial hemorrhage, and necrotizing enterocolitis
Opiates	(1) No known teratogenic effects, and it may be more dangerous to have the mother undergo withdrawal while pregnant than to continue exposure to the drug (2) Enroll the mother in a methadone maintenance program throughout the pregnancy

2. Oxytocin causes uterine contractions. It has a short half-life, and its effects stop shortly after the IV flow is stopped.
3. Amniotomy (breaking of the amniotic sac) facilitates contraction strength by decreasing the stretching of the muscle fibers of the myometrium. Do *not* elevate the fetal head from the pelvis when doing this, since it can cause prolapse of the umbilical cord as the fluid rushes out.

IV. Stages of Labor
  A. Cardinal Movements of Labor
    1. Engagement: Presenting part enters the pelvis.
    2. Flexion of the head.
    3. Descent of the head into the pelvis.
    4. Internal rotation from the occiput transverse (OT) presentation so that the sagittal suture is parallel to the anteroposterior diameter of the pelvis.
    5. Extension: As the vertex passes beyond the symphysis pubis.
    6. External rotation: Allows delivery of the shoulders. The anterior shoulder is delivered before the posterior shoulder.
  B. First Stage of Labor: From the Onset of Labor to Full Dilation of the Cervix
    1. Can last for 10 to 12 hours in a nulliparous or 6 to 8 hours in a multiparous patient. The duration of each phase will be longer in nulliparous women than in multiparous women.
    2. Phases
      a. Latent: A period of slow cervical change that lasts from the onset of labor until dilation to 3 or 4 cm.
      b. Active: A period of rapid cervical change from dilation of 4 to 9 cm. The cervix changes by 1 to 1.2 cm/hr.
      c. Deceleration/transition: The period in which the dilation progresses from 9 cm to fully dilated (10 cm).
  C. Second Stage of Labor: From Full Dilation to Delivery of the Infant
    1. Can last for up to 2 hours in a nulliparous or 1 hour in a multiparous patient. The duration of stage 2 can be lengthened by the use of epidural anesthesia.
    2. On fetal heart rate monitoring, repetitive early and variable decelerations of the fetal heart rate are often seen but are not worrisome if they end at the same time as the contractions. Repetitive late decelerations, bradycardia, and loss of variability are signs of fetal distress.
    3. Fetal distress can be managed by the following strategies:
      a. Give oxygen by face mask.
      b. Turn the patient on her left side to avoid compression of the inferior vena cava.
      c. Stop oxytocin until the fetal heart monitor shows a more reassuring pattern.
      d. If uterine hyperstimulation is suspected, terbutaline can be given to relax the uterus.
      e. If reassuring patterns do not result from these measures, then the position of the infant should be assessed to determine whether to deliver through an operative vaginal delivery or cesarean section.

D. Types of Delivery
   1. Vaginal delivery: Encourage pushing of the fetus until crowning occurs. If necessary, an episiotomy can be performed. Once the head is delivered, bulb suction the mouth and upper airway. If meconium is present, use a DeLee suction tube to suction the mouth and nares and prevent meconium aspiration. Also check for a nuchal cord before delivering the shoulders.
   2. Operative vaginal delivery
      a. Indications include a prolonged second stage of labor, maternal exhaustion, or a need to hasten delivery.
      b. In a forceps-assisted delivery, the blades are placed around the infant's head and the mother's efforts are aided by guiding the head of the infant.
         (1) Full dilation of the cervix, an engaged head with at least +2 station, absolute knowledge of the fetal position, and an empty bladder are necessary before attempting a forceps delivery.
         (2) Complications can include bruising of face and head, lacerations to the fetal head and birth canal, facial nerve palsy, and intracranial damage (rare).
      c. Vacuum extraction: The indications are same as for forceps-assisted extraction, and the most common complication is cephalohematoma. This can take weeks or months to resolve.

E. Third Stage of Labor: From Delivery of the Infant to Delivery of the Placenta
   1. Delivery of the placenta should occur within 30 minutes (usually within 5) of delivery of the infant.
   2. Oxytocin can be used to induce contractions, facilitate shearing of the placenta, and prevent uterine atony.
   3. Signs of placental separation include cord lengthening, a gush of blood, and uterine fundal rebound. Suprapubic pressure should be applied during delivery of the placenta to prevent uterine inversion.
   4. Removal of a retained placenta can be performed if the placenta has not been delivered within 30 minutes of the infant. This is done either manually or via curettage, to prevent retention of the products of conception.

F. Fourth Stage of Labor: After the Delivery of the Placenta
   1. Assess uterine contraction: Uterine massage and oxytocin can be used to contract the uterus and minimize uterine bleeding. In cases of uterine atony, additional measures to contract the uterus include the following.
      a. Prostaglandins: carboprost, misoprostol.
      b. Surgery: Ligation or embolization of the uterine or internal iliac arteries. The obstetrician can also attempt to contract uterus mechanically with sutures. Hysterectomy is a last resort.
   2. All lacerations should be repaired. Degrees of laceration are as follows:
      a. First degree—Involves mucosa or skin.
      b. Second degree—Extends into the perineal body but does not involve the sphincter.
      c. Third degree—Extends into or through the anal sphincter.
      d. Fourth degree—Anal mucosa is torn.

V. Cesarean Section ("C-Section")

A. Indications for cesarean section over normal spontaneous vaginal delivery (NSVD) include cephalopelvic disproportion, prolonged second stage of labor, breech or compound presentation, fetal distress, cord prolapse, active herpes lesions, failed operative vaginal delivery, or previous cesarean section. In addition, certain critical situations (abruption, fetal bradycardia, hemorrhage from placenta previa) require cesarean section as an emergency intervention.

B. Disadvantages of Cesarean Section: Compared with NSVD there is increased operative morbidity and mortality and a longer recovery time.

C. Vaginal Birth after Cesarean Section (VBAC): This can be performed if the previous cesarean section used a low transverse incision without any extensions into the cervix and uterine upper segment. Complications include rupture through a prior uterine scar, which will cause abdominal pain, decelerations of the fetal heart rate, and decreased uterine pressure.

VI. Complications in the Perinatal Period

A. Preterm Labor: Labor that occurs before 37 weeks GA. This requires the presence of both contractions and cervical change.

1. Risk factors for preterm labor include maternal **d**isease, preterm **r**upture of membranes, **a**bruption, maternal **w**eight less than 50 kg, **m**ultiple gestations, **u**terine anomalies, **c**horioamnionitis, and a **h**istory of preterm delivery (mnemonic—DRAW MUCH).

2. Complications associated with preterm labor include low birth weight, respiratory distress syndrome (RDS), intraventricular hemorrhage (IVH), sepsis, and necrotizing enterocolitis (NEC).

3. Indications for immediate delivery include chorioamnionitis, nonreassuring fetal testing, and significant placental abruption.

4. In more stable cases, tocolytic measures can be used to delay or stop the progression of labor.

a. Hydration can work by decreasing antidiuretic hormone (ADH) level (which cross-reacts with oxytocin receptors and can induce contractions).

b. Pharmacotherapy often can only prolong gestation for 48 hours, but this allows time to induce lung maturity. Tocolytic agents include

(1) Beta-mimetics (ritodrine and terbutaline): Side effects include pulmonary edema.

(2) $MgSO_4$: Acts as a Ca^{++} antagonist and a membrane stabilizer. Toxic levels can produce respiratory depression, pulmonary edema, hypoxia, and cardiac arrest. Patients with impaired renal function will accumulate Mg^{++} levels quickly. Mg^{++} levels can be monitored by looking for loss of deep tendon reflexes (indicates Mg^{++} level 1 mg/dL).

(3) Calcium channel blockers (e.g., nifedipine).

(4) Prostaglandin inhibitors (e.g., indomethacin). Side effects in the fetus include premature constriction of the ductus arteriosus, pulmonary hypertension, oligohydramnios, and a risk of NEC and IVH.

c. Lung maturity can be induced using betamethasone. This will decrease the likelihood of RDS in the fetus.

B. Preterm and Premature Rupture of Membranes (ROM)

1. Patients may have experienced a recent gush of fluid from the vagina or increased vaginal discharge.

2. Pooling, nitrazine, or ferning tests may be positive. In addition, ultrasonography may demonstrate oligohydramnios.

3. Types

a. Preterm ROM: ROM at less than 37 weeks GA. Complications include preterm labor, preterm delivery, and chorioamnionitis.

b. Premature ROM: ROM before the onset of labor.

c. Prolonged ROM: ROM that lasts for more than 18 hours.

d. Prolonged premature ROM: ROM before the onset of labor lasting for more than 18 hours. Complications include chorioamnionitis, abruption, and cord prolapse.

4. Treatment

a. Premature ROM: Tocolysis can to allow time to induce lung maturity (see preterm labor section).

b. Prolonged premature ROM: Treat with corticosteroids to induce lung maturity. Wait for week 36 or for evidence of fetal lung maturity and then deliver. Ampicillin with or without erythromycin should also be given.

c. If ROM occurs from 34 to 36 weeks GA, labor is usually induced.

C. Chorioamnionitis: Infection of the amniotic fluid surrounding the fetus

1. The major risk factor is preterm and/or prolonged ROM.

2. Patients may have fever, uterine tenderness, and fetal tachycardia.

3. Evaluation

a. Complete blood count (CBC) will show maternal leukocytosis.

b. Amniotic fluid culture is diagnostic. Chorioamnionitis is commonly caused by organisms that colonize the vagina and rectum. Infection with group B β-hemolytic streptococci (GBBS) causes a substantial risk of neonatal mortality from sepsis. Patients are tested for GBBS status at weeks 36–37.

4. Treat with broad-spectrum antibiotics, and hasten delivery with induction, augmentation, or cesarean section (if fetal tracings are nonreassuring).

D. Antepartum Hemorrhage (Table 9-4)

E. Obstruction and Malposition (Table 9-5)

F. Amniotic Fluid Disorders

1. Measured using ultrasonography to determine the amniotic fluid index (AFI). Oligohydramnios has an AFI of less than 5, while polyhydramnios has an AFI of greater than 20.

2. Oligohydramnios

a. Can be caused by rupture of membranes, growth restriction, or congenital anomalies (especially of the genitourinary system).

b. Treat by induction of labor in patients with ROM. Amnioinfusion may be required if signs of fetal distress are present.

3. Polyhydramnios

Congenital anomalies associated with oligohydramnios include polycystic kidney disease, genitourinary tract obstruction, and renal agenesis (Potter's syndrome).

TABLE 9-4 Causes of Antenatal Hemorrhage

Disorder	Symptoms and Signs	Treatment
Placenta previa	(1) Types include complete previa (placenta completely covers the internal os), partial previa (placenta partially covers the internal os), and marginal previa (when the edge of the placenta reaches the margin of the internal os). (2) Patients have painless vaginal bleeding during the third trimester. Diagnosis can be confirmed by ultrasonography. (3) Risk factors include multiparity, advanced maternal age, smoking, abnormal placentation, and a history of previous previa or cesarean section. (4) Abnormalities of placentation include circumvallate placenta (membranes double back over the edge of the placenta and form a dense ring around it), vasa previa (velamentous cord insertion causes the fetal vessels to pass over the internal cervical os), velamentous placenta (vessels insert between the amnion and the chorion), and succenturiate placenta (extra lobe of the placenta that is implanted away from the rest of the placenta). These all carry a high risk of fetal death owing to fetal vessel rupture and exsanguination.	(1) Stabilize patients in whom previa is suspected, and monitor their complete blood count (CBC) to assess for blood loss. (2) Marginal previa or low-lying placenta in the second trimester may resolve spontaneously if the placenta moves up as the lower uterine segment develops. (3) In emergency cases (unstoppable labor, fetal distress, life-threatening bleeding), perform an emergency cesarean section. (4) In stable patients who are preterm, treat with expectant management and try to take to term. Prepare for preterm delivery by giving betamethasone and tocolysis (if <34 weeks of gestational age), and deliver by cesarean section at 36 weeks if fetal lung maturity is present or bleeding recurs.
Placenta accreta	(1) Abnormal invasion of the placenta into the uterine wall. Types include accreta (superficial invasion of the placenta up to the uterine myometrium), increta (invasion into the myometrium), and percreta (invasion through the myometrium into the uterine serosa). (2) Patients have a placenta that will not separate from the uterine wall following delivery. This can produce hemorrhage, shock, and maternal death. Hematuria or hematochezia may be present if the placenta invades the bladder or rectum.	If the mother's life is in danger, then a puerperal hysterectomy can be performed.

TABLE 9-4 Causes of Antenatal Hemorrhage—cont'd

Disorder	Symptoms and Signs	Treatment
Placental abruption	(1) Premature separation of the placenta from the uterine wall that most frequently occurs between week 30 of gestational age and delivery. (2) Types of blood loss include concealed hemorrhage (bleeding is confined to the uterine cavity and will cause retroplacental clots) and external hemorrhage (which presents with vaginal bleeding). (3) Symptoms include third-trimester vaginal bleeding, abdominal pain, uterine contractions, uterine tenderness, and fetal distress. (4) Ultrasound can be done to rule out placenta previa, but it may not visualize the abruption. (5) Risk factors include maternal hypertension, maternal trauma, rapid uterine decompression, and a prior history of abruption.	(1) Treat by stabilizing the patient, preparing for future hemorrhage, and preparing for preterm delivery. Deliver at 36 weeks of gestational age if fetal lung maturity is present and bleeding remains controlled. (2) Complications include premature delivery, uterine hyperstimulation, DIC, hypovolemic shock, acute renal failure, fetal death, and maternal death.
Uterine rupture	(1) Causes include uterine scarring (from prior cesarean section or uterine surgery), abdominal trauma or surgery, labor-induction (especially with excessive oxytocin administration), and spontaneous (associated with placenta accreta, multiple gestation, grand multiparity, invasive mole, or choriocarcinoma). (2) Symptoms include sudden onset of abdominal pain and bleeding. Fetal distress, regression of the presenting fetal part, and sudden cessation of uterine contractions may also be present.	(1) Treat with immediate laparotomy with either hysterectomy or primary closure of the rupture. (2) Future pregnancies should be discouraged.
Nonobstetric causes	May be due to cervical factors (severe cervicitis, polyps, benign masses, or malignancy), vaginal factors (including lacerations, varices, benign masses, or malignancy), or other causes (hemorrhoids, congenital bleeding disorder, or trauma).	Maintain hemodynamic stability, and treat the cause.

DIC, disseminated intravascular coagulation.

TABLE 9-5 Obstructions and Malpresentations

Disorder	Symptoms and Signs	Treatment
Cephalopelvic disproportion	(1) Occurs when there is a problem with the size of the fetus or the pelvis. (2) Pelvic shapes include gynecoid (round), android (triangular), anthropoid (long anteroposterior diameter), and platypelloid (long transverse diameter).	(1) NSVD can be tried. (2) Cesarean section may be necessary if failure to progress occurs.
Malpresentation of vertex	(1) Normally presenting fetuses should be vertex and in occiput anterior (OA) positioning at the time of delivery. (2) Types include facial presentation, brow presentation, shoulder presentation, compound presentation (fetal extremity presents alongside the vertex or breech), or persistent occiput transverse (OT) or occiput posterior (OP).	(1) Fetuses with face and brow presentations may be rotated and delivered vaginally. (2) Deliver shoulder or compound presentation by cesarean section owing to the increased risk of cord prolapse, uterine rupture, and the difficulty of vaginal delivery. (3) Other presentations often require vacuum or forceps delivery owing to a prolonged second stage of labor. Perform cesarean section in cases of excessive difficulty.
Breech presentation	(1) Fetus presents with the buttocks (instead of the vertex) facing the birth canal. (2) Risk factors include previous breech delivery, uterine anomalies, polyhydramnios, oligohydramnios, multiple gestations, preterm rupture of membranes, hydrocephalus, and anencephalus. (3) Types of breech include frank (flexed hips and extended knees with the feet near the head), footling (foot or knee lies below the breech in the birth canal) and complete (flexion of both hips and knees making the fetus sit cross-legged). (4) Diagnose with Leopold's maneuvers, cervical examination (palpation of the gluteal cleft), or ultrasonography.	(1) External version to vertex position is usually only performed after 37 weeks of gestational age. (2) Breech vaginal delivery can be attempted. Contraindications include nulliparity, fetal weight >3800 g, or incomplete breech presentation. Cesarean section should be performed if vaginal delivery is difficult. (3) Complications include cord prolapse and entrapment of the fetal head.

TABLE 9-5 Obstructions and Malpresentations—cont'd

Disorder	Symptoms and Signs	Treatment
Shoulder dystocia	(1) Results from difficulty in delivering anterior shoulder owing to its impaction behind the pubic symphysis. (2) Risk factors include fetal macrosomia, gestational diabetes, previous shoulder dystocia, maternal obesity, postdate pregnancy, and prolonged second stage of labor.	(1) Deliver the infant, which may require widening of the birth canal or fracture of the infant's clavicle (2) Complications include fractures of the humerus and clavicle, brachial plexus nerve injuries (Erb's palsy), hypoxic brain injury, and death.

NSVD, normal spontaneous vaginal delivery.

a. Can be caused by congenital and chromosomal anomalies, diabetes, hydrops, and multiple gestations.

b. During labor, evaluate the patient for cord prolapse during rupture of membranes.

Congenital anomalies associated with polyhydramnios include GI obstruction and neural tube defects.

G. Post-term Pregnancy

1. May be caused by inaccurate dating, anencephaly, fetal adrenal hypoplasia, or an absent fetal pituitary.

2. Management includes a nonstress test at 41 weeks GA with induction of labor if testing is nonreassuring. Otherwise, a biophysical profile and nonstress test should be repeated at 42 weeks. Labor should be induced if the pregnancy exceeds 42 weeks.

VII. Postpartum Care and Complications

A. Routine Postpartum Care

1. NSVD: Pain can be managed with NSAIDs or acetaminophen. Patients with episiotomies can be given perineal ice packs around the clock to reduce swelling. Also check them for hematomas and for the quality of the repair.

2. Cesarean section: Pain can be managed with narcotics and NSAIDs. Administer local wound care, and monitor for infection.

3. Breast care: Onset of lactation occurs 24 to 72 hours after delivery. Non-breast-feeding patients can be managed with ice packs, tight brassiere, and anti-inflammatories. Breast-feeding patients are relieved by breast-feeding.

4. Postpartum contraception: Diaphragms, cervical caps, and IUDs should not be used. Hormonal contraceptives can decrease the amount of milk produced by breast-feeding mothers. This happens to the least extent with progesterone-only pills and medroxyprogesterone.

B. Postpartum Hemorrhage: Blood loss greater than 500 mL in NSVD or greater than 1 L in cesarean section

1. Occurs within the first 24 hours (but can happen for several weeks postpartum in patients with retained products of conception).

2. Causes (Table 9-6).

3. Treatment

TABLE 9-6 Causes of Postpartum Hemorrhage

Disorder	Description
Lacerations	Include those occurring during delivery and episiotomy sites.
Uterine atony	(1) Leading cause of postpartum hemorrhage. (2) Risk factors include chorioamnionitis, exposure to $MgSO_4$, multiple gestations, macrosomic fetus, history of atony in other pregnancies, multiparity, and uterine abnormalities.
Placenta accreta	Bleeding is unresponsive to contractile agents and requires surgical management.
Vaginal hematoma	(1) May not be immediately apparent in the case of a retroperitoneal hematoma. (2) Retroperitoneal hematomas will present with lower back pain and a large drop in the patient's hematocrit, in the absence of an obvious location for hemorrhage.
Retained products of conception (POC)	(1) Evaluate for retained POC through hysteroscopy. (2) Dilation and curettage (D&C) is indicated if POC are found. If no POC are present, then suspect placenta accreta.
Uterine inversion	(1) Risk factors include fundal implantation of the placenta, uterine atony, placenta accreta, and excessive cord traction during labor. (2) Give relaxants such as nitroglycerin, and attempt to manually replace the uterus. If that fails, then surgically reorient the uterus or perform hysterectomy.
Uterine rupture	(1) Risk factors include previous uterine surgery, breech extraction, obstructed labor, and high parity. (2) Treat by surgical uterine repair or hysterectomy.

a. Fluid resuscitation.
b. Investigate cause of hemorrhage.
(1) Repair lacerations.
(2) For uterine atony, try oxytocin with uterine massage. Then try methylergonovine maleate (except in hypertensive patients). Then try dinoprostone (except in asthmatic patients). Then try surgery.
c. Give coagulation factors and platelets if blood loss exceeds 2–3 L.

4. Complications include Sheehan's syndrome (pituitary infarction). Patients will have an absence of lactation or failure to restart menstruation secondary to the absence of gonadotropins.

C. Endomyometritis: Polymicrobial infection of the uterine wall
1. Occurs 1–2 weeks after delivery.
2. Symptoms include fever, elevated WBCs, and uterine tenderness. It is more likely to occur following cesarean section.
3. Retained products of conception are a possible cause, so perform a careful evaluation for products of conception in these patients.
4. Treat with broad-spectrum IV antibiotics or triple antibiotic therapy.

Septic pelvic thrombophlebitis can occur in association with endometrial infection. Suspect this when there is persistent fever and tachycardia despite several days of antibiotic treatment for presumed endomyometritis. These patients should be treated with heparin for 7–30 days.

D. Mastitis
1. Occurs 1–2 weeks after delivery and is most likely due to breast-feeding.

2. Symptoms include focal tenderness, erythema, and differences in temperature from one region of the breast to the other.
3. Treat with oral antibiotics (commonly dicloxacillin). The patient can continue breast-feeding or breast-pumping. If an abscess develops, treat it with incision and drainage.

E. Postpartum Depression
1. Postpartum "blues" refer to mood swings, changes in appetite, changes in sleep in the postpartum period, and can be found in up to half of patients. Symptoms begin shortly after delivery and resolve spontaneously within 2 weeks.
2. Postpartum depression presents with low energy level, anorexia, insomnia, hypersomnolence, extreme sadness, and other depressive symptoms that last for more than a few weeks. These patients often do not care for their infants and may have suicidal ideation. Symptoms can occur anytime in the first year postpartum. Postpartum depression usually resolves on its own, but antidepressants can be used in severe cases.

VIII. Fetal Complications of Pregnancy
A. Disorders of Fetal Growth (Table 9-7)
B. Rh Incompatibility: Occurs when the mother is Rh– and the fetus is Rh+
1. The first pregnancy with Rh incompatibility is usually uneventful, but the mother's immune system sensitizes to the Rh antigen following exposure to fetal red blood cells (usually during delivery). Once antibodies have been generated, future pregnancies are at risk for immune-mediated hemolysis.
2. Erythroblastosis fetalis presents with a hyperdynamic state, heart failure, diffuse edema, ascites, and pericardial effusion. Bilirubin accumulation can result in CNS damage following birth (it is cleared by the placenta before birth).
3. Treatment
a. Unsensitized Rh– mothers should be given RhoGAM any time that the mother may be exposed to fetal blood. A Kleihauer-Betke test can be used to evaluate possible exposures to fetal blood and to calculate the dose of RhoGAM.
b. Sensitized Rh– mothers: If the baby is Rh+, monitor the antibody titer. If it becomes greater than 1:16, then perform serial amniocentesis to assess severity of disease. Severe disease can be treated with percutaneous umbilical transfusions.

Other immune-mediated hemolytic anemias can be found with ABO incompatibility (mild hemolysis), Lewis antigens (mild hemolysis), and the Kell and Duffy antigens (severe hemolysis and fetal hydrops).

C. Fetal Demise and Spontaneous Abortion
1. Patients experience a decrease in fetal movement and cessation of the symptoms associated with pregnancy. Retention of a fetal demise for 3–4 weeks can result in hypofibrinogenemia and disseminated intravascular coagulation (DIC).
2. Types of spontaneous abortion
a. Complete: Expulsion of all fetal and placental tissue prior to 20 weeks GA.
b. Incomplete: Expulsion of some, but not all, fetal and placental tissue prior to 20 weeks GA.

TABLE 9-7 Disorders of Fetal Growth

Size Disorder	Symptoms and Signs	Evaluation	Treatment
Small for gestational age (SGA)	(1) Estimated fetal weight is <10th percentile. (2) Causes of SGA include decreased growth potential (congenital anomalies, intrauterine infections, or teratogen exposure), intrauterine growth retardation (IUGR) (associated with maternal hypertension, anemia, chronic renal disease, autoimmune disease, malnutrition, or placental disease), small parental stature. (3) Growth disorders can be symmetric (fetus is proportionally small) or asymmetric (usually with wasting of the abdomen and extremities with sparing of the brain).	(1) Follow with serial ultrasounds. Fetus with decreased growth potential starts and stays small. Fetus with IUGR starts within the normal range and then falls off the growth curve. (2) After 20 weeks, the fundal height should be approximately equal to the gestational age as an indicator of degree of growth.	(1) Fetuses with decreased growth potential do not need to have delivery expedited. (2) IUGR fetuses require assessment weekly with a nonstress test, oxytocin challenge test, and biophysical profile. Nonreassuring testing indicates delivery. (3) SGA infants have a better outcome than premature infants of the same weight.
Large for gestational age (LGA)	(1) Estimated fetal weight is >90th percentile. (2) Macrosomia is the term used for babies with a birth weight >4500 g. (3) Risk factors for LGA include diabetes, maternal obesity, postterm pregnancy, multiparity, advanced maternal age, and a history of LGA infants.	Same as for SGA.	(1) Treatments are focused on minimizing the risk factors. Maternal diabetes can be treated with glycemic control. Obese patients can be encouraged to lose weight before conception or gain less weight during pregnancy. (2) Labor should be induced before macrosomic status is reached. Prepare for shoulder dystocia, and avoid the use of forceps or vacuum. (3) Complications include shoulder dystocia, birth trauma, low Apgar scores, hypoglycemia, polycythemia, hypocalcemia, and jaundice. There is also an increased childhood risk of leukemia, Wilms' tumor, and osteosarcoma.

c. Missed abortion: Fetal demise before 20 weeks GA without expulsion of fetal or placental tissue.

d. Threatened: Uterine bleeding prior to 20 weeks GA without cervical dilation or effacement.

e. Inevitable: Uterine bleeding prior to 20 weeks GA with cervical dilation but no expulsion of fetal or placental tissue.

3. Patients have an abnormal ultrasound image, low human chorionic gonadotropin (hCG) levels, and an absent fetal heartbeat.

4. Treat with dilation and evacuation (if <20 weeks) or induction of labor (if >20 weeks). Possible causes can be assessed with coagulation testing, fetal karyotype, TORCH (*Toxoplasma*, rubella, cytomegalovirus, herpes simplex virus) infection titers, and fetal autopsy.

D. Multiple Gestations: Rate of natural twinning is 1 in 80

1. Uterine arrangements

a. Dichorionic, diamniotic: Separation occurs before differentiation of the trophoblast.

b. Monochorionic, diamniotic: Separation occurs after trophoblast differentiation and before amnion formation.

c. Monochorionic, monoamniotic: Separation occurs after the amnion has formed.

2. Patients show rapid uterine growth, excessive maternal weight gain, and palpation of multiple fetuses on Leopold's maneuvers.

3. hCG, α-fetoprotein, and human placental lactogen will all be abnormally high. Diagnosis can be confirmed with ultrasound.

4. Delivery method depends on the presentation of the fetuses.

a. Vertex/vertex: Trial of delivery.

b. Vertex/nonvertex: Can undergo trial of NSVD if the twins are concordant or the first twin is larger.

c. Nonvertex/nonvertex: Perform cesarean section.

5. Complications

a. Mothers are at risk for preterm labor, placenta previa, cord prolapse, postpartum hemorrhage, cervical incompetence, gestational diabetes, and preeclampsia.

b. Fetuses are at risk for congenital abnormalities, small size for gestational age (SGA), and malpresentation.

c. Twin-twin transfusion syndrome: Occurs in monochorionic diamniotic twins, and can result in one twin being large and the other being small.

d. Monochorionic monoamniotic twins have a high mortality rate owing to cord entanglements.

GYNECOLOGY

IX. Reproductive Medicine

A. Female Reproductive Cycle (Fig. 9-3)

1. Consists of 28-day intervals in healthy women unless interrupted by pregnancy, lactation, or hormone-based contraceptives. The cycle is

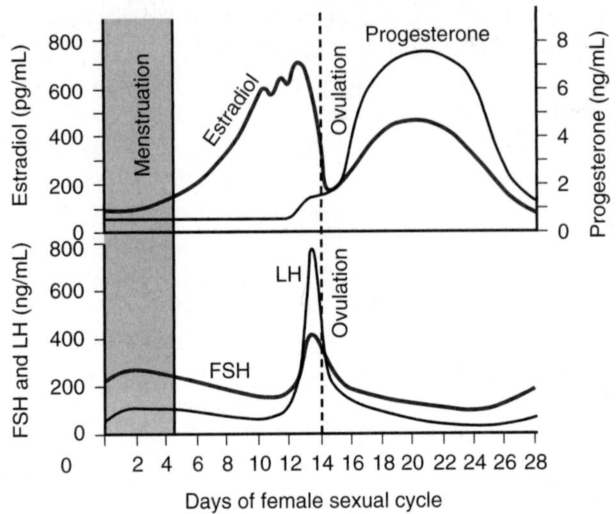

9-3: *Hormonal changes during the female reproductive cycle. Diagrammatic representation of the cyclic pattern of hormone release during the menstrual cycle. FSH, follicle-stimulating hormone; LH, luteinizing hormone.*

produced by the interaction between hypothalamic gonadotropin-releasing hormone (GnRH), pituitary gonadotropins (FSH and LH), and ovarian sex steroid hormones (estradiol and progesterone).

2. Phase 1: Menstruation and follicular phase.
   a. First day of menstrual bleeding is day 1 of the cycle.
   b. Plasma estradiol, progesterone, and LH are low. FSH is high, which leads to estrogen secretion, the maturation of ovarian follicles, and the selection of a dominant follicle. FSH levels will decrease and LH levels will increase as estrogen levels rise.
   c. An average menstruation is 3–5 days with loss of approximately 30–50 mL of blood. Uterine cramps may occur owing to liberation of prostaglandins (mainly PGF_{2a}) from the endometrium.
   d. The endometrium is sloughed early in phase 1 because of withdrawal from progesterone. As estrogen levels increase, the endometrium will enter the proliferative phase and the lining will thicken.
   e. An LH surge at day 11–13 causes ovulation. The oocyte is expelled, and the follicle becomes the corpus luteum to facilitate progesterone production.
3. Phase 2: Ovulation—the oocyte is expelled from the ovary and patients may feel a twinge of pain (mittelschmerz). Patients also have a slight increase in body temperature.
4. Phase 3: Luteal phase.
   a. High levels of progesterone are present and maintained by the corpus luteum. The corpus luteum has fixed life span of 13–14 days unless pregnancy occurs.
   b. The progesterone will cause the endometrium to transition from the proliferative phase to the secretory phase (phase 4).

c. In the absence of fertilization, the corpus luteum will involute near the end of the monthly cycle and cause a drop in estrogen and progesterone levels. This brings about sloughing of the endometrium, and menstruation ensues.

5. Pregnancy

a. Fertilization and implantation will cause hCG secretion to sustain the corpus luteum for 6–7 more weeks. hCG levels peak near week 12 GA and then decrease, but remain at elevated levels throughout pregnancy.

b. Estrogen and progesterone levels also rise in pregnancy but at a slower rate than hCG. Levels of progesterone peak shortly before parturition, and estrogen continues to rise until parturition occurs.

6. Perimenopause/menopause

a. As a woman ages, ovarian follicles decrease in number and become less sensitive to FSH.

b. Ovulation becomes increasingly inefficient, and the patient becomes anovulatory.

c. Cyclic hormone production ceases after the cessation of ovulation. The endometrium becomes atrophic.

d. Patients may experience hot flushes, irritability, fatigue, anxiety, decalcification of bone, and occasionally psychosis. The use of estrogen replacement to treat these symptoms was previously common but is currently controversial.

B. Amenorrhea: Absence of menstruation

1. Types

a. Primary amenorrhea: Occurs in young women who have never menstruated. This condition accounts for less than 1% of amenorrhea.

b. Secondary amenorrhea: Occurs in menstrual-aged women who have previously menstruated but have failed to do so within the past 6 months.

2. Causes (Fig. 9-4)

a. Pregnancy: Most common cause of secondary amenorrhea. This can be ruled out with a pregnancy test.

b. Hypothalamic-pituitary dysfunction: May cause amenorrhea through an altered or disrupted pulsatile release of GnRH or through alterations in catecholamine secretion. This can be diagnosed by low serum FSH and LH in the presence of a normal prolactin level.

c. Ovarian failure: The ovarian follicles are exhausted or are resistant to stimulation by LH and FSH.

(1) Causes may be genetic (Turner's syndrome), iatrogenic (alkylating chemotherapy) menopausal, autoimmune (Blizzard's syndrome), or idiopathic.

(2) Symptoms can include hot flashes, mood changes, sleep disturbances, or dyspareunia.

(3) Serum FSH and LH are high.

d. Obstruction of the genital outflow tract.

3. Treatment can be attempted using clomiphene to induce ovulation.

C. Dysfunctional Uterine Bleeding: Irregular menstruation without anatomic lesions of the uterus (Fig. 9-5)

The progesterone challenge test is an important tool in the evaluation of amenorrhea. It involves administration of a progesterone bolus and subsequent evaluation for any spotting or bleeding 5–7 days later. A positive test shows spotting or bleeding within this period and indicates that the anterior pituitary, endometrium, and genital outflow tract are functioning normally. Amenorrhea in the face of a positive progesterone challenge is most likely due to hypothyroidism, hyperprolactinemia, or ovulatory failure.

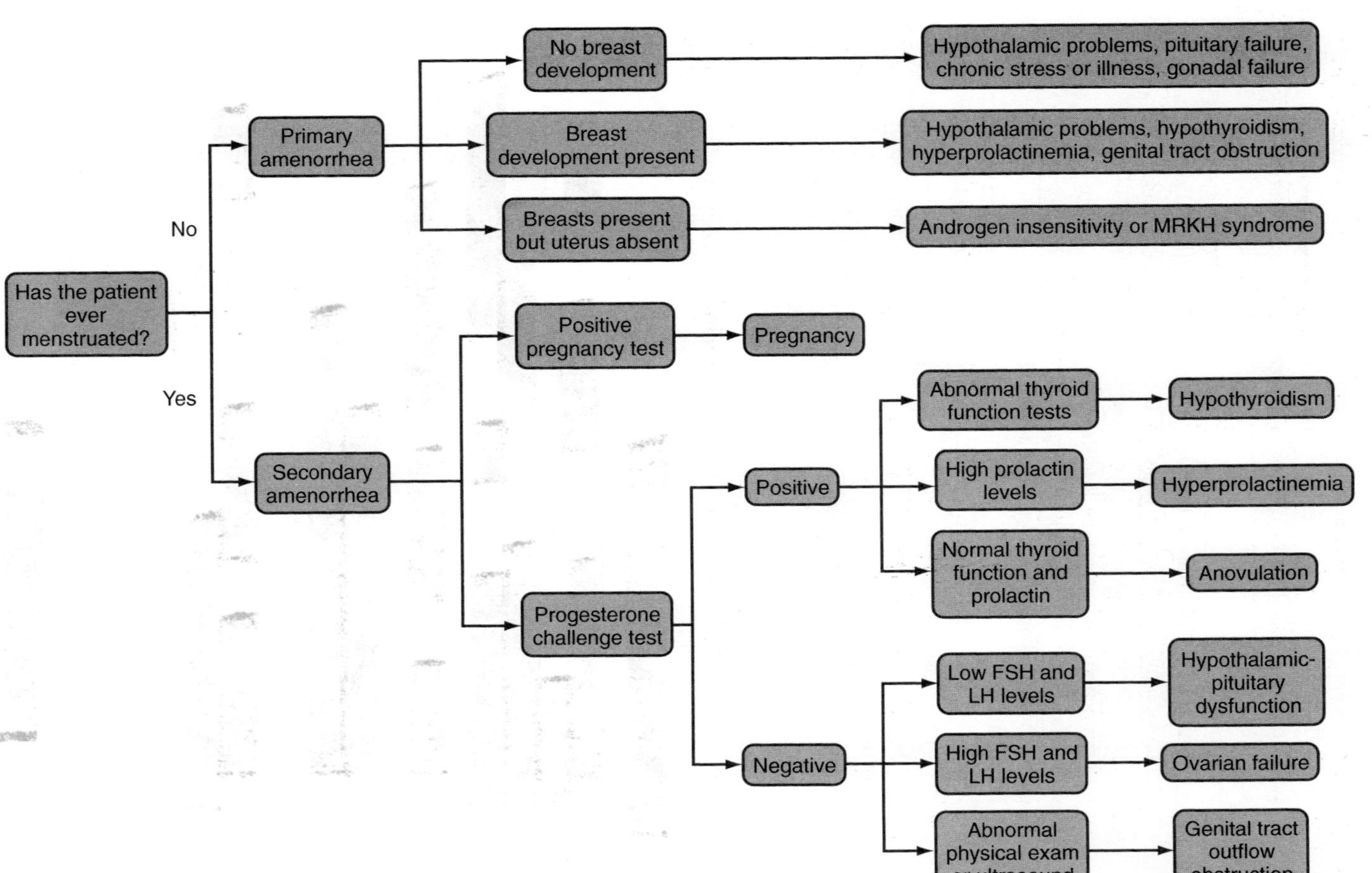

9-4: *Algorithm for the evaluation of amenorrhea. MRKH, Mayer-Rokitansky-Küster-Hauser syndrome.*

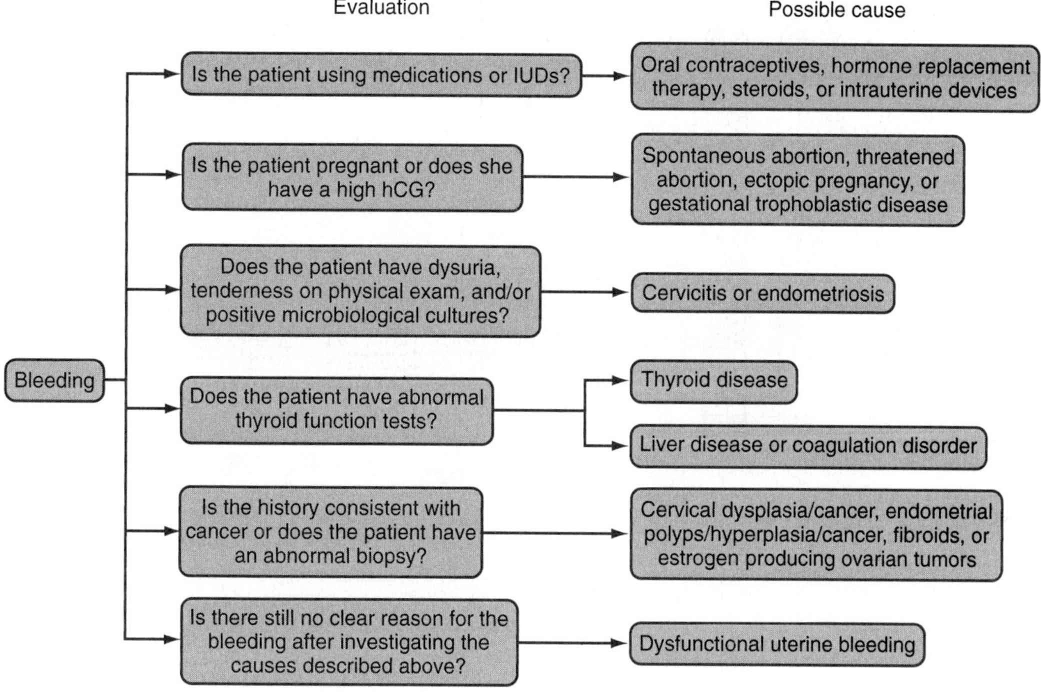

9-5: *Evaluation of dysfunctional uterine bleeding.*

1. Most likely to occur in association with anovulation as found in polycystic ovary disease, exogenous obesity, and adrenal hyperplasia.
2. Bleeding can occasionally occur with ovulation, which is called a luteal phase defect (ovulation occurs and the corpus luteum is not fully developed to secrete adequate progesterone to support a pregnancy).
3. Anatomic causes include fibroids, cervical lesions, vaginal lesions, and endometrial or cervical cancer.
4. Treat by converting the proliferative endometrium into secretory endometrium with the use of progestational agents such as medroxyprogesterone acetate.

D. Hirsutism and Virilism
   1. Hirsutism: Increase in terminal hairs on the face, chest, back, lower abdomen, and inner thighs in a woman. Pubic hair may develop a male (diamond shaped) escutcheon.
   2. Virilism: Development of male features, such as deepening of the voice, frontal balding, increased muscle mass, clitorimegaly, breast atrophy, and male body habitus.
   3. Causes and mechanisms are described in Table 9-8.

E. Contraception and Sterilization (Table 9-9)

F. Elective Termination of Pregnancy
   1. First-trimester abortion
      a. Suction curettage: Highly effective with minimal complications.

TABLE 9-8 Causes of Hirsutism and Virilism

Cause	Description
Pathologic production of androgens	ACTH stimulates the production of cortisol, aldosterone, and androgens. In cases where cortisol or aldosterone cannot be made, the pathway is shunted into production of more androgens.
Cushing's syndrome	(1) Increases in androgens are present in conditions in which ACTH is elevated. Cortisol will also be elevated. (2) Causes include pituitary adenoma, ectopic ACTH production, and tumors of the adrenal gland (see Chapter 3). (3) Patients can have hirsutism, acne, and menstrual irregularities. Other symptoms include moon face, buffalo hump, and truncal obesity with relatively thin extremities. (4) Androgen suppression can be achieved with glucocorticoids (prednisone) or antiandrogens (spironolactone).
Congenital adrenal hyperplasia	(1) Causes include deficiencies of enzymes involved in sex steroid synthesis (most common is 21α-hydroxylase). (2) Patients have adrenal insufficiency and salt wasting (due to lack of mineralocorticoids). They also have ambiguous genitalia. (3) Other deficiencies include 3β-hydroxysteroid dehydrogenase deficiency (causes accumulation of DHEA and DHEA-S and causes feminization of males and virilization of females) and 11β-hydroxylase deficiency. (4) Androgen suppression can be achieved with glucocorticoids (prednisone) or antiandrogens (spironolactone).
Theca lutein cysts	(1) Theca cells are stimulated by LH to produce androstenedione and testosterone androgens, which are then aromatized in granulosa cells to produce estrogens. Theca lutein cysts produce excess androgens and can cause hirsutism and virilization. (2) Ovarian androgen suppression can be achieved with oral contraceptive pills.
Polycystic ovary syndrome	(1) Caused by excess LH stimulation (LH/FSH >2 : 1) leading to cystic changes in the ovaries and excess ovarian androgen production. (2) Symptoms include hirsutism, virilization, anovulation, amenorrhea, obesity, and an increased incidence of diabetes. (3) Ovarian androgen suppression can be achieved with oral contraceptive pills.
Stromal hyperplasia and hyperthecosis	(1) The ovaries are enlarged and fleshy and can produce excess androgens. (2) Androgen suppression can be achieved with oral contraceptive pills.
Neoplasia	Causes include Sertoli-Leydig cell tumors, granulosa-theca cell tumors, hilar cell tumors, germ cell tumors, and luteomas.
Exogenous effectors	(1) Drugs (androgens and corticosteroids) can increase testosterone by decreasing levels of SHBG. Other drugs that increase androgens include minoxidil, phenytoin, diazoxide, cyclosporin. (2) Drug-induced hirsutism can be treated by discontinuation of the drugs.

ACTH, adrenocorticotropic hormone; DHEA, dehydroepiandrosterone; DHEA-S, dehydroepiandrosterone sulfate; FSH, follicle-stimulating hormone; LH, luteinizing hormone; SHBG, sex hormone–binding globulin.

TABLE 9-9 Methods of Contraception and Sterilization

Category	Method	Description
Natural methods	Periodic abstinence	(1) Emphasizes fertility awareness and abstinence before and after ovulation. Effectiveness is 55% to 80%. (2) Relatively unreliable and requires a lot of effort. Good for religiously motivated couples.
	Coitus interruptus	Withdrawal before ejaculation. Effectiveness is 75%.
	Lactational amenorrhea	(1) Nursing induces hypothalamic suppression of ovulation. Effectiveness is highly variable. (2) Should not be used in excess of 6 months after delivery.
Barrier methods	Condoms	(1) Male condoms are 98% effective, Female condoms are 80% to 85% effective. (2) Prevents sexually transmitted disease (STD) transmission. (3) Allergic reactions due to latex sensitivity may occur.
	Diaphragm	(1) Covers the cervix. Spermicidal jelly is placed in the cup. Should be placed before intercourse and left in 6–8 hours after intercourse. Effectiveness is 94%. (2) Protects against some STDs. (3) Can lead to cystitis and toxic shock syndrome. (4) Needs to be replaced every 5 years or when the patient gains or loses 10 lb.
	Cervical cap	Soft rubber cap that fits directly over the cervix. Efficacy is 85%, but dislodgement can be a problem.
	Sponge	Soft sponge embedded with a spermicide called nonoxynol 9. Poor efficacy in parous women is due to dislodgement during intercourse.
	Spermicides	(1) The most widely used are nonoxynol 9 and octoxynol 9. They should be placed at least 30 minutes before intercourse to allow dispersion. (2) Nonoxynol 9 can protect against STDs. (3) Can cause irritation.
Intrauterine devices (IUDs)		(1) Thought to act through a sterile spermicidal inflammatory response. Decreases likelihood of an ectopic pregnancy. (2) No protection against STDs. (3) Good for patients in whom OCPs are contraindicated, and those at low risk for STDs. (4) Contraindications include pregnancy, abnormal bleeding, suspected gynecologic malignancy, acute genital infection, and history of pelvic inflammatory disease (PID). An IUD should be removed if a patient becomes pregnant. (5) Side effects can include infection, bleeding, and perforation. Infection usually occurs within 20 days of initial implantation of the device.

continued

TABLE 9-9 Methods of Contraception and Sterilization—cont'd

Category	Method	Description
Hormonal methods	Oral contraceptive pills (OCPs)	(1) Composed of progesterone alone or a combination of progesterone and estrogen. (2) Places the body in a pseudopregnancy state by interfering with the pulsatile release of FSH and LH and thus suppressing ovulation. OCPs also change the cervical mucus to render it less penetrable to sperm and by changing the endometrium to make it unsuitable for implantation. (3) Types include fixed combination pills (fixed dose of estrogen/progesterone for 21 days and then 7 days off), dose varying pills (vary the dose of progestin at lower levels during the 21 days of hormone pills), and progestin-only pills (taken every day of the cycle). (4) Advantages are high efficacy and noncontraceptive health benefits, such as reduced incidence of ovarian cancer, endometrial cancer, ectopic pregnancy, PID, and benign breast disease. (5) Disadvantages include a large number of drug interactions and the side effects of hypercoagulability, benign hepatic tumors, and an increase in gallbladder disease. They are contraindicated in patients >35 years of age who smoke.
	Levonorgestrel	(1) Sustained release system for the progestin levonorgestrel over 5 years. Efficacy rate >99%. (2) Side effects include irregular bleeding, headaches, weight change, and mood changes. Major disadvantages are that it is expensive and that it requires a physician to remove the rods.
	Medroxyprogesterone acetate	(1) Medroxyprogesterone is injected intramuscularly and released slowly for 3 months. Efficacy rate >99%. (2) Side effects include spotting, irregular menses (for the first year), and depression. Ovulation may take 18 months to return after discontinuation.
Surgical sterilization	Tubal ligation	(1) Banding, clipping, coagulating, or ligating both fallopian tubes to prevent unity of ovum and sperm. More than 99% effective. (2) Reversible in only ~50% of cases. The patient can still become pregnant via in vitro fertilization.
	Vasectomy	(1) Ligation of the vas deferens. More than 99% effective. (2) Other forms of contraception should continue to be used until 6 weeks after the procedure. (3) Success rate of reversal is 65%.

b. RU-486 (mifepristone): Synthetic hormone that binds to progesterone receptors in the endometrium to block the actions of progesterone. Side effects include incomplete abortion, failed abortion, and uterine cramping.

c. Postcoital pill: High dose of estrogen to prevent pregnancy after intercourse has taken place. Equivalent to a double dose of birth control pills in 2 doses 12 hours apart. Must be taken within 72 hours of coitus and is usually given with an antiemetic. May produce teratogenic effects in fetuses that are not aborted.

2. Second-trimester abortion: Can be performed by reason of congenital anomalies, complications of pregnancy, or undesired pregnancy.

a. Induction of labor: Using dinoprostone, amniotomy, and oxytocin. Complication rates and emotional stress are high.

b. Dilation and evacuation: Gradual dilation of the cervix using laminaria tents or metal dilators followed by large suction cannulas to extract the fetal tissue.

G. Infertility and Assisted Reproduction

1. Infertility is the inability to conceive after 1 year of unprotected intercourse.

2. Male factor infertility: Accounts for 40% of cases.

a. May be caused by endocrine disorder, anatomic defects, abnormal sperm production or mobility, or sexual dysfunction.

b. Risk factors include environmental exposure (chemicals, irradiation, excessive heat), varicocele, history of mumps, pituitary tumor, anabolic steroid use, or impotence.

c. Evaluate with semen analysis, endocrine evaluation, and a postcoital test (to evaluate sperm-mucus interaction).

d. Treatment

(1) Improvements in coital practice: Have intercourse every 2 days with female on the bottom. The female should lie on her back and hold knees to chest for 15 minutes afterward.

(2) Low semen volume can be treated using washed sperm for intrauterine insemination.

(3) Hypothalamic failure can be treated with injections of human menopausal gonadotropins (hMGs).

(4) Varicocele and anatomic abnormalities may be correctable through surgery.

(5) Assisted reproductive technologies (see later discussion).

3. Female factor infertility: Responsible for 40% of overall infertility (the remaining 20% is of unknown cause).

a. May be caused by peritoneal factors (endometriosis, adhesions), ovulatory factors (ovulatory failure, endocrine abnormalities, polycystic ovary disease), uterine tubal factors (scarring, endometriosis, pelvic inflammatory disease), or cervical factors (structural abnormalities, abnormal cervical mucus).

b. Evaluation

(1) Progestin challenge test: Administer a progestin over 5–10 days to build up the endometrium, and abruptly stop it. This should

cause a withdrawal bleed within a week if the endometrium is normal. If not, the patient may have ovulatory failure.

(2) Routine imaging and blood testing for other endocrine and structural causes.

c. Treatment

(1) Correct any endocrine abnormalities.

(2) Ovulation can be induced using clomiphene citrate.

(3) Surgery may be required to correct anatomic abnormalities, endometriosis, or scarring.

(4) Assisted reproductive technologies (see later discussion).

4. Assisted reproduction technology

a. Induction of ovulation

(1) Clomiphene citrate: Binds hypothalamic estrogen receptors and increases GnRH release. This is usually effective within 3–6 cycles. If not, then proceed to more extreme measures.

(2) hMG: Directly increases FSH and LH. Menotropins are most commonly used (Pergonal). Pergonal is more effective than clomiphene but also can produce ovarian hyperstimulation and multiple gestation pregnancy.

Both clomiphene and hMG cause development of multiple follicles, but hMG is more likely to result in multiple gestations.

b. Advanced techniques

(1) In vitro fertilization (IVF): Fertilization occurs in vitro, and the zygote is placed into the uterus using a catheter.

(2) Gamete intrafallopian transfer (GIFT): Mature eggs are laparoscopically placed into the fallopian tube with washed sperm.

(3) Zygote intrafallopian transfer (ZIFT): Zygotes are placed laparoscopically into the fallopian tube after being fertilized in vitro.

X. Benign Disorders of the Lower Genital Tract

A. Congenital Genitourinary Anomalies (Table 9-10)

B. Vulvar Dystrophies

1. Hypertrophic lesions: Often the result of chronic vulvar irritation.

a. Most common form is lichen simplex chronicus.

b. Patients with acute disease display erythematous lesions, but these may develop into raised white lesions over time.

c. Treat with hydrocortisone cream to decrease pruritus and local inflammation.

2. Atrophic lesions: Usually result from decreased estrogenization of vulvar tissues (common in postmenopause).

a. Most common form is lichen sclerosus et atrophicus.

b. Patients are postmenopausal and have dysuria, dyspareunia, vulvodynia, and pruritus. The lesions can be erythematous or hyperkeratotic secondary to chronic scratching and rubbing. Fusion of the labia minora and majora and thinning of the local tissues may also be seen.

c. All suspicious lesions should be sampled for biopsy.

d. Treat with hydrocortisone topically (to decrease itching) and with testosterone cream (to build up the atrophic epithelium) for 6 weeks. Patients may require corticosteroid injections if a stronger effect is needed.

TABLE 9-10 Congenital Anomalies of the Genitourinary Tract

Disorder	Description	Treatment
Labial fusion	(1) Associated with excess androgens (exogenous androgens or endogenous androgens due to an enzymatic error). 21α-hydroxylase deficiency, causing congenital adrenal hyperplasia, is the most common congenital cause. (2) Patients have ambiguous genitalia. Most will also have an adrenal crisis with salt wasting (see Chapter 3).	(1) Cortisol decreases the secretion of ACTH. (2) Give a mineralocorticoid (fludrocortisone acetate) for salt wasting. (3) Perform reconstructive surgery for anatomic abnormalities.
Imperforate hymen	(1) The hymen is located between the sinovaginal bulbs and the urogenital sinus, and should have an opening. (2) Imperforate hymen usually presents as primary amenorrhea in the setting of menstrual cramps resulting from lack of outflow. Patients can also experience abdominal pain and an increase in lower abdominal girth as fluid accumulates. (3) Physical examination reveals hematocolpos (build-up of blood behind the hymen), hydrocolpos, or mucocolpos.	Treat with surgery.
Transverse vaginal septum	(1) The vagina forms as the müllerian system joins the sinovaginal bulb at the müllerian tubercle, which then must be canalized for a normal vagina to form. Lack of canalization results in a transverse vaginal septum between the lower two thirds and the upper one third of the vagina. (2) Patients have primary amenorrhea and cramping, but the hymen is normal.	Treat with surgery.
Mayer-Rokitansky-Küster-Hauser-(MRKH) syndrome	(1) Müllerian agenesis or dysgenesis with aberrant development. The vagina may be present as a rudimentary pouch. (2) The patient has ovaries and a 46,XX karyotype.	Treat with surgery using serial dilatation or a split-thickness skin graft from the GI tract. "Vagina" must be kept open by dilation or intercourse.
Testicular feminization	(1) Patients have a 46,XY karyotype but are insensitive to testosterone. (2) They may have a rudimentary vagina as in MRKH syndrome, and undescended testicles may be palpable on physical examination.	(1) Treat with surgery. (2) Undescended testicles must be removed.

C. Cervical Abnormalities
1. Cervical cysts
a. Most are dilated retention cysts called nabothian cysts that arise from blockage of endocervical glands. These do not require treatment.
b. Mesonephric cysts are remnants of the mesonephric (wolffian) ducts that tend to lie deeper in the cervical stroma and on the external surface of the cervix.
c. Endometriosis also can cause cysts in the cervix (see later discussion).
2. Cervical polyps: Produce symptoms only if they are occluding the os. These have minimal malignant potential, but they are usually removed to prevent later confusion.
3. Cervical fibroids: Can produce symptoms of intermenstrual bleeding, dyspareunia, or bladder and rectal pressure. They are usually removed only if they are symptomatic.
4. Cervical stenosis
a. Can be congenital, the product of scarring, or secondary to obstruction by a neoplasm, polyp, or fibroid.
b. Symptoms of cervical obstruction may occur.
c. Removal of obstructive lesions and dilation may allow better outflow.

XI. Vulvar and Vaginal Neoplasia
A. Preinvasive Vulvar Disease
1. Extramammary Paget's disease: Intraepithelial neoplasia that can be associated with underlying adenocarcinoma with high metastatic potential.
a. Patients (usually >60 years of age) have long-standing pruritus that accompanies velvety-red lesions of the skin. These skin lesions can become eczematous and scar into white plaques.
b. Evaluation includes vulvar biopsy.
c. Treat with wide local excision. Recurrence rate is high.
2. Vulvar intraepithelial neoplasia (VIN): Premalignant disease of the vulva most commonly found in patients in their 50s and 60s.
a. Risk factors include human papillomavirus (HPV) infection, cigarette smoking, and immunosuppression.
b. Patients have vulvar pruritus or vulvodynia unresponsive to treatments for candidiasis. Younger women may have multifocal lesions that can rapidly become invasive and more aggressive. Older women have single lesions that are usually slower to become invasive.
c. Treatment
(1) Wide local excision.
(2) Laser ablation can be done, but it does not allow pathologic evaluation.
(3) Follow up with colposcopies every 3 months until the patient has been disease free for 2 years. The interval can then be extended to 6 months.
B. Vulvar Carcinoma
1. Risk factors include a history of vulvar dysplasia, low socioeconomic status, and smoking. HPV infection is present in over half of cases, but it may not be a true risk factor.

2. Squamous cell is the most common type, but melanoma, sarcoma, and undifferentiated types also occur.
3. Patients have pruritus, palpable mass, ulceration, or dysuria in the vulvar region for several months with a failure of antifungal treatment.
4. Diagnosis is made by vulvar biopsy.
5. Treat with wide excision or radical local excision. Groin dissection may be required for lesions that invade more than 1 mm, or that are greater than 2 cm in width. Radiation therapy can be used for locally advanced disease, and chemotherapy is used only for metastasis outside the pelvis.

XII. Cervical Cancer

A. The major risk factor for cervical cancer is HPV infection. Certain subtypes of HPV can lead to cervical intraepithelial neoplasia (CIN) and eventually to cancer. Current screening for cervical cancer evaluates cervical cells for changes consistent with dysplasia or HPV infection, and more specific tests are available to specifically screen for the high-risk types of HPV infection.
B. Patients typically are asymptomatic but may have irregular vaginal bleeding.
C. Most are squamous cell carcinomas, but adenocarcinomas, sarcomas, neuroendocrine tumors, and melanoma can also occur.
D. Cervical cancer cannot be diagnosed by Pap smear, but cytologic changes indicative of atypical or dysplastic cells are sufficient to justify cervical biopsy. Low-grade intraepithelial lesions (often called ASCUS lesions owing to the presence of atypical squamous cells of undetermined significance) can be further evaluated by colposcopy. Cervical biopsy using a cold knife, loop electrosurgical excision procedure (LEEP), or a carbon dioxide laser can be performed in cases of an abnormal or insufficient colposcopic sample, or evidence of high-grade cells or invasive disease on cytologic examination. Cervical biopsy allows the definitive diagnosis of cervical cancer.
E. Staging: Cystoscopy, proctoscopy, bimanual examination, and biopsy are required.
1. Stage I: Tumor is confined to the cervix.
2. Stage II: Tumor is beyond the cervix but has not extended to the pelvic wall.
3. Stage III: Tumor has extended to the pelvic wall.
4. Stage IV: Metastasis outside the pelvis.
F. Treatment
1. Surgery is indicated only when the entire lesion can be removed. Local excision can be done for microscopic disease, or hysterectomy can be performed for larger lesions.
2. Radiation therapy can be used for disease confined to the pelvis.
3. Chemotherapy can be used for metastasis outside the pelvis.

XIII. Uterine Disease

A. Anatomic Anomalies of the Uterus
1. Usually result from problems during fusion of the paramesonephric (wolffian) ducts. There may also be urinary tract abnormalities.

2. Types include septate uterus, bicornuate uterus (with or without double cervix), or uterus didelphys with a double cervix and possibly a septate vagina.
3. Symptoms and signs
   a. Patients have dysmenorrhea, dyspareunia, cyclic pelvic pain, and infertility.
   b. Uterine septa are fibrous and may interfere with implantation or pregnancy. Patients may have recurrent first-trimester pregnancy loss.
   c. Bicornuate uterus usually causes problems in pregnancy due to size restriction. These are associated with second-trimester abortion, premature labor, and malpresentation.
4. Treat with surgical repair if the patient is symptomatic.

B. Uterine Leiomyoma (Fibroid)
1. These tumors are usually hormonally responsive to estrogen, which means that they may grow quickly during pregnancy or during exposure to exogenous estrogens. They may also atrophy during menopause.
2. Symptoms and signs
   a. Patients are usually asymptomatic, but the fibroids can become large enough to cause a mass effect on pelvic structures, with pain and pressure.
   b. Abnormal uterine bleeding, anemia, and infertility are other common complaints of patients with fibroids. A uterine mass may be palpable on bimanual examination.
   c. In pregnant patients, fibroids can cause IUGR, malpresentation, premature labor, and shoulder dystocia.
3. Treatment
   a. Surgical excision with myomectomy (if the patient wants to retain fertility) or hysterectomy.
   b. If the patient is pregnant, the infant must be delivered by cesarean section to prevent malpresentation and shoulder dystocia.
   c. Pharmacologic therapies: Medroxyprogesterone, danazol, GnRH agonists (nafarelin acetate, leuprolide) can be effective.

C. Endometrial Hyperplasia: Abnormal proliferation of glandular and stromal elements of the endometrium resulting in histologic alteration and/or cellular atypia
1. Risk factors are consistent with unopposed estrogen exposure (obesity, nulliparity, late menopause, and exogenous estrogen use without progesterone, chronic anovulation, polycystic ovary syndrome, and estrogen producing tumors).
2. Patients have abnormal or excessive uterine bleeding, and they may have an enlarged uterus.
3. Evaluation includes ultrasonography and endometrial biopsy. Dilation and curettage (D&C) is indicated in patients with a history of atypical complex hyperplasia, or in whom biopsy is difficult.
4. Treat with progestin therapy (medroxyprogesterone or megestrol) for 3 months with a follow-up endometrial biopsy. Atypical complex hyperplasia has a significant risk of developing into endometrial carcinoma, so it can be treated by hysterectomy in patients who are not interested in future fertility.

D. Endometriosis: Presence of endometrial tissue and stroma outside the endometrial cavity

1. Risk factors include family history and a history of adenomyosis.
2. Symptoms and signs
   a. Patients have dysmenorrhea, dyspareunia, cyclic pelvic pain, and infertility. Other symptoms include premenstrual and postmenstrual spotting, menorrhagia, ovulatory pain, and midcycle bleeding.
   b. Uterosacral nodularity, tender ovaries, or a fixed or retroverted uterus may be detected on physical examination.
3. Laparoscopy allows visualization of the lesions. Look for dark brown "powder burns" or raised, blue-colored "mulberry" or "raspberry" lesions.
4. Treatment
   a. Expectant management for patients with minimal symptoms.
   b. Medical treatment with medroxyprogesterone, oral contraceptives, danazol, or leuprolide.
   c. Surgical treatments include conservative therapy (using laser ablation or electrocautery) and hysterectomy with bilateral salpingo-oophorectomy.

The most common sites of endometriosis are the ovary and the pelvic peritoneum.

"chocolate cysts"

E. Adenomyosis: Extension of the endometrial glands and stroma into the uterine musculature

1. Risk factors include endometriosis and leiomyomas.
2. Patients have dysmenorrhea, menorrhagia, and pressure symptoms. Signs include a symmetrically enlarged uterus with a softer consistency than found in a uterine myoma.
3. Evaluate with MRI and postoperative pathologic studies following hysterectomy.
4. Treatment
   a. Women near menopause with minimal symptoms may be treated with analgesics alone.
   b. Hysterectomy is the only definitive treatment.

The uterus becomes diffusely enlarged and globular owing to hypertrophy and hyperplasia of the myometrium adjacent to ectopic tissue. It does not undergo cyclic changes induced by the ovary.

F. Endometrial Cancer

1. Risk factors are related to age and unopposed estrogen exposure (estrogen replacement therapy, obesity, anovulatory cycles, early menarche, late menopause, nulliparity, and tamoxifen use).
2. Patients have abnormal uterine bleeding, usually postmenopausally.
3. Evaluate with endometrial biopsy. D&C should be performed on patients with persistent bleeding or suspicious findings on biopsy.
4. Types include adenocarcinoma, and mucinous, serous carcinoma, and clear cell and squamous cell carcinomas. Metastatic tumors from breast, ovarian, gastric, colonic, and pancreatic cancers can occur.
5. Treatment
   a. Local disease can be treated with hysterectomy and bilateral salpingo-oophorectomy. Patients with high-risk histologic characteristics and involvement of the ovaries, serosa, cervix, or vagina should also receive pelvic and periaortic lymph node sampling.
   b. Advanced disease can be treated with chemotherapy (cisplatin and doxorubicin).

XIV. Ovarian Disease

A. Ovarian Cysts

1. Follicular cysts: Most common functional cysts
   a. Arise after failure of the follicle to rupture.
   b. These are usually asymptomatic and unilateral, but they may cause a tender and palpable ovarian mass or ovarian torsion.
   c. Most spontaneously disappear within 60 days.
2. Corpus lutein cysts
   a. Occur during the luteal phase of the menstrual cycle and may fail to regress.
   b. Can cause a delay in menstruation and a dull, lower quadrant pain.
   c. Corpus hemorrhagicum can cause acute pain and signs of hemoperitoneum.
3. Theca lutein cysts: Small bilateral cysts filled with clear, straw-colored liquid. They usually result from stimulation by abnormally high hCG from a molar pregnancy, choriocarcinoma, or clomiphene therapy.
4. Treatment for the preceding cysts is dependent on age.
   a. Prepubertal or postmenopausal patient: Exploratory laparotomy.
   b. Reproductive-age patient: Exploratory laparotomy or laparoscopy if the cyst is greater than 8 cm or is present for longer than 60 days. Otherwise only observation and follow-up ultrasonography are required. Oral contraceptive pills can be used to suppress gonadotropin secretion.

B. Ovarian Cancer

1. Ovarian cancer is thought to be related to chronic uninterrupted ovulation. Oral contraceptives are thought to be protective. Risk factors include family history, history of uninterrupted ovulation (nulliparity, decreased fertility, delayed childbearing, late menopause), and a history of breast cancer.
2. Symptoms and signs
   a. Patients are usually asymptomatic, but some will have lower abdominal pain or enlargement. Symptoms of advanced disease include gastrointestinal complaints, urinary frequency, dysuria, pelvic pressure, and ascites.
   b. Physical examination findings include ascites and a solid, fixed pelvic mass.
3. Types (Table 9-11)
4. Evaluation
   a. Pelvic ultrasonography: Signs of malignancy include size greater than 8 cm, solid or mixed consistency (not cystic), multilocular septation, and bilateral findings.
   b. CT scan to evaluate metastatic disease.
   c. Tumor markers can be used to follow some cancers.
      (1) CA-125 can be expressed by epithelial cell tumors.
      (2) α-Fetoprotein (AFP) and hCG can be expressed by germ cell tumors.
5. Treatment (see Table 9-11)

Ovarian cancer tends to spread to lymph nodes, peritoneum, lung, and brain.

TABLE 9-11 Types of Ovarian Tumors

Type	Symptoms and Signs	Evaluation	Treatment
Epithelial tumors	(1) Derived from the surface mesothelial cells of the ovary. Types include serous, mucinous, endometrioid, clear cell, Brenner's, and undifferentiated. (2) Typically slow growing and not diagnosed until very late.	Marker is CA-125; more often used to evaluate progression/ regression instead of as a diagnostic tool (not specific).	(1) Surgical treatment with hysterectomy and bilateral salpingo-oophorectomy. (2) Chemotherapy with cisplatin and paclitaxel (Taxol). (3) Associated with poor prognosis.
Germ cell tumors	(1) Arise from totipotent germ cells. (2) Usually occur in women in their teens and 20s. (3) 95% are benign. (4) Patients have a rapidly enlarging adnexal mass and abdominal pain. (5) The most common types are dysgerminomas and immature teratomas. Other types include embryonal cell carcinoma, endodermal sinus (yolk sac) tumors, nongestational choriocarcinoma, and mixed germ cell tumors.	Tumor markers expressed include LDH (dysgerminomas), AFP (embryonal sinus), and hCG (choriocarcinomas).	(1) Surgical removal of involved ovary. (2) Multidrug chemotherapy using platinum-based therapy. (3) Whole abdominal irradiation is useful for dysgerminomas.
Sex cord–stromal tumors	(1) Arise from either the sex cords of the embryonic ovary or the stroma of the ovary. (2) Rare and typically bilateral. (3) Typically affect women in their 40s to 70s. (4) Types (a) Granulosa–theca cell tumors: resemble fetal ovaries and produce excessive estrogen. Symptoms include feminization, precocious puberty, and postmenopausal bleeding.	Serum hormone levels may be helpful in distinguishing the hormone-secreting tumors.	Chemotherapy is ineffective, so the only treatment is hysterectomy and bilateral salpingo-oophorectomy.

continued

TABLE 9-11 Types of Ovarian Tumors—cont'd

Type	Symptoms and Signs	Evaluation	Treatment
	(b) Sertoli-Leydig cell tumors: resemble fetal testis and produce testosterone and other androgens. Symptoms include hirsutism, deepened voice, acne, and clitorimegaly. (c) Ovarian fibromas: Develop from mature fibroblasts. Patients can have ascites and/or Meigs' syndrome (ovarian tumor, ascites, and right hydrothorax).		
Fallopian tube cancers	(1) Bilateral in 10% to 20% of cases and often the result of metastasis. (2) Tumor can spread to the peritoneum and cause ascites.	Usually diagnosed incidentally.	Treatment includes hysterectomy with bilateral salpingo-oophorectomy, adjunct chemotherapy, and possible total abdominal irradiation.

AFP, α-fetoprotein; hCG, human chorionic gonadotropin; LDH, lactic dehydrogenase.

XV. Gestational Trophoblastic Disease: Can produce high levels of hCG (Table 9-12)

The pelvis is supported by muscles (levator muscles), fascia (urogenital diaphragm, endopelvic fascia), and ligaments (uterosacral and cardinal ligaments).

XVI. Pelvic Relaxation and Incontinence

A. Causes: May be caused by birth trauma, chronic increases in intra-abdominal pressure (obesity, chronic cough, heavy lifting), intrinsic weakness, or atrophic changes due to aging or estrogen deficiency.

B. Herniations: Herniations into the vaginal vault may involve the bladder (cystocele), urethra (urethrocele), rectum (rectocele), small bowel (enterocele), or uterus (uterine prolapse).

C. Degrees of Pelvic Relaxation

1. First degree: Structure is in the upper two thirds of the vagina.
2. Second degree: Structure has descended to the level of the introitus.
3. Third degree: Structure protrudes out of the vagina.

D. Symptoms: Symptoms include pelvic pressure and pain, dyspareunia, bowel and bladder dysfunction, and urinary incontinence

E. Types of Urinary Incontinence (Table 9-13)

TABLE 9-12 Types of Gestational Trophoblastic Disease

Disorder	Description	Treatment
Molar pregnancy	(1) Also called hydatidiform mole. (2) Types include complete mole (trophoblastic proliferation and the absence of fetal parts) and incomplete mole (molar degeneration in association with an abnormal fetus). (3) Patients have irregular or heavy vaginal bleeding early in pregnancy. Patients may also have uterine contractions, hypertension, hyperemesis, hyperthyroidism, and trophoblastic pulmonary emboli. (4) Physical examination may reveal large grapelike clusters in the vagina, large bilateral theca-lutein cysts, and the absence of fetal heart sounds. (5) hCG levels are abnormally high, and pelvic ultrasound shows a snowstorm pattern with no fetus in the uterus.	(1) Remove uterine contents by suction dilation and evacuation (D&E) or hysterectomy. (2) Follow up with hCG testing until normal for 1 year. Prevent pregnancy during the testing period. (3) Complete mole has more malignant potential than incomplete mole.
Invasive mole	(1) Result from a malignant transformation of benign disease or a recurrence of gestational trophoblastic disease. (2) The molar villi and trophoblasts penetrate locally into the myometrium and can reach through the peritoneal cavity.They do not often metastasize. (3) Presentation is the same as for molar pregnancy, but it may happen during the follow-up period of a previous molar pregnancy. (4) hCG is high, and ultrasound results are similar to those seen in a molar pregnancy.	Sensitive to chemotherapy. Treat nonmetastatic disease with methotrexate or actinomycin D. Treat metastatic disease with **m**ethotrexate, **a**ctinomycin D, and **c**hlorambucil (MAC).
Choriocarcinoma	(1) Malignant necrotizing tumor that can arise from trophoblastic tissue weeks to years after any type of gestation (50% after molar pregnancy, 25% after term pregnancy, 25% after abortion or ectopic pregnancy). It invades the uterine walls and venous channels with trophoblastic cells. (2) It is often metastatic and spreads hematogenously to the lungs, vagina, pelvis, brain, liver, intestines, and kidneys. (3) Patients have symptoms and signs of metastatic disease. (4) Evaluate with hCG and ultrasonography. Evaluate for metastases.	Sensitive to chemotherapy using the regimens described for invasive moles.
Placental site trophoblastic tumor (rare)	(1) Arise from the placental implantation site and subsequently invade the myometrium and blood vessels. (2) Common symptoms include bleeding that can occur weeks to years after an antecedent pregnancy. (3) These tumors are rarely metastatic and produce only low levels of hCG.	Not sensitive to chemotherapy. Treatment of choice is hysterectomy.

TABLE 9-13
Types of Urinary Incontinence

Disorder	Symptoms and Signs	Diagnostic Tests	Treatment
Stress incontinence	(1) Increases in abdominal pressure are distributed more to the bladder than to the urethra, which results in the expulsion of urine. (2) Associated with pelvic relaxation and displacement of the urethrovesical junction. (3) Patients have urine loss when they exert or strain themselves.	Standing stress test or cotton swab test (while coughing).	(1) Kegel exercises to increase urethral closing pressure. (2) Pharmacotherapy with estrogen replacement, alpha-adrenergic agonists (prazosin, terazocin, phenoxybenzamine, pseudoephedrine) to increase urethral sphincter tone. (3) Pessaries or surgery to support the bladder neck and restore anatomic relationships.
Urge incontinence (detrusor instability)	(1) Leakage due to involuntary bladder contractions. (2) Causes include bladder wall irritation (from stones, foreign body, UTI, or tumor) or neurologic dysfunction. (3) Patients have urgency, frequency, and nocturia.	Ultrasonography.	(1) Pharmacotherapy with cholinergics (bethanechol), alpha-adrenergic agonists, smooth muscle relaxants (diazepam, dantrolene). (2) Behavioral training with Kegel exercises, bladder training, and psychotherapy.
Total incontinence	(1) Usually caused by fistula formation due to pelvic surgery, radiation therapy, endometriosis, pelvic inflammatory disease, or ectopic ureters. (2) Patients present with painless, continuous loss of urine.	(1) Methylene blue infusion to the bladder to diagnose vesiculovaginal fistula. (2) Indigo carmine infusion to the bladder to diagnose ureterovaginal fistula. (3) Cystourethroscopy or intravenous pyelography (IVP) can be used to further localize the fistulas.	Give antibiotics, estrogen (if patient is postmenopausal), and corticosteroids for 3–6 months postoperatively to prevent infection and decrease inflammation. After this period, fix surgically.

TABLE 9-13 Types of Urinary Incontinence—cont'd

Disorder	Symptoms and Signs	Diagnostic Tests	Treatment
Overflow incontinence	(1) Occurs owing to absent bladder contractions. (2) Can be caused by neurologic dysfunction, urethral obstruction, medications, psychogenic factors, or fecal impaction. (3) Patients have frequent or constant urinary dribbling with symptoms of stress and urge incontinence.	Imaging as necessary to rule out fistula, stress incontinence, and urge incontinence.	(1) Treat with alpha-adrenergic agents, cholinergics, and muscle relaxants. (2) Symptoms can be managed with self-catheterization. (3) Surgical correction can be performed.

F. Treatment
1. Kegel exercises to strengthen the pelvic musculature.
2. Mechanical support devices: Pessaries can support the pelvis in patients in whom surgery is contraindicated or relaxation may be temporary (postpartum).
3. Surgical repair: Varies from suspension to colorrhaphy to hysterectomy, depending on the cause of the problem.
4. Estrogen replacement: Can reverse atrophic changes and increase tone.

10 CHAPTER

Oncology

Esophageal cancer most commonly occurs in men over age 50. It has an incidence of 5 in 100,000.

Barrett's esophagus increases the risk of developing adenocarcinoma by 40 times. Patients with Barrett's esophagus require esophagoscopy and biopsy yearly, and patients with low-grade dysplasia should have a biopsy every 6 months.

I. Esophageal Cancer

A. Symptoms: Patients often have progressive dysphagia and greater difficulty swallowing solids than liquids.

B. Types

1. Squamous cell cancer is the most common type. Risk factors include smoking, alcohol, and nutritional deficiencies.
2. Adenocarcinoma is another common type. Risk factors include gastroesophageal reflux disease and Barrett's esophagus (columnar metaplasia of the distal esophagus).

C. Evaluation

1. Barium swallow evaluation should be performed before other tests to define the anatomy of the esophagus and possibly identify the cause of dysphagia.
2. Esophagoscopy allows direct visualization of the lesion and biopsy of any abnormal regions.
3. Bronchoscopy may be performed in patients with concurrent pulmonary symptoms.
4. Endoscopic ultrasonography can be useful for clinical staging.

D. Treatment

1. Surgical procedures include Ivor-Lewis esophagectomy (in which the esophagus is resected using an approach from the right chest) or transhiatal esophagectomy (in which the esophagus is approached from the abdomen and the neck for resection). Pyloroplasty or pyloromyotomy also are performed because both vagus nerves are removed. The colon or jejunum can be used as a conduit if the stomach needs to be removed. The risk of anastomotic leak is higher for cervical anastomosis than for intrathoracic anastomosis, but intrathoracic leaks are a more serious complication.
2. Contraindications to surgery include advanced age, severe illness, tumor invasion of vital structures (aorta), malignant esophagorespiratory fistula, and metastatic disease.
3. Radiation therapy can be performed in patients unsuitable for surgery.
4. Chemotherapy using cisplatin-based combination therapy can be effective. Specialized forms of chemotherapy include brachytherapy (which uses intracavitary radioactive materials to locally treat the tumor) and phototherapy (which uses photoactivated compounds to produce singlet oxygen in the area exposed to light).

E. Prognosis: Of patients who have disease limited to the esophagus and are candidates for surgery, 25% can be cured. The prognosis is poorer for disease outside the esophagus.

Gastric cancer most commonly occurs in men over age 40. The incidence is especially high in Japan, Chile, and Iceland.

II. Gastric Cancer

A. Risk Factors

1. Gastric polyps (adenomatous, not hyperplastic).
2. Chronic atrophic gastritis and intestinal metaplasia.
3. Pernicious anemia: These patients have gastric mucosal atrophy, low levels of intrinsic factor, and vitamin B_{12} deficiency in association with autoantibodies that bind gastric parietal cells and intrinsic factor.
4. Ménétrier's disease: Hyperplasia of the gastric mucosal folds.
5. Benign gastric ulcer.
6. *Helicobacter pylori* infection.
7. Diet: Nitrates, alcohol.
8. Smoking.

B. Symptoms and Signs

1. Patients can have weight loss, nausea, abdominal pain, and anorexia.
2. Proximal gastric tumors often cause dysphagia, whereas distal gastric cancers often cause gastric outlet obstruction.
3. Blood loss from gastric tumors may manifest with anemia, melena, occult blood in the stool, or coffee-ground emesis.
4. Signs of metastatic gastric cancer include Virchow's node (palpable left supraclavicular node), Irish's node (palpable left axillary node), Sister Mary Joseph's sign (periumbilical mass from nodal metastasis), Krukenburg's tumor (ovarian tumor associated with metastatic gastric cancer), and Blumer's shelf (shelf found on pelvic or rectal examination indicating peritoneal metastasis).

C. Adenocarcinomas make up 95% of gastric cancers. Other tumor types include leiomyosarcoma, lymphoma, and rarely adenosquamous, squamous, and carcinoid tumors.

D. Evaluation

1. An upper GI imaging series should be done first to define the anatomy of the GI tract.
2. Endoscopy allows direct visualization and biopsy sampling of lesions. A biopsy should be taken of all ulcerative lesions.
3. CT scans can be used to evaluate for metastases and local invasion.
4. Endoscopic ultrasound allows an assessment of the depth of penetration and lymph node involvement.

E. Treatment

1. Laparoscopy can be performed for staging and jejunostomy tube insertion, if necessary.
2. Neoadjuvant therapy (irradiation or chemotherapy before surgery) can be effective in gastric cancers.
   a. Advantages of neoadjuvant therapy:
      (1) Better blood flow to the tumor.
      (2) Postoperative complications might have delayed the initiation of therapy.
      (3) Preoperative therapy may cause shrinkage of the tumor and increase the likelihood of excision of all tumor cells.

b. Disadvantages of neoadjuvant therapy:
(1) It may cause an increase in surgical morbidity or mortality.
(2) The delay of surgery may allow tumor growth or metastasis.

3. For proximal gastric cancer, a radical total gastrectomy can be performed. This involves the removal of the omentum, stomach, and the first portion of the duodenum.
4. For distal gastric cancer, a radical distal gastrectomy can be performed. This involves removal of the omentum, most of the stomach, and the first portion of the duodenum.
5. Reconstruction can be done with a Roux-en-Y esophagojejunostomy.
6. Palliative therapy (using surgical bypass or dilation techniques, chemotherapy, or radiation) can be performed for patients with dysphagia and metastatic disease.
7. Complications of surgery for gastric cancer are shown in Table 10-1.

F. Prognosis: Prognosis is extremely variable and depends on the portion of the stomach involved, depth of invasion locally, and presence of spread outside the stomach. No cure is available for patients with spread outside the stomach.

III. Pancreatic Cancer

A. Risk Factors: Smoking, diabetes, alcohol use, benzidine or β-naphthylamine exposure, and others

B. Symptoms and Signs

1. Patients can have decreased food intake and pruritus (due to bile salt deposition in the skin). Tumors of the pancreatic head often cause painless obstructive jaundice. Tumors of the body or tail of the pancreas may cause more general symptoms of weight loss and pain in the absence of jaundice.
2. Physical examination findings include a palpable nontender gallbladder (Courvoisier's sign), acholic stools, and dark urine.
3. Patients may have bleeding problems due to coagulation defects (as a result of vitamin K deficiency or hepatocellular dysfunction).

C. Types (Table 10-2)

D. Evaluation

1. Liver function tests (LFTs) may show increased direct bilirubin and alkaline phosphatase as indicators of biliary obstruction.
2. Prothrombin time (PT) may be prolonged and nutritional studies (total protein, albumin, and prealbumin) may be abnormal owing to liver dysfunction.
3. Spiral CT scanning with oral and IV contrast is the preferred imaging modality.
4. Ultrasonography can be used to evaluate for biliary obstruction.
5. Percutaneous biopsy is not done, because of the risk of seeding the peritoneum with tumor cells.

E. Treatment

1. Surgery can be performed starting with diagnostic laparoscopy to determine the resectability of the tumor.

TABLE 10-1 Complications Encountered Following Gastrectomy

Complication	Description
Anastomotic leak	(1) A leak of the surgical anastomosis of two segments of the GI tract. (2) Patients have fever, abdominal tenderness, and leukocytosis. (3) Check for anastomotic leaks on postoperative day 5 or 6 with an oral contrast radiograph. (4) Small leaks may be treated with drain placement by an interventional radiologist. Large leaks require immediate surgery for correction.
Dumping syndrome	(1) Early symptoms include vasomotor (diaphoresis, weakness, dizziness, and palpitations) and gastrointestinal (nausea, abdominal fullness, pain, cramping, and diarrhea) symptoms within 30 minutes of eating. These symptoms are caused by a high osmotic load in the GI tract. (2) Late symptoms appear 2–4 hours after eating. These mainly consist of vasomotor symptoms caused by insulin hyperresponsiveness to a carbohydrate load. (3) Dumping syndrome can be avoided by eating small daily meals that are high in protein and low in carbohydrate. Fluid intake should also be restricted. (4) Cases unresponsive to dietary management can be treated with octreotide.
Postvagotomy gastroparesis	(1) Poor gastric emptying can result in recurrent bezoar formation in the stomach. (2) Delayed gastric emptying can be documented using radionuclide gastric emptying studies. (3) Can be treated with prokinetic agents (erythromycin) or resection of the atonic areas.
Postvagotomy diarrhea	(1) Patients have rapid small intestinal transit and numerous liquid stools per day. (2) May resolve with time or may require surgical intervention to slow small intestinal transit.
Alkaline reflux gastritis	Can present with epigastric pain and bilious vomiting.
Afferent loop syndrome	(1) Patients have postprandial epigastric fullness and pain that is relieved by bilious vomiting. (2) CT scan demonstrates dilation of the proximal small intestine. (3) Surgical correction is necessary for treatment.
Megaloblastic anemia	Can occur due to a lack of intrinsic factor following gastrectomy, which impairs vitamin B_{12} absorption. Give vitamin B_{12} as treatment.

2. Evidence of metastasis, advanced cardiac or pulmonary disease, and portal hypertension make the tumor nonresectable. In these cases, endoscopic stenting can be performed to relieve obstructive jaundice and minimize the side effects of hyperbilirubinemia (pruritus). Opioids can be given for pain.
3. For resectable tumors of the pancreatic head, a Whipple procedure (resection of the gastric antrum, gallbladder, duodenum, head of the

TABLE 10-2
Common Types of Pancreatic Cancer

Type	Description
Ductal adenocarcinoma	(1) Most of these tumors arise in the head and neck of the pancreas. (2) The resectability rate is low and prognosis is poor because of advanced disease at diagnosis. However nonadenocarcinoma types of pancreatic cancer have a better prognosis.
Cystic tumors	(1) Serous cystoadenomas are found in the head area, and they have the characteristic "honeycomb" appearance of cysts <2 cm. Removal is indicated if the mass is rapidly enlarging or the patient is symptomatic. (2) Mucinous cystic neoplasms usually occur in the body and tail areas and are composed of cysts that are >2 cm in size and may have papillary or solid components in the walls. These have a higher malignant potential than cystoadenomas and should always be removed.
Islet cell tumor (insulinoma)	Patients present with Whipple's triad (hypoglycemia, mental status changes/vasomotor instability, and relief of symptoms with the administration of glucose). Treat symptoms with glucose, and remove the mass.
Somatostatinoma	(1) Somatostatin inhibits gallbladder contraction, so these tumors are associated with gallstone formation. (2) Patients often also have diabetes and steatorrhea.
Glucagonoma	Patients have diabetes and a characteristic dermatitis (necrotizing migratory erythema).
Gastrinoma	Associated with Zollinger-Ellison syndrome (gastrinoma with peptic ulcer disease due to excessive gastric acid production).

pancreas, and common bile duct) or pylorus-preserving Whipple procedure can be performed. Anastomoses are made between the stomach, common hepatic duct, and the pancreatic duct with the small intestine. Complications are frequent and can include pancreatic fistula, anastomotic leak, and postgastrectomy syndromes (see Table 10-1).

4. For tumors of the body or tail of the pancreas, distal resection of the pancreas can be performed. Irradiation and chemotherapy are still experimental for these types of tumors.

F. Prognosis

1. Patients with localized, surgically resectable disease may be cured in 50% of cases.
2. Patients with inoperable tumors have a mean survival of less than 1 year.

The differential diagnosis of lower GI bleeding includes diverticular disease, cancer, inflammatory bowel disease, polyps, vascular ectasias, ischemic colitis, rectal ulcers, hemorrhoids, and upper GI bleeding.

IV. Liver Cancer (Table 10-3)

V. Colorectal Cancer

A. Risk factors include high-fat, low-fiber diets, inflammatory bowel disease, smoking, polyps (adenomatous polyps and familial polyposis, but not hyperplastic polyps), and a family history of colon cancer.

TABLE 10-3
Tumors of the Liver

Type	Description	Evaluation	Treatment
Hemangioma	(1) Most common benign tumor. (2) Patients have right upper quadrant abdominal pain, bruits, congestive heart failure, or shock with bleeding (in cases of rupture).	Diagnose with CT, ultrasonography, or MRI.	Treat by observation, and resect if the patient is symptomatic.
Hepatic adenoma	(1) The main risk factor is oral contraceptive use. Anabolic steroid use and glycogen storage disease are also risk factors. (2) Patients may have abdominal fullness, or rupture of the tumor may cause hemoperitoneum and shock (more common in pregnancy).	(1) Ultrasound and CT scans show a solid tumor with cystic areas of hemorrhage or necrosis. (2) Histologically, the tumor will look like normal hepatocytes without bile ducts.	Discontinue oral contraceptives. Employ surgical resection for subcapsular lesions or if pregnancy might occur, because of the risk of rupture.
Focal nodular hyperplasia	Patients may have abdominal pain and right upper quadrant abdominal mass.	CT scan shows a liver mass with a central scar.	Surgery is needed only for rapidly growing or symptomatic lesions.
Hepatocellular carcinoma	(1) Associated with hepatitis B, cirrhosis, aflatoxin (from *Aspergillus*), schistosomiasis, and glycogen storage disease. (2) 10% of patients with cirrhosis progress to hepatocellular carcinoma. (3) Patients have right upper quadrant abdominal pain, hepatomegaly, constitutional signs, and splenomegaly. (4) The most common site of metastasis is the lung.	(1) Alpha-fetoprotein is elevated. (2) CT or MRI imaging can visualize the tumor.	Possible therapies include resection, transplantation, and interventional radiologic techniques.

continued

TABLE 10-3 Tumors of the Liver—cont'd

Type	Description	Evaluation	Treatment
Cholangiocarcinoma (intrahepatic)	(1) Risk factors include liver fluke infection (from Southeast Asia), sclerosing cholangitis, biliary atresia, cholelithiasis, and exposure to Thorotrast. (2) Patients may have abdominal pain, pruritus, and constitutional symptoms.	(1) Alkaline phosphatase and gamma-glutaryltransferase (GGT) will be increased. (2) Use CT or MRI for localization.	(1) Resection or palliative stent placement can be performed. Half of cases are nonresectable. (2) Chemotherapy using 5-fluorouracil, doxorubicin, or mitomycin C can also be used.
Angiosarcoma	Rare tumor associated with vinyl chloride, arsenic, or Thorotrast contrast exposure.	CT, MRI, and angiography detect lesions.	Perform surgical resection, but most patients die within 6 months.
Metastatic	(1) The patient may have symptoms indicating the primary tumor. (2) Metastatic tumors are 20 times more common than primary tumors of the liver.	Imaging (CT or MRI) and biopsy may help determine the primary tumor location.	Depends on primary tumor type.

B. Patients have weight loss, rectal bleeding, bowel obstruction, diarrhea, tenesmus, change in stool caliber, or perineal pain. Physical examination findings include ascites, hepatomegaly, palpable mass or blood on digital rectal examination, and signs of anemia.

C. Evaluation
   1. Fecal occult blood test, colonoscopy, and sigmoidoscopy can be used as screening tools.
   2. Chest radiograph to evaluate for lung metastases.
   3. CT scan to evaluate for abdominal metastases.
   4. Endorectal ultrasonography allows for tumor staging.
   5. Serum carcinoembryonic antigen (CEA) is a marker for colon cancer.

D. Types of colorectal cancer include adenocarcinoma (most common), carcinoid, leiomyosarcoma, lymphoma, squamous cell carcinoma (in the anal canal), and metastases.

E. Treatment
   1. Surgical removal.
   2. Chemotherapy with 5-fluorouracil and levamisole or leucovorin.
   3. Irinotecan can be used in patients with metastatic disease or tumors unresponsive to 5-fluorouracil therapy.

F. Prognosis
   1. Patients with stage I, II, and III disease are considered curable in most cases.
   2. Patients with stage IV disease have a mean survival of 1–2 years.

VI. Lung Cancer
   A. Risk factors include cigarette smoking and exposure to asbestos or radon. A history of smoking is present in 90% of cases of lung cancer.
   B. Symptoms and Signs
      1. Patients may have cough, dyspnea, hemoptysis, anorexia, and weight loss.
      2. Complications associated with lung cancer include **s**uperior vena cava syndrome, **P**ancoast's tumor, **H**orner's syndrome, **e**ndocrine disorders (paraneoplastic syndromes), **r**ecurrent laryngeal nerve injury, and **e**ffusions (mnemonic—SPHERE).
         a. Superior vena cava syndrome: Usually occurs owing to compression of the superior vena cava by tumor (lung cancer or lymphoma). Symptoms can include cyanosis, edema, venous engorgement of the head and upper body, airway obstruction, and effusions (pleural and pericardial). Superior vena cava thrombosis has a similar presentation and may occur following the use of a subclavian catheter.
         b. Pancoast's tumors cause Horner's syndrome and brachial plexopathy via direct spread of the lung tumor from the lung apex.
         c. Paraneoplastic syndromes can occur in small cell lung cancer and squamous cell lung cancer.
            (1) Small cell lung cancer can produce endocrine symptoms (Cushing's syndrome or SIADH) and neurologic symptoms (weakness due to Lambert-Eaton myasthenic syndrome).
            (2) Squamous cell lung cancer can produce hypercalcemia owing to secretion of a parathyroid hormone–related peptide.
         d. Recurrent laryngeal nerve injury can cause hoarseness.
      3. Signs of metastasis to liver, adrenal, bone, and brain may also be present.
   C. Types
      1. Small cell lung cancer: Highly associated with smoking. It can produce a variety of paraneoplastic syndromes (see previous discussion).
      2. Non–small cell lung cancer.
         a. Squamous cell cancer: Tends to have centrally located endobronchial lesions and may be associated with hypercalcemia.
         b. Adenocarcinoma: Presents with peripheral lung nodules. This type is not associated with smoking.
         c. Large cell lung cancer: Cytologic studies display large, undifferentiated cells. Subtypes include giant cell carcinomas and clear cell carcinomas.
   D. Evaluation
      1. Chest radiograph may show masses, atelectasis, infiltrates, or effusion.
      2. Bronchoscopy may be performed to obtain a biopsy specimen.
      3. Sputum cytology may be performed to characterize tumor cells.
   E. Staging
      1. Stage I: Isolated lesion.
      2. Stage II: Spread to hilar nodes.
      3. Stage IIIa: Resectable mediastinal spread.
      4. Stage IIIb: Nonresectable mediastinal spread.
      5. Stage IV: Metastatic disease.

F. Treatment: Indications for therapy are dependent on stage
1. Stage I: Surgery.
2. Stage II: Surgery with or without radiation therapy.
3. Stage IIIa: Neoadjuvant chemotherapy and radiation therapy followed by surgery.
4. Stage IIIb: Radiation therapy with or without chemotherapy (paclitaxel + carboplatin) and/or surgery. Alternative chemotherapy includes cyclophosphamide, vinorelbine, gemcitabine, or etoposide.
5. Stage IV: Supportive measures; possibly surgery or radiation therapy for brain metastases.

Most lung cancers are unresectable at the time of presentation.

G. Prognosis: Depends on the type of lung cancer.
1. Non–small cell cancers are curable in over half of patients with stage I or II disease and in fewer patients with stage III disease.
2. Small cell lung cancers are curable in up to 25% of cases if the disease is caught early.
3. Advanced-stage small cell lung cancer is curable in less than 5% of cases.

Renal cell cancer most commonly occurs in men over age 55. It has an incidence of 3 in 10,000.

VII. Renal Cancer
A. Risk factors include smoking and von Hippel–Lindau disease.
B. Symptoms and Signs
1. Patients can have hematuria, flank pain, and abdominal mass. Bilateral lower extremity edema can occur if the inferior vena cava is blocked.
2. Paraneoplastic syndromes can include fever, polycythemia, and hypercalcemia.
C. CT and MRI should be performed to assess metastatic spread and inferior vena cava involvement.
D. Treatment
1. Treat with resection and immunomodulation with IL-2 and interferon alpha.
2. Radiation therapy and chemotherapy are not effective.
E. Prognosis
1. Patients with disease confined to the kidney have a 5-year survival rate of up to 75%.
2. Metastasis to lymph nodes lowers the 5-year survival to 15%, and other organ metastases lower the 5-year survival to 5%.

The lifetime risk of a woman developing breast cancer is 10%.

VIII. Breast Cancer
A. Risk factors and Associated Conditions (Table 10-4)
B. Symptoms and Signs
1. Patients can present asymptomatically, or with symptoms of breast pain, breast asymmetry, or nipple discharge.
2. Physical examination signs can include breast dimpling, erythema, and edema (orange peel appearance).
C. Types of Breast Cancer (Table 10-5)
D. Evaluation

TABLE 10-4 Risk Factors for Breast Cancer

Condition	Description
Ductal carcinoma in situ (DCIS)	(1) There are malignant cells in the ducts but no evidence of invasion through the basement membrane. (2) Accounts for 30% of neoplasms diagnosed by mammography, and 30% of these patients will develop invasive ductal carcinoma if left untreated. (3) Spread to axillary nodes is rare enough that axillary node dissection is not recommended.
Lobular carcinoma in situ (LCIS)	(1) There are carcinoma cells in the lobules without invasion. (2) 30% of people with LCIS will develop cancer in either breast. The cancer will not necessarily be in the same breast, and the most common type is infiltrating ductal carcinoma. (3) Treat with intense follow-up.
Papilloma	Most common cause of bloody discharge in young women. It rarely progresses to papillary carcinoma.
History of other breast disease	Including previous breast cancer, hyperplasia, or atypia.
Family history of breast cancer	(1) 5% to 10% of breast cancers are inherited. (a) *BRCA1* gene: 80% of people who have it will get breast cancer, and 40% will get ovarian cancer. (b) *BRCA2* gene: increases breast cancer risk. (2) Genetic testing and prophylactic measures (mastectomy or intense follow-up) are options for women at high risk.
Nulliparity or late first pregnancy	These conditions increase the risk of breast cancer as a result of the increased length of time of unopposed estrogen exposure in the patient's life.
Radiation exposure	Irradiation has mutagenic effects.

1. Mammography
   a. Guidelines vary, but most professional associations advise obtaining a baseline mammogram somewhere after age 40 years (or earlier if there is a positive family history of breast cancer) and then yearly mammograms after age 50.
   b. Indicators of malignancy include stellate or dominant masses and architectural distortion. Invasive cancer is found in 30% of microcalcific lesions after excision.
   c. Mammography misses 10% to 15% of cancers.
2. Ultrasound is useful for at-risk patients under 30 years of age.
3. Breast biopsy can be performed using one of several techniques (wire localized breast biopsy, stereotactic core biopsy, or fine-needle aspiration biopsy).

Common sites of metastasis for breast cancer are lymph nodes, lung, pleura, liver, bone, and brain.

TABLE 10-5 Disorders Associated with Breast Mass

Type	Disorder	Description
Benign	Fibrocystic disease	(1) Causes a green, straw-colored, or brown nipple discharge. (2) Patients present with pain in breast that varies with menstrual cycle. (3) Treat by stopping stimulants and taking NSAIDs. Cysts can be drained. Recurrence requires biopsy.
	Fat necrosis	Most common cause of breast mass after breast trauma.
	Cystosarcoma phyllodes	(1) Benign breast tumor arising from mesenchymal lobular tissue. (2) Presents as mobile, smooth breast mass in a patient over 30 years of age.
	Fibroadenoma	(1) Most common type of breast tumor in people under 30 years of age. (2) Can also present as a solid mobile breast mass.
	Mastitis	(1) Infection of the breast (cellulitis). (2) Commonly associated with *Staphylococcus aureus* and breast-feeding. (3) Rule out inflammatory breast cancer, and treat by discontinuing breast-feeding and administering local heat and antibiotics.
Malignant	Invasive ductal or lobular carcinoma	(1) Diagnosis requires biopsy and histologic evaluation. (2) Patients may have one of several risk factors for the development of breast carcinoma (see Table 10-4).
	Inflammatory carcinoma	(1) Symptoms include breast enlargement, erythema, and edema (orange peel appearance). (2) Treat with chemotherapy preoperatively. (3) Treat aggressively with multiagent chemotherapy. Five-year survival is 50%.
	Paget's disease of the breast	Scaling dermatitis of the nipple caused by invasion of skin by cells from a ductal carcinoma.

E. Treatment

1. For localized disease, excisional biopsy (lumpectomy) with radiotherapy is usually performed. Recurrence rates of lumpectomy alone are approximately 30%. Pregnancy is an absolute contraindication to the use of irradiation.
2. The use of chemotherapy depends on the characteristics on the tumor and whether lymph nodes are involved.
   a. Estrogen receptor–expressing tumors can respond to tamoxifen.

b. For multiagent chemotherapy, combinations of cyclophosphamide/methotrexate/5-fluorouracil, or doxorubicin/cyclophosphamide can be given.

3. Lymph nodes should be tested to assess nodal metastases. If nodal involvement is found, proceed with a total axillary lymph node dissection. For localized disease, the first node in the local lymphatic chain (sentinel node) can be tested to determine whether additional nodes require excision and testing.

4. Reconstruction surgeries, often involving saline implants or transverse rectus abdominis myocutaneous (TRAM) flaps, can be performed to alleviate patient concerns about appearance.

5. Prophylactic bilateral mastectomy is offered to women with the BRCA1 or BRCA2 gene because of their high risk for the development of breast cancer.

6. Complications of surgery include ipsilateral arm lymphedema, infection, and nerve injury.

F. Prognosis

1. Patients with stage 0 or I disease have a 5-year survival rate of 88% to 95%.

2. Patients with stage II, III, and IV disease have 5-year survivals of 66%, 36%, and 7%, respectively.

IX. Prostate Cancer

A. Symptoms and Signs

1. Patients may have hematuria, sudden impotence, perineal pain, and symptoms of bladder outlet obstruction.

2. The patient may have an enlarged and nodular prostate on digital rectal examination.

B. Evaluation

1. Prostate-specific antigen (PSA).

a. PSA greater than 4 units is possible malignancy.

b. PSA greater than 10 units is probably malignancy.

2. Transrectal ultrasound and biopsy will show foci of adenocarcinoma within the gland.

3. Abdominal and pelvic CT scans will assist in staging.

4. Bone scans are indicated to search for bone metastases if PSA is greater than 10 units.

C. Grading is more important than staging. Grading is classified using the Gleason system.

1. Grade A: Incidental finding.

2. Grade B: Cancerous cells confined to the prostate.

3. Grade C: Extracapsular periprostatic spread.

4. Grade D1: Spread to pelvic lymph nodes.

5. Grade D2: Metastatic skeletal disease.

D. Treatment: Surgery is recommended in patients under 65 years old. Patients with locally advanced disease, seminal vesicle involvement, or bone metastases are given hormonal treatment instead of surgery.

Prostate cancer most frequently occurs in men over age 50. It has an incidence of 179 in 100,000 men.

Digital rectal examination is recommended yearly in men after age 50.

1. Grades A and B: Radical prostatectomy or close follow-up.
2. Grade C: Radiation therapy.
3. Grade D: Hormone therapy.
   a. Orchiectomy.
   b. Leuprolide.
   c. Antiandrogen compounds include synthesis inhibitors (ketoconazole or aminoglutethimide) and antagonists (flutamide, cyproterone).

E. Prognosis: Highly variable depending on the patient's comorbidities.

X. Testicular Cancer

A. Most commonly found in men between ages 15 to 40 years.
B. The primary risk factor is cryptorchidism.
C. Symptoms and Signs
   a. Most commonly presents with painless swelling of the testicle.
   b. Hormone-secreting tumors can produce gynecomastia.
   c. Metastases to lung can produce respiratory distress.
D. Evaluation
   a. CT scans for staging.
   b. Serum hCG and AFP can help classify the tumor. Both markers may be present in nonseminomatous germ cell tumors and will be absent in seminomas.
E. Treatment
   1. Tumors restricted to the testicle can be treated with radical orchiectomy.
   2. Seminomas can be cured with radiation therapy.
   3. Nonseminomatous germ cell tumors or metastatic tumors can be treated with chemotherapy using cisplatin, etoposide, and bleomycin.
F. Prognosis: Depends on the type of tumor, but patients with stage I tumors have a survival rate greater than 95% and patients with stage III tumors have a 70% cure rate.

XI. Bladder Cancer

A. The primary risk factor for bladder cancer is smoking. Others are hydrocarbon exposure, long-term cyclophosphamide treatment, and chronic *Schistosoma haematobium* infection.
B. Patients have hematuria and may have bladder spasms. Local spread may cause pelvic bone and leg swelling.
C. Most common type is transitional cell cancer.
D. Evaluation
   1. Cystoscopy for direct visualization.
   2. Routine urine cytologic examination in those occupationally exposed to hydrocarbons.
   3. IV pyelogram is used if cystoscopy fails to localize the lesion.
E. Treatment
   1. Superficial tumors
      a. Transurethral resection of the bladder (TURB).
      b. Cystoscopy every 3 months to assess recurrence.

c. Relapses can be treated with intravesicular bacille Calmette-Guérin (BCG) or thiotepa.

2. Tumors that invade the muscle wall can be treated with cystoscopy and ileal conduit placement.

3. Tumors that invade through the bladder wall should not be treated surgically. Treat with irradiation and multiagent chemotherapy.

F. Prognosis

1. Prognosis is good for stage I and II bladder cancers, but the recurrence rate is high.

2. Patients with stage III disease have a 50% cure rate, and patients with stage IV disease are rarely cured.

XII. Melanoma

A. Patients may have lesions of the skin that show abnormal **a**symmetry, **b**orders, **c**olor, or **d**iameter (>6 mm; mnemonic—ABCD). Men tend to have lesions on the trunk, whereas women have them on the lower limbs, which is consistent with the sun-exposure patterns of each sex.

B. Types include superficial spreading, lentigo maligna, acral lentiginous, and nodular.

C. Evaluate with a punch biopsy, which provides a full thickness sample. Shave biopsies are not so useful, because the depth of the lesion cannot be assessed.

D. Staging: Uses the Breslow system

1. Tis: Melanoma in situ, not invasive.

2. T1: Tumor less than 0.75 mm invading papillary dermis.

3. T2: Tumor 0.75–1.5 mm or invading the papillary-reticulodermal interface.

4. T3: Tumor 1.5–4 mm thick or invading the reticular dermis.

5. T4: Tumor greater than 4 mm thick or invading subcutaneous tissue or satellites within 2 cm of primary tumor.

E. Treatment: Surgical excision

1. Use 1 cm margins for melanoma in situ or tumor less than 1 cm.

2. Use 2 cm margins for tumor greater than 2 cm.

3. Elective lymph node dissection can be performed if micrometastases are a concern.

4. Regional hyperthermic perfusion, in which a chemotherapeutic agent (melphalan) is infused at 40°C, can be used for advanced lesions of the extremities.

F. Prognosis: Depends on degree of spread.

1. Patients with deep lesions or with lymph node spread have a high rate of recurrence.

2. Patients with metastatic spread to other organs have a poor outcome.

One in 85 people in the United States will develop melanoma at some point in their life. Although the risk increases with age, melanoma frequently occurs in young people. It is the most common cause of cancer death in women aged 25 to 30.

XIII. Adult Neuro-oncology (see Chapter 8)

TABLE 10-6 Central Nervous System Tumors Found in Children

Type	Description
Cerebellar astrocytoma	(1) Occurs in children 5–8 years of age. (2) Patients have increased intracranial pressure, nystagmus, and intention tremor. (3) Treat with surgical excision, radiotherapy, and corticosteroids (to decrease tumor edema).
Medulloblastoma	(1) Occurs in children 3–5 years of age. (2) Patients have increased ICP and obstructive hydrocephalus in the fourth ventricle. (3) Can metastasize through the CSF. (4) Treat with surgical excision, radiotherapy, chemotherapy, and corticosteroids.
Ependymoma	(1) Patients have increased ICP and obstructive hydrocephalus in the fourth ventricle. (2) Rarely metastasizes through the CSF. (3) Treatment is the same as for medulloblastoma.
Brainstem glioma	(1) Occurs in children 5–7 years of age. (2) Patients have a triad of multiple cranial nerve deficits (VII, IX, X, V, and VI), lesions in the pyramidal tracts, and cerebellar lesions. (3) ICP will increase late in the course of disease. (4) Treatment includes palliative radiotherapy and experimental chemotherapy.
Pinealoma	(1) Patients have paralysis of upward gaze, eyelid retraction, precocious puberty. Signs of increased ICP may also be present. (2) Metastasis through the CSF may occur.
Hypothalamic glioma	(1) Occurs in children 2–5 months of age. (2) Patients have an alert, euphoric, emaciated appearance, with emesis and optic atrophy. (3) Treat with radiotherapy, which may cause posttreatment obesity.
Cerebral astrocytoma	(1) Occurs in children between 5 and 10 years of age. (2) Patients have personality changes, weakness, seizures, and late increases in ICP. (3) Treat with surgical resection or radiotherapy, anticonvulsants, corticosteroids, and chemotherapy.
Optic glioma	(1) Occurs in children <2 years of age. (2) Patients have poor vision, exophthalmos, increased ICP, and optic atrophy. (3) 25% of patients have neurofibromatosis. (4) Treat with resection or radiation therapy and chemotherapy.
Craniopharyngioma	(1) Occurs in children between 7 and 12 years of age. (2) Patients may have bitemporal hemianopsia and retardation of sexual and physical development. (3) Treat with preoperative cortisol replacement followed by tumor excision.

CSF, cerebrospinal fluid; ICP, intracranial pressure.

XIV. Pediatric Oncology

A. Wilms' Tumor

1. Mean age at diagnosis is approximately 3 years.
2. Can be associated with hemihypertrophy, sporadic aniridia (absence of an iris), and structural genitourinary abnormalities.
3. Patients usually have a palpable abdominal mass that may be associated with pain, fever, hypertension, and hematuria.
4. Diagnostic tests include routine blood tests and ultrasonography to visualize the mass and differentiate Wilms' tumor from an adrenal mass.
5. Treatment
   a. Surgical removal.
   b. Chemotherapy with vincristine, actinomycin D, and doxorubicin.
   c. Radiation therapy is indicated for metastatic disease.

Five percent of Wilms' tumors are bilateral, and 5% recur.

B. Osteosarcoma

1. Usually occurs in adolescents.
2. Patients with a history of retinoblastoma have 500 times the risk of osteosarcoma.
3. Tumors are usually located in the epiphysis or metaphysis of bones associated with maximal growth velocity.
4. Patients have pain at a bony site and maybe a palpable mass.
5. A radiograph of the affected bone will show lytic lesions. Bone scan and chest CT should be performed to screen for metastatic disease.
6. Treat with preoperative chemotherapy followed by either limb salvage or amputation. Postoperative chemotherapy should then also be used.

C. Ewing's Sarcoma

1. Small, round, blue cell tumor of the bone, most commonly involving the femur and pelvis.
2. Evaluate for metastatic disease with bone scans and CT. MRI of the primary lesion can help assess the degree of bone involvement.
3. Treat with irradiation. Chemotherapy is not usually used.

D. Central Nervous System Tumors of Children (Table 10-6)

11 CHAPTER

Pediatrics

I. Pediatric Cardiology (Table 11-1)

II. Pediatric Pulmonology
  A. Asthma (see Chapter 13)
  B. Cystic Fibrosis
    1. Autosomal recessive inheritance (1/2500 in Caucasian population).
    2. Disorder of exocrine gland function that affects the lungs, sinuses, pancreas, sweat/salivary glands, intestines, and reproductive system.
    3. Symptoms include cough, steatorrhea, meconium ileus, infertility, and hypochloremic acidosis due to Cl^- loss in sweat.
    4. Can be diagnosed by an elevated sweat chloride test (>60 mEq/L) on two occasions or through DNA analysis for mutation of the CFTR gene.
    5. Treat with supportive nutritional therapy, antibiotic prophylaxis (tobramycin plus a penicillin or cephalosporin), and DNase, pancreatic enzyme replacement, and surgery for meconium ileus.
  C. Lymphocytic Interstitial Pneumonitis
    1. Indicates immunodeficiency.
    2. Dyspnea is the presenting complaint with fluffy diffuse infiltrates in chest radiograph.
    3. Treat with corticosteroids.
  D. Pulmonary Hemosiderosis
    1. Accumulation of hemosiderin in lung macrophages due to diffuse alveolar hemorrhage.
    2. Patients have cough, dyspnea, and microcytic, hypochromic anemia.
    3. Associated with cow milk allergy or Goodpasture's syndrome (see Chapter 14).
    4. Treat with supportive therapy for bleeding and hypoxia and corticosteroids for immunosuppression.

III. Gastroenterology
  A. Appendicitis (see Chapter 4)
  B. Intussusception
    1. Telescoping of one part of the intestine into another, most often at the ileocecal valve.
    2. Symptoms include violent episodes of irritability, colicky pain, and emesis interspersed with nonsymptomatic periods. Rectal bleeding may also occur with "currant jelly" stools. Affects children 2 months to 2 years of age.
    2. Treat with hydrostatic reduction using barium enema or by pneumatic reduction with air enema.

Appendicitis is the most common indication for surgery in childhood.

TABLE 11-1 Common Congenital Cardiac Anomalies

Condition	Symptoms and Signs	Tests	Treatment
Ventricular septal defect (VSD) *(most common congenital heart lesions)*	(1) Large VSD with Eisenmenger physiology presents with shortness of breath, dyspnea on exertion, chest pain, a holosystolic murmur, and cyanosis. (2) As pulmonary vascular resistance increases, the holosystolic murmur shortens and the pulmonary component of S_2 increases in intensity. The patient may also have poor feeding.	(1) Chest radiograph shows increased pulmonary vascularity with cardiomegaly. (2) Echocardiogram.	Symptoms are indications for surgery.
Atrial septal defect (ASD)	Acyanotic heart disease with a widely split S_2 and a diastolic rumble.	(1) ECG shows right ventricular enlargement. (2) Radiograph shows increased pulmonary vascularity.	Will cause arrhythmias and heart failure in adults. Correct between 2 and 5 years of age.
Truncus arteriosus	(1) Causes cyanosis with harsh holosystolic murmur, a single loud second heart sound, and a wide pulse pressure. (2) CHF develops as the peripheral vascular resistance exceeds pulmonary resistance (3) A large VSD is always present.	(1) Echocardiogram. (2) Radiograph may have no thymic shadow if the patient has DiGeorge syndrome.	Surgery to correct anatomy.
D-transposition of the great arteries	(1) Circulation is in parallel rather than in series. Great arteries arise from the wrong chambers. Requires either a septal defect or a patent ductus arteriosus for survival. (2) Cyanosis noted in first day of life and progresses rapidly, and the upper body has a lower O_2 saturation than the lower body.	(1) Radiograph shows an egg-shaped heart. (2) Echocardiogram and Doppler show abnormal vessel arrangement.	(1) Give PGE1 to keep the ductus arteriosus patent. (2) Arterial switch operation (ASO). Mortality without intervention is 90% in the first year. Mortality after ASO is 5%.
Total anomalous pulmonary venous connection (TAPVC)	Right ventricular heave, wide fixed and split S_2 with a systolic ejection murmur at the left upper sternal border.	(1) Echocardiogram. (2) Radiograph shows a small heart with increased pulmonary vascularity. (3) ECG shows severe right ventricular hypertrophy.	Treat CHF initially, then surgically correct the heart.
Tricuspid atresia	(1) Tricuspid valve and right ventricle are underdeveloped. (2) Both a VSD and an ASD are usually present. The patient has a harsh holosystolic murmur of a VSD, and the patient's condition worsens as the VSD gets smaller after birth. (3) Cyanosis and poor feeding over the first 2 weeks of life.	ECG shows prominent left ventricular hypertrophy.	Give PGE1 to keep the ductus arteriosus patent if the VSD is small.

continued

TABLE 11-1 Common Congenital Cardiac Anomalies—cont'd

Condition	Symptoms and Signs	Tests	Treatment
Tetralogy of Fallot	(1) Heart anomaly with four components: (a) Anterior malalignment VSD (b) Right ventricular outflow tract obstruction (c) Right ventricular hypertrophy (d) Overriding large ascending aorta (2) Anything that reduces peripheral vascular resistance will cause cyanosis as blood is shunted systematically. Patients can have "tet spells" in which periodic episodic cyanosis and agitation occur due to an increase in right ventricular outflow tract resistance and an increase in right-left shunting.	(1) Boot shaped heart on radiograph. (2) ECG shows right ventricular hypertrophy.	(1) Total surgical correction at <6 months of age. Surgical mortality is 5%. (2) Treat "tet spells" with O_2, putting the child in the "knees to chest" position, and giving morphine.
Ebstein's anomaly	(1) Oversized tricuspid valve leaflets extend far into the right ventricle. (2) Patients display cyanosis, CHF, and arrhythmia due to Wolff-Parkinson-White syndrome.	(1) Severe cardiomegaly on radiograph. (2) Echocardiogram.	Give PGE1 for ductus arteriosus patency and propranolol for arrhythmia.
Hypoplastic left heart syndrome	Signs of CHF (edema, poor peripheral pulses, S_3) as the ductus closes.	ECG shows severe right ventricular hypertrophy.	Give PGE1 and perform surgery in the first week of life.
Common atrioventricular canal *(common in Down syndrome)*	(1) CHF in infancy with tachypnea, dyspnea, and poor feeding. (2) S_2 with widely fixed split from the ASD. (3) Blowing holosystolic murmur at the left lower sternal border from the VSD.	(1) Radiograph shows increased pulmonary vascularity with cardiomegaly. (2) Echocardiogram.	Surgical repair by 3 months of age.
Patent ductus arteriosus (PDA)	Acyanotic heart disease with a continuous machinery murmur.	(1) Radiograph shows increased pulmonary vascularity with cardiomegaly. (2) Echocardiogram.	Give indomethacin or do a ligation procedure.
Coarctation of the aorta	(1) Usually occurs at the level of the ductus arteriosus. (2) There is hypertension in the upper extremities, and the pulses in the lower extremities are weak and delayed.	Early ECG may show right ventricular hypertrophy, but later will show left ventricular hypertrophy.	Surgical correction at the time of diagnosis.

CHF, congestive heart failure.

C. Pyloric Stenosis
   1. Presents as gastric outlet obstruction with emesis in children 2 weeks to 2 months of age.
   2. Symptoms include projectile nonbilious vomiting with an olive-like mass on abdominal palpation.
   3. Visualize with ultrasonography.
   4. Treat with fluid resuscitation and pyloromyotomy.

D. Malrotation and Volvulus
   1. Due to malposition of the intestines in the abdomen and abnormal posterior fixation of the mesentery, which can impinge on its vascular supply (volvulus). Peak incidence is under 1 month of age.
   2. Principal symptom is bilious emesis, but you also see abdominal distention and shock.
   3. Upper GI radiologic examination will show abnormal positioning of the ligament of Treitz and the cecum.
   4. Treat with surgical correction.

E. Hirschsprung's Disease
   1. Results from the failure of myenteric plexus ganglion cells to migrate down the developing colon. The colon then remains contracted in this region and causes intestinal obstruction.
   2. Suspect it if an infant fails to pass meconium within 24 hours or requires repeated rectal stimulation to induce bowel movements.
   3. Symptoms in first month of life include poor feeding, bilious vomiting, and abdominal distention.
   4. Rectal biopsy reveals no ganglion cells and hypertrophied nerve trunks.
   5. Treat through surgical correction.

F. Meckel's Diverticulum
   1. This vestigial remnant of the omphalomesenteric duct is the most common anomaly of the GI tract.
   2. Presents as painless rectal bleeding, with a peak incidence around 2 years of age.
   3. There are usually ectopic gastric cells in this region, which can be seen on a Meckel scan (Tc99m).
   4. Treat with surgical resection.

G. Gastroesophageal Reflux (see Chapter 4)

H. Diarrhea (see Chapter 6)

I. Constipation
   1. Infrequent passage of hard, dry stools. Incomplete stooling can result in intestinal stretching and a functional ileus.
   2. In infancy, constipation is commonly associated with an anal fissure.
   3. Beyond neonatal period, the most common cause is voluntary withholding, or functional constipation.
   4. Treat through dietary changes or with a mild stool softener.

IV. Nephrology

A. Nephrotic Syndrome

1. Presents with proteinuria, hypoalbuminemia, hyperlipidemia, and edema. Most common in ages 2 to 6 years (boys > girls). Cause is noninflammatory.

2. Variants and treatment

a. Minimal change disease (80%): Can treat without renal biopsy if the patient is less than 7 years of age. Use prednisone for up to 4 weeks.

b. Focal segmental glomerulosclerosis (FSGS) (10%): Looks like minimal change disease but is not responsive to corticosteroids. Try immunosuppressive agents for treatment (methylprednisolone, cyclophosphamide).

c. It is useful to restrict water and salt (<2 g/day) intake. ACE inhibitors can also be used.

B. Glomerulonephritis

1. Inflammatory: Presents with hematuria (tea colored), azotemia (increased BUN and creatinine), oliguria, edema, and hypertension.

2. Types

a. Poststreptococcal: Most common type.

(1) Follows throat infection by 8 to 12 days.

(2) High IgG antistreptococcus antibodies and depressed complement levels will be found in the blood. IgG and complement deposition will be found in the kidney (glomerular humps).

b. IgA nephropathy: Shows renal mesangial IgA deposits.

c. Alport's syndrome: Progressive inherited nephritis in which the glomerular basement membrane is weak and tends to rupture and scar. Bilateral hearing loss is usually present.

d. Rapidly progressive glomerulonephritis: Crescent formation is seen in the glomeruli, and patients progress rapidly to renal failure. This is rare in children.

3. Treatment: Corticosteroid therapy, cytotoxic agents with or without plasmapheresis if antiglomerular basement membrane antibodies are present.

C. Renal Tubular Acidosis (RTA)

1. Children will have growth failure and acidosis.

2. Types

a. Type I: Distal RTA

(1) Deficiency in the distal H^+ secretion, which causes inability to acidify urine.

(2) Systemic acidosis is due to inability to clear H^+ in urine.

(3) Urine has a pH greater than 6.0.

b. Type II: Proximal RTA

(1) Reduced HCO_3 absorption. Distal H^+ ion secretion is normal, so the urine can be acidified. Systemic acidosis results from low HCO_3.

(2) Fanconi syndrome is one cause of type II RTA. Fanconi syndrome is a generalized disorder of proximal tubule transport with excessive losses of HCO_3, proteins, glucose, electrolytes, and water. Calcium loss may lend to the development of rickets.

Calculation of urine anion gap (AG) allows distinction of RTA types. Urine anion gap = Na + K − Cl

Negative AG indicates proximal RTA.

Positive AG with hyperkalemia indicates distal RTA type 4.

Positive AG without hyperkalemia indicates distal RTA type 1.

c. Type IV RTA
   (1) Associated with mineralocorticoid deficiency or decreased distal tubular responsiveness. Most common type in children is distal RTA type IV, which results from hyperkalemia that interferes with ammonia production.
   (2) Causes hyperkalemic, hyperchloremic acidosis.
   (3) Can be caused by obstructive uropathy.
   (4) Symptoms include growth failure and acidosis, and hyperkalemia may cause muscle weakness and polyuria.
   (5) Tests: Urine pH under 5.5 and low HCO_3 are consistent with proximal RTA.
   (6) Treatment
      (a) Alkalinizing agents (bicarbonate or citrate).
      (b) Correction of any obstructive uropathy that may be causing the type IV RTA.

D. Diabetes Insipidus (DI)
   1. Results from the inability to produce or respond to antidiuretic hormone (ADH).
   2. Presents with polyuria, polydipsia, and growth retardation with repeated episodes of hypernatremic dehydration.
   3. Nephrogenic (the inability to respond to ADH) and neurogenic (the inability to produce ADH) diabetes insipidus can be differentiated by administering synthetic ADH (DDAVP, a.k.a. desmopressin). Patients with nephrogenic diabetes insipidus show no response to DDAVP, while patients with neurogenic diabetes insipidus have decreased urine output after DDAVP treatment.
   4. Treatment
      a. Slow correction of electrolytes.
      b. Central DI: ADH replacement.
      c. Nephrogenic DI: Low-salt, high-water diet.
      d. Thiazide diuretics may decrease intravascular volume and increase proximal water and salt reabsorption.

E. Acute Renal Failure (see Chapter 7)

F. Chronic Renal Failure
   1. Cause
      a. Most common cause in children 0 to 10 years of age is obstructive uropathy.
      b. After 10 years of age, acquired disease is the most common cause.
   2. Patients frequently have growth failure.
   3. Treatment
      a. High-calorie, high-protein, low-phosphate diet.
      b. HCO_3/citrate to buffer acidosis.
      c. Renal transplantation, if possible.
      d. Hemodialysis or peritoneal dialysis can be used but is not completely adequate. Dysequilibrium syndrome is a dangerous complication of hemodialysis.

Adult polycystic disease has autosomal dominant inheritance and typically presents with cysts in the glomerulus, renal tubules, liver, and pancreas in adult patients (30- to 50-year-olds). Cerebral aneurysms can also be found in these patients.

G. Infantile Polycystic Kidney Disease
   1. Autosomal recessive inheritance.
   2. Kidneys are normal but the collecting tubes (as well as the hepatic bile ducts) are dilated.
   3. Usually presents as a palpable renal mass, hepatomegaly, pneumothorax, proteinuria, or hematuria.
   4. Diagnosis made by ultrasound in utero.
   5. Treatment is supportive, although renal transplantation and liver shunting/transplantation may be beneficial. Many patients die in the neonatal period of pulmonary hypoplasia.
H. Ureteropelvic Junction Obstruction
   1. Causes hydronephrosis, urinary stasis, infection, hematuria, and gradual destruction of the renal parenchyma.
   2. Evaluate with the aid of renal ultrasound and voiding cystourogram (VCUG).
   3. Treat with surgical pyeloplasty.
I. Vesicoureteral Reflux
   1. Causes recurrent urinary tract infections (UTIs).
   2. Can lead to renal scarring and failure.
   3. VCUG is used to evaluate and grade the reflux.
   4. Treatment
      a. Prophylactic antibiotic therapy with trimethoprim/sulfamethoxazole (TMP/SMX) and serial urine cultures.
      b. Ureteral reimplantation if UTIs recur despite antibiotic therapy or if structural damage is occurring.
J. Posterior Urethral Valves
   1. Only in males, found in the prostatic urethra. Results in partial bladder obstruction and weak or dribbling urine steams. May also present as a palpable bladder or renal mass or as a UTI.
   2. Evaluate with ultrasound and VCUG.
   3. Treat with transurethral ablation.
K. Hypospadias
   1. The urethral meatus is located below and proximal to its normal position. Can be associated with hernias and undescended testes.
   2. Do not circumcise the patient. Treat with gradual extension of the urethral opening to correct placement.
L. Cryptorchidism
   1. Undescended testes are found in 0.7% of children after 1 year of age. Bilateral cryptorchidism in adults causes infertility.
   2. Surgical correction at an early age increases the chances for fertility as an adult.
   3. Risk of malignancy in an undescended testis is 20% to 44% by the third or fourth decade of life.
M. Hydrocele
   1. Fluid-filled sac that is the result of lack of closure of the processus vaginalis.

2. Repair if it communicates with the peritoneal cavity because of the risk of hernia incarceration.

N. Testicular Torsion

1. Presents as unilateral scrotal pain, vomiting, and scrotal edema. Cremasteric reflex is absent on the affected side.

2. Surgical intervention must occur within 6 hours of onset.

O. Enuresis

1. Involuntary loss of bladder control in children above 5 years of age. Usually due to a delay in the maturation of sphincter control rather than to an organic disease process.

2. Organic causes include UTI, ectopic ureter or tract obstruction, diabetes mellitus, diabetes insipidus, or pelvic masses.

3. Treatment

a. Counseling

b. Audio alarm clock that goes off when the child starts to urinate.

c. Desmopressin acetate to concentrate urine and make it more likely that the child will last through the night without wetting.

d. Imipramine: Dangerous to use because of tricyclic antidepressant (TCA) side effects and the risks of accidental ingestion and overdose.

P. Urinary Tract Infection (UTI)

E. coli is the most common cause of urinary tract infections in children.

1. Most result from genitourinary (GU) contamination with fecal flora.

2. Patients with fever, chills, vomiting, and flank pain probably have kidney involvement.

3. Rule out anatomic abnormalities in children less than 2 years of age and in male patients with recurrent UTIs.

4. Pyelonephritis can cause scarring and decreased renal function.

5. Treat with ampicillin or cotrimoxazole if the patient does not look very ill. Add an IV aminoglycoside if the patient looks ill.

V. Pediatric Neurology

A. Assessment of Infantile Reflexes (Table 11-2)

B. Common Developmental Milestones (Table 11-3)

C. Neural Tube Defects

1. Incidence is decreased in mothers with folic acid supplementation.

TABLE 11-2 Common Infantile Reflexes

Reflex	Description
Moro	Abrupt head extension causes extension and flexion of the limbs.
Grasp	Placing finger in child's hand causes child to grasp it.
Rooting	Perioral stimulation causes the infant to move its mouth toward the stimulus.
Placing	Placing child feet-first on a surface cause child to place feet on it.
Tonic neck	Turning child's head results in the extension of the ipsilateral arm and leg (fencing posture).

All of these reflexes appear at birth and can disappear at 4–6 months.

TABLE 11-3 Commonly Used Developmental Milestones

Task	Normal Age of Acquisition
Smile spontaneously	1–2 mo
Hold head up	2–4 mo
Sit without support	4–7 mo
Thumb and finger grasp	9–11 mo
Stand alone	11–14 mo
Speak one word	11–15 mo
Use spoon or fork	12–19 mo
Walk up steps	15–20 mo
Two-word sentences	2 yr
Three-word sentences	3 yr

2. Screen for maternal serum α-fetoprotein at 16–18 weeks.
3. Caudal end of the cord can be tethered in spina bifida, which prevents cord ascension and growth. This results in scoliosis, lower extremity deformities, and the Arnold-Chiari malformation (which can cause hydrocephalus).

D. Hydrocephalus
1. Can be either noncommunicating (cerebral aqueduct is blocked) or communicating (subarachnoid villi are blocked) and will cause an increase in intracranial pressure.
2. Symptoms include Cushing's triad (bradycardia, hypertension, and respiratory changes) late in the development of hydrocephalus.
3. Treatment consists of ventriculoperitoneal shunting.

E. Cerebral Palsy
1. Disorder of movement and posture, which can be spastic, ataxic, choreoathetoid, and dystonic. Symptoms can vary in distribution from spastic diplegia (affecting both lower limbs) to hemiplegia (affecting a single side) or quadriplegia (affecting all limbs).
2. Patients may also have strabismus, visual field defects, mental retardation, and seizures.

F. Seizures
1. Generalized seizures are associated with loss of consciousness. EEG will show symmetrical bilateral activity. Seizures can be managed with carbamazepine, phenobarbital, phenytoin, or valproate.
2. Petit mal seizures show a characteristic 3 per second spike and wave pattern on EEG. These are brief staring episodes with alterations of consciousness. Treat with ethosuximide or valproate.

3. Infantile spasms are flexor/extensor spasms that may happen hundreds of times in a row. Treat with corticotropin and corticosteroids.
4. Febrile seizures: Occur in children between the ages of 6 months and 7 years. Febrile seizures are complex if they last longer than 15 minutes, recur within 24 hours, or show signs of focalization. The risk of development of epilepsy is usually no greater than in the general population (1%). Most children require no treatment, and rectal diazepam can be used during a seizure to prevent a prolonged event.
5. Patients requiring seizure medications can be treated with phenobarbital or valproic acid, but serious side effects (fatal hepatic necrosis with valproic acid and behavioral disturbances with phenobarbital) can occur with long-term use. Regular serum drug monitoring is also recommended with seizure medications owing to bone marrow suppression.

G. Reye's Syndrome
1. An encephalopathy associated with liver dysfunction that has been observed in children with a viral illness who have been treated with aspirin.
2. Symptoms include mental status changes, hyporesponsiveness, lethargy, stupor, or coma with hyperammonemia.
3. Treat with supportive care, and treat fulminant liver failure (with lactulose, vitamin K, and liver transplantation if possible). Mortality is 80% to 90%.

H. Congenital Neurologic Syndromes (Table 11-4)

VI. Pediatric Immunology and Rheumatology

A. Complement Defects
1. Patients will be susceptible to *Neisseria* species (meningitides and gonorrhea). May present as recurrent pyogenic infection, infection with *Neisseria,* lupus-like disease, or vasculitis.
2. C1 esterase inhibitor deficiency (hereditary angioedema).
a. Recurrent episodes of angioedema that occur in response to stress. These episodes can occur in any tissue and may obstruct airways.
b. Treat with stanozolol or danazol (these have androgenic side effects), vaccination, and antibiotic prophylaxis. In addition, purified C1 esterase inhibitor can be given shortly before surgery.

B. Allergic Disorders
1. Atopic Dermatitis
a. Erythematous papules typically found on extensor surfaces (before 2 years of age) and on flexor surfaces (after 2 years of age) because of environmental contact. The rash may be associated with sensitivity to specific substances.
b. Treat with skin hydration, the avoidance of chemical triggers, topical corticosteroids, and antihistamines.
2. Food allergies: Most common allergies are to peanuts, eggs, milk, soy, wheat, and fish.
a. Signs include colic, diarrhea, and failure to thrive.
b. Evaluate with a double-blind placebo food challenge.

Patients with humoral deficiencies (Table 11-5) will be more sensitive to infection with encapsulated organisms (*Haemophilus influenzae, Streptococcus pneumoniae*). Patients with T cell deficiencies (Table 11-6) will be more susceptible to fungal infections or opportunistic infections, such as *Pneumocystic carinii* pneumonia.

The allergic triad includes allergic rhinitis, reactive airway disease, and atopic dermatitis, which are frequently found together.

TABLE 11-4 Congenital Neurologic Syndromes

Disorder	Description
Adrenoleukodystrophy	Adrenal problems in combination with CNS demyelination. Spasticity and extensor posturing are often seen.
Acute cerebellar ataxia	An autoimmune disease that presents with horizontal nystagmus, postural ataxia, vomiting, and dysarthria.
Ataxia telangiectasia	A hereditary disorder (autosomal recessive inheritance) that presents in toddlers as telangiectasias with immunodeficiency and ataxia.
Friedreich's ataxia	Occurs in late childhood and presents with progressive ataxia, weakness, and muscle wasting. Patients also have a cardiomyopathy-like heart disease which kills them before the age of 30 years.
Tuberous sclerosis	A congenital syndrome (autosomal dominant inheritance) that causes facial angiofibromas and cerebral cortical dysplasia with mental retardation and epilepsy. Other skin abnormalities include flat hypopigmented macules (ash-leaf spots), shagreen patches (abnormal skin thickening in lumbar regions), sebaceous adenomas, and hyperpigmented forehead lesions.
von Hippel–Lindau disease	Patients have retinal vascular hamartomas and CNS vascular abnormalities with associated renal and adrenal carcinomas.
Sturge-Weber syndrome	Patients have a port wine stain near the eye and hemangiomas of the meninges. Patients may experience seizures and glaucoma. The skin lesions can be treated with laser surgery, and seizures are often controlled with standard anticonvulsant agents.
Spinal muscular atrophy	(1) Caused by degeneration of anterior horn cells. Infants exhibit progressive proximal weakness, decreased spontaneous movement, and floppiness. Eye movements are spared. Lower motor neuron injury findings are present on electromyography. (2) The fulminant form (Werdnig-Hoffmann syndrome) presents as quadriplegia with respiratory failure and death within the first year. (3) The milder form (Kugelberg-Welander syndrome) begins in late childhood with proximal weakness in the legs and progresses slowly.
Neurofibromatosis	See Chapter 8.
Hereditary neuropathy	See Chapter 8.

TABLE 11-5 Humoral Congenital Immunodeficiencies

Disorder	Symptoms and Signs	Treatment
X-linked agammaglobulinemia	(1) Deficiency of B cells that appears early in infancy as maternal antibody levels fall. The patient has no endogenously produced antibodies. (2) Patients are prone to infection by encapsulated bacteria (*S. pneumoniae, H. influenzae*, staphylococci, and *Pseudomonas*) and enteroviruses.	Treat with IVIg for protection.
Selective IgA deficiency*	Patients react normally to viral infections but are more susceptible to bacterial infections of the respiratory, GI, and urinary tracts.	Treat with IVIg for protection.
Hyper IgM syndrome	(1) Defect in B cell affinity maturation and class switching causes elevated IgM but normal IgG and IgA. (2) Patient has recurrent pulmonary infections (especially due to *P. carinii* and intracellular pathogens). (3) Thrombocytopenia, hemolytic anemia, hypothyroidism, and neutropenia may also be present.	Treat with IVIg and prophylactic antibiotic therapy if needed.
Common variable immunodeficiency	(1) Normal initial immune function followed by a severe reduction in IgG, IgM, and IgA. (2) Patient has recurrent sinus and pulmonary infections. (3) Many may also have GI symptoms (malabsorption, diarrhea), hemolytic anemia, thrombocytopenia, and neutropenia. (4) Some cases may be due to adverse reaction to phenytoin.	Treat with IVIg and prophylactic antibiotic therapy if needed.

IVIg, intravenous immunoglobulin.
*Most common immunodeficiency syndrome.

c. Treatment with antihistamines, bronchodilators, and epinephrine as needed. The patients should be instructed to avoid the food product in the future.

3. Asthma (see Chapter 13).
4. Allergic Rhinitis

a. Usually an IgE-dependent response to pollens, dust mite allergen, pet dander, or mold spores.

b. Patients experience recurrent sneezing, nasal congestion, clear rhinorrhea, and pruritus of nose and eyes. Symptoms may worsen in late fall and early spring.

TABLE 11-6 Cell-mediated Congenital Immunodeficiencies

Disorder	Symptoms and Signs	Treatment
Severe combined immunodeficiency (SCID)	(1) Usually associated with lack of T cell lines but normal B cell numbers. (2) Patients have failure to thrive, severe bacterial infections within the first month of life, chronic candidiasis, *P. carinii* infection, and intractable diarrhea. (3) Associated with a variety of mutations, including adenosine deaminase deficiency (ADA).	(1) Treat with bone marrow or stem cell transplant. (2) Give IVIg if humoral deficiencies exist. (3) PEG-ADA (IM injection) and gene therapy have been useful in ADA deficiency.
DiGeorge syndrome	(1) Hypoplasia of the thymus, which results in the lack of a thymic shadow and the inability to stimulate T cells. (2) Infant has congenital heart disease, hypocalcemic tetany, and immune dysfunction ranging from mild abnormalities to SCID. Facial abnormalities can occur.	Degree of immunodeficiency is highly variable, so treatments range from observation to treatment for severe immunodeficiency.
Chronic granulomatous disease	(1) Results in defective intracellular killing of bacteria and intracellular pathogens by phagocytes and neutrophils. (2) Associated with chronic or recurrent infections by catalase-positive bacteria or fungi. (3) Patients may have failure to thrive, chronic diarrhea, and persistent candidiasis.	Trimethoprim-sulfamethoxazole prophylaxis, interferon gamma administration, or recombinant granulocyte colony-stimulating factor and granulocyte-maerophage colony-stimulating factor.
Wiscott-Aldrich syndrome	(1) X-linked disorder that causes thrombocytopenia, eczema, immunodeficiency, and a predisposition to lymphoproliferative disease. (2) Patients get recurrent infection with bacteria, cytomegalovirus, *P. carinii* pneumonia, or herpes simplex virus, and often die of hemorrhage due to thrombocytopenia.	Bone marrow or stem cell transplantion.

c. Physical examination shows clear nasal discharge, enlarged pale turbinates, injected sclera, cobblestoning of the posterior pharynx, and geographic tongue.

d. Evaluate using include skin tests or in vitro serum testing (RAST).

e. Treatment includes avoidance of allergens and the use of

(1) Intranasal steroids (fluticasone, mometasone, budesonide) for treating congestion.

(2) Antihistamines for treating pruritus and rhinorrhea. Sedating (diphenhydramine, hydroxyzine) or nonsedating (loratadine, cetirizine, fexofenadine) types can be used.
(3) Oral decongestants (pseudoephedrine).
(4) Ipratropium bromide for decreasing rhinorrhea.
(5) Allergen immunotherapy: Suitable for children with severe rhinitis due to identified allergens. Patients are given increasing doses of allergen periodically. Treatment for more than 3 years has been associated with long-term alleviation or cure of the allergy.

5. Anaphylaxis
   a. Can be caused by any allergen, but frequent ones include antibiotics (penicillin), latex, insect stings, and food (peanuts, egg, seafood, milk).
   b. Symptoms include urticaria, stridor, laryngeal edema, wheezing, diarrhea, and hypotension.
   c. Treatment
      (1) Discontinue exposure to antigen.
      (2) Give SC or IM epinephrine.
      (3) If the cause is an injection or insect bite, apply more epinephrine locally and place a tourniquet around the extremity.
      (4) Give IV fluids for hypotension and intubation for airway maintenance if necessary.
      (5) Patients with egg allergy should not get vaccines containing egg protein (influenza and yellow fever).
6. Serum sickness
   a. Follows administration of large doses of antigen: 7–14 days after first antigen administration or 2–4 days after repeated exposure.
   b. Symptoms include pruritus, fever, polyarticular arthritis, lymphadenopathy, urticaria, and angioedema. Patients may also have a characteristic serpiginous rash on hands and feet.
   c. Evaluation: Increased ESR; complement C3 and C4 may be depressed; thrombocytopenia, proteinuria, microhematuria, and hyaline casts may be seen.
   d. Treatment
      (1) Avoidance of the antigen.
      (2) Antihistamines may help pruritus and prevent further immunocomplex deposition.
      (3) NSAIDs for joint pain.
      (4) Prednisone if other organs are involved.

C. Autoimmune and Inflammatory Disorders
   1. Juvenile rheumatoid arthritis
      a. Patients may show morning stiffness, night pain, rheumatoid nodules, and refusal to bear weight. Usually presents between 1 and 3 years of age or in the early teenage years.
      b. Can be classified as pauciarticular (<5 joints involved) or polyarticular (>5 joints involved).

(1) The pauciarticular type frequently involves the knees, ankles, and elbows in young children and also the hips in older ones (8 years of age).
(2) The polyarticular type frequently involves the large joints, cervical spine, temporomandibular joint (TMJ), sternocleidomastoid joint, and distal interphalangeal (DIP) joints.

c. Patients can also develop uveitis, which is often asymptomatic but can lead to blindness.

d. Evaluation: More young children have antinuclear antibodies (ANAs) than rheumatoid factor (RF), and older patients usually have normal tests.

e. Treatment
(1) NSAIDs can decrease swelling and inflammation.
(2) Methotrexate for severe disease. Use etanercept in cases of methotrexate failure or intolerance.
(3) Systemic corticosteroids for life-threatening inflammation.
(4) Treat uveitis with corticosteroids eyedrops and dilating agents.

2. Henoch-Schönlein purpura
a. Patients have URI symptoms, followed by characteristic rash, GI bleeding, and possibly glomerulonephritis by 2 months after onset.
b. Nonthrombocytopenic purpura will be seen over the buttocks and lower extremities.
c. Most recover without therapy, but corticosteroids may help edema. Renal transplant can treat irreversible renal insufficiency if it develops.

3. Kawasaki disease
a. Multisystem vasculitis including coronary artery aneurysms that occurs most commonly in those of Japanese ancestry.
b. Acute phase: 10 days with fever, conjunctivitis, extremity edema, and rash. Aseptic meningitis, pericarditis, and myocarditis may also occur.
c. Subacute phase (days 11–21): Fever decreases, nonpainful desquamation of hands and feet occurs. Patients have a risk of coronary artery aneurysm rupture or myocardial infarction during this period.
d. Convalescent phase (day 21 until acute-phase reactants subside): Coronary artery aneurysms may be detected, and the risk of coronary artery aneurysm rupture or myocardial infarction still exists.
e. Treat with aspirin or IVIg. This is the only indication for aspirin in children. Corticosteroids are contraindicated because they worsen the aneurysms.

VII. Pediatric Dermatology

A. Varicella (see Chapter 6)
1. Children with chickenpox are contagious from 24 hours before rash onset until all lesions have crusted over.
2. A vaccine is available to protect against varicella.

B. Bacterial Skin Infections (see Chapter 6)
   1. *Staphylococcus aureus* and group A beta-hemolytic streptococci are the most frequent bacterial skin infections.
   2. *S. pneumoniae* is the most common pathogen in hematogenously spread cellulitis (in children immunized against *H. influenzae*).
C. Scabies
   1. Linear burrows and extreme pruritus. These burrows are more often seen in the skin creases, but face and scalp can be involved in infants.
   2. All family members and bed linens need to be treated.
   3. Treatment: 5% permethrin cream for 12 hours. Itching can persist for 2 weeks.
D. Pediculosis (Lice)
   1. The louse resides in the hair or the clothing and periodically bites the child.
   2. Diagnose by direct visualization.
   3. Suspect sexual abuse in children with pubic lice.
   4. Treat close contacts, and notify school in cases of head lice. Treat with 1% permethrin cream or pyrethrin.
E. Acne
   1. Caused by *Propionibacterium acnes.*
   2. Lesions can be comedonal, pustular, or cystic. Cystic lesions have the greatest risk of scarring. Usually lasts for 3 to 5 years.
   3. Treatment
      a. Topical keratolytic agents (benzoyl peroxide)
      b. Topical antibiotics (clindamycin)
      c. Oral tetracyclines
      d. Patients unresponsive to therapy can be given oral isotretinoin. This requires frequent follow-up for side effects. It is highly teratogenic, so measures to prevent conception should be taken in young women.
F. Psoriasis (see Chapter 14)
G. Urticaria (hives)
   1. Hives are usually part of an allergic or stress reaction, and patients have wheals with edema that evolves over several hours.
   2. Treat with antihistamines and avoidance of the allergenic stimulus.
H. Erythema Multiforme
   1. Frequently found in HSV-infected patients.
   2. Erythematous macules evolve into papules, which evolve into plaques, which evolve into vesicles, which develop into target lesions. Whole evolution happens over several days.
   3. Most severe form is Stevens-Johnson syndrome (SJS) with general systemic signs followed by sudden onset of high fever, erythema multiforme, and inflammatory bullae of two or more mucous membranes.
   4. Most commonly caused by medications (NSAIDs, sulfonamides, anticonvulsants, penicillin, tetracycline) or mycoplasma pneumonia infection.
   5. Treatment
      a. Simple erythema multiforme: Antihistamines.
      b. SJS: Barrier isolation and electrolyte support. Ophthalmologic complications are common. There is a 5% to 15% mortality.

I. Toxic Epidermal Necrolysis
   1. Most severe form of cutaneous hypersensitivity (>30% of body surface involved) with sheetlike desquamation.
   2. Acute onset of high fever and burning of the mucus membranes. Patients can also have skin erosions.
   2. Most cases are secondary to medications (sulfa drugs, NSAIDs, anticonvulsants).
   4. Can lead to sepsis and death. Mortality is 30% to 50%.
   5. Treat with barrier isolation and wound care as for a second-degree burn.

VIII. Pediatric Endocrinology
   A. Juvenile Diabetes Mellitus (DM)
      1. Most children have type 1 (insulin-dependent) DM due to autoimmune destruction of the pancreas. Type 2 (non-insulin-dependent) DM is rising with childhood obesity. Treat these patients similarly to adult type 2 diabetics.
      2. Patients have polyuria, polydipsia, abdominal cramping, nausea, and vomiting. Patients in diabetic ketoacidosis will have tachypnea with deep (Kussmaul) respirations and fruity odor of breath with mental status changes.
      3. Tests include fasting glucose (>126 mg/dL) or 2-hour postprandial glucose (>200 mg/dL on two occasions).
      4. Treatment
         a. Diabetic ketoacidosis: Fluid replacement and correction of acidosis. Use isotonic glucose-free fluid. Give insulin to correct hyperglycemia. Acidosis usually responds to insulin treatment. Only use HCO_3 in severe cases.
         b. Outpatient management of type 1 DM: Glucose level goals depend on age.
            (1) Children less than 5 years of age: 100–200 mg/dL
            (2) School-aged children: 80–180 mg/dL
            (3) Adolescents: 70–150 mg/dL
         c. Insulin injection: Scheduling and dosing varies with the child's needs and lifestyle (see Chapter 3).
         d. Diet: 50% carbohydrates, 20% protein, and less than 30% fat.
         e. Daily blood glucose testing and HbA_{1c} every 3 months.
         f. Annual ophthalmologic and urine analysis.
         g. Give an ACE inhibitor if microalbuminuria develops.
      5. Complications of diabetic ketoacidosis include mental status changes, pupillary dilation, and hypertension with bradycardia. Cerebral edema develops in 1% to 5%, and it has a mortality of 20% to 80%.
   B. Hyperthyroidism (see Chapter 3)
   C. Hypothyroidism (see Chapter 3)
   D. Congenital Adrenal Hyperplasia
      1. Autosomal recessive disease with mutated 21-hydroxylase.
      2. Types
         a. Virilizing type: Boys will look normal, girls will be virilized.

b. Salt-wasting type: Patients have emesis, salt wasting, dehydration, and shock in the first 2–4 weeks of life. Laboratory tests show an increase in 17-hydroxyprogesterone.

3. Treat with cortisol and mineralocorticoids, along with fluid resuscitation.

E. Precocious Puberty

1. Secondary sex characteristics develop before 7.5 years of age in girls or before 9 years of age in boys. Short stature may be present owing to premature closure of the epiphyseal plates.

2. Testicular enlargement suggests increased GnRH, while isolated virilism suggests an exogenous or adrenal source.

3. Gonadotropin-dependent type: Girls more than boys. Usually idiopathic in girls and due to CNS tumor in boys.

4. Evaluation

a. LH and hCG levels in boys: To detect overproduction by secretory tumors.

b. Thyroid function tests: Hypothyroidism can lead to precocious puberty.

c. Sex steroid levels: Testosterone, estradiol, DHEAS.

5. Treatment

a. Gonadotropin-dependent type is treated with long-acting GnRH injections. Exogenous GnRH analogs will suppress endogenous secretion.

b. GnRH-independent type in boys can be treated with antiandrogens (spironolactone), ketoconazole, or aromatase inhibitors (testolactone).

c. GnRH-independent type in girls can be treated with tamoxifen.

d. Prognosis for precocious puberty due to neoplasia is dependent on the type of neoplasm.

(1) Dysgerminomas of the pineal gland are radiosensitive.

(2) Hepatoblastomas lead to death within months.

IX. Pediatric Electrolyte Management (see Chapter 7)

X. Pediatric Infectious Disease (see Chapter 6)

XI. Pediatric Emergency Management

A. Poisoning and Overdose (see Chapter 2)

B. Foreign Body Aspiration

1. Full obstruction will cause one-sided atelectasis (usually on the right side).

2. Partial obstruction will show trapped air (the inflated lung film will look normal, but the expiratory film will appear hyperinflated on one side).

C. Burns (see Chapter 2)

D. Abuse: Pathognomonic lesions include fractures prior to ambulation, bruising in low-trauma areas, spiral fractures, and retinal hemorrhages.

XII. Pediatric Ophthalmology (Table 11-7)

Grading of burns: first degree—only the epidermis (blisters); second degree—epidermis and dermis; third degree—skin and fascia, muscle, bone or joint tissue

Prevent with smoke detectors and by lowering hot water setting.

Children above 8 years of age can be screened for visual acuity according to adult guidelines.

TABLE 11-7 Common Conditions in Pediatric Ophthalmology

Condition	Symptoms	Treatment
Strabismus	Deviation of the eye, which is testable by corneal light reflection or cover tests.	Early recognition and treatment can prevent amblyopia and allow permanent realignment.
Amblyopia	(1) Reduced vision that develops in early childhood in an otherwise normal eye. (2) Can be caused by suppression of retinal images by strabismus, and also by opacities of the cornea or lens.	Early recognition of problems that cause amblyopia can prevent its development.
Nasolacrimal duct obstruction	Common cause of tearing in infants and neonates.	Refer to specialist if it persists beyond 9 months of age.
Leukokoria	(1) White pupil, absence of the red reflex. (2) Most common cause is congenital cataract, but can also be due to retinoblastoma or retinopathy of prematurity.	Remove cataract or tumor.
Red eye in the infant	(1) May be due to chemical irritation or infection. (2) *Chlamydia* and gonorrhea are the most common infections. (3) Gonorrheal infection can cause blindness.	(1) Chemical cause: Do nothing. (2) *Chlamydia*: Give tetracycline ointment and erythromycin. (3) Gonorrhea: Give penicillin or ceftriaxone.

XIII. Pediatric Orthopedics
   A. Structural Abnormalities Presenting in Childhood (Table 11-8)
   B. Traumatic Bone Injury
      1. Types of fracture
         a. Salter classification of limb fractures (Fig. 11-1).
         b. Greenstick fracture: The force of the injury breaks one side of the bone and bends the other side.
      2. Treatment
         a. Salter types I and II fractures can be managed by closed reduction techniques unless they are in the distal femur.
         b. Salter types III, IV, and distal femur fractures require anatomic alignment and internal fixation.
         c. Fractures through the growth plate may result in deformity or limb-length discrepancy.
      3. Subluxation of radial head (nursemaid's elbow)
         a. The patient holds the arm flexed with the hand pronated and has limited movement at the elbow.
         b. Treatment: Hold the elbow at 90 degrees and manipulate the forearm into supination.

TABLE 11-8 Orthopedic Abnormalities Present in Childhood

Condition	Symptoms	Treatment
Slipped capital femoral epiphysis	(1) Separation of the proximal femoral growth plate that is more common in obese male patients and typically occurs during the adolescent growth spurt. (2) Patients display a limp, pain, limited internal rotation, and limb shortening.	(1) Observe whether younger children have full range of motion. (2) Older patients or those with bone changes require orthotic bracing or surgery.
Legg-Calvé-Perthes disease	(1) Avascular necrosis of the femoral head. (2) Patients have intermittent pain and limping in the anterior thigh and restricted range of motion of the hip on abduction and internal rotation.	Treat with casting or surgery to contain the femoral head in the acetabulum.
Osgood-Schlatter disease	Inflammation of the tibial tuberosity that occurs in patients 10–17 years of age.	Treat with rest or casting.
Idiopathic scoliosis	Painless curvature of the spine (usually to the right).	Curvature of <25 degrees requires observation. More severe curvatures can be treated with orthoses or surgery.
Congenital scoliosis	Curvature of the spine that is due to a defect in the formation of vertebrae or disks and may be associated with structural genitourinary abnormalities and cardiac problems.	Treat with spinal fusion surgery if severe.
Neuromuscular scoliosis	Curvature of the spine due to weakening of muscles in progressive neuromuscular disorders (Duchenne muscular dystrophy, cerebral palsy, superior mesenteric artery syndrome, spina bifida). The curvature is progressive due to progression of weakness.	Requires surgery for correction and stabilization.
Kyphosis	(1) Increased angulation of the spine forward. (2) Can be due to poor posture (postural round back), to structural abnormality (Scheuermann's disease), or to congenital abnormalities of the vertebral bodies. (3) Patients may have symptoms of nerve compression.	(1) Patients with Scheuermann's disease may require orthosis or casting. (2) Congenital kyphosis can lead rapidly to progression to paraplegia. Surgical correction is indicated.
Spondylolysis and spondylolisthesis	(1) Spondylolysis: Defect in the pars interarticularis without forward slippage of the involved vertebrae. This can produce symptoms of nerve compression. (2) Spondylolisthesis: Forward slippage of the vertebra in which the pars interarticularis is abnormal. Most common site is L5. This can produce symptoms of nerve compression, and the vertebral displacement may be palpable.	(1) Spondylolysis: Periodic evaluation, orthotics if painful. (2) Spondylolisthesis: Either orthotics for nerve compression symptoms or spinal fusion.

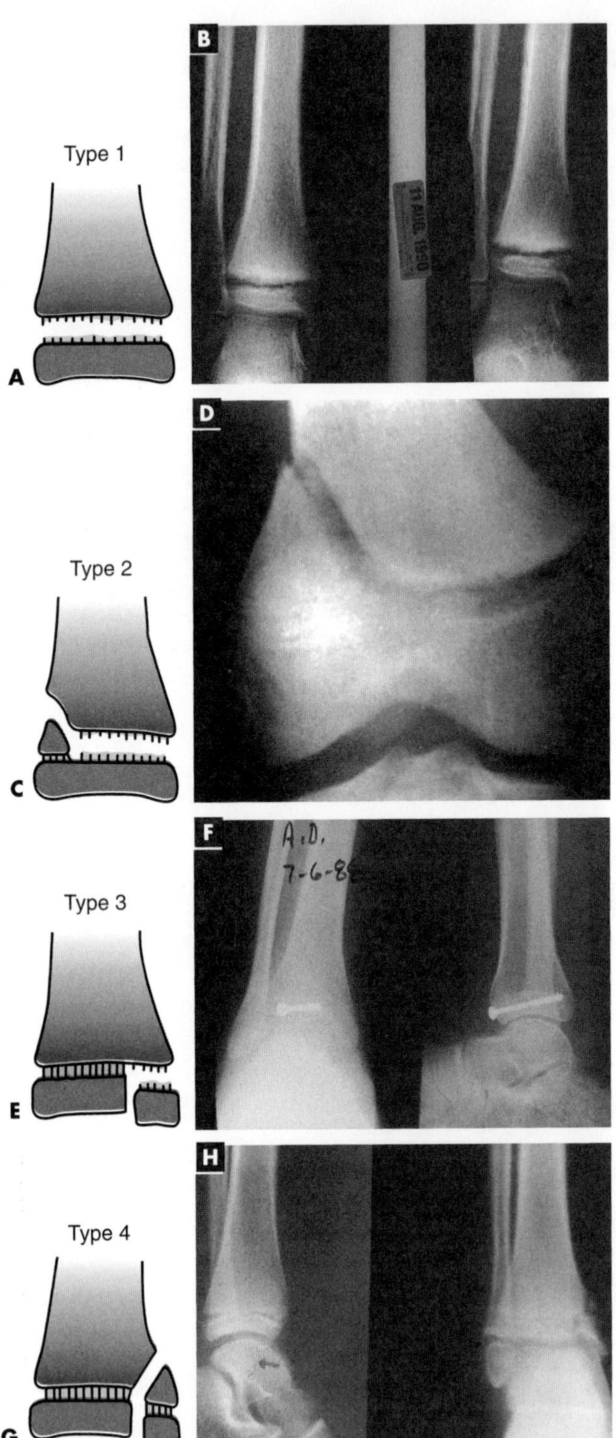

11-1: *Salter classification of limb bone fractures. A and B, Type I: through growth plate entirely. C and D, Type II: through growth plate and proximal bone. E and F, Type III: through growth plate and distal bone. G and H, Type IV: through both proximal and distal.*

C. Osteomyelitis

1. Symptoms include fever, refusal to move the involved limb, and localized bone pain.
2. Bone aspirate should be sent for culture (*S. aureus* is the most common pathogen).
3. Treat with oxacillin for staphylococci (add ampicillin and gentamycin for group B beta-hemolytic *Streptococcus* in neonates).

D. Septic Arthritis

1. Presents as a painful swollen joint accompanied by fever, irritability, and refusal to bear weight.
2. The most common cause is *S. aureus*, but consider *N. gonorrhoeae* in a sexually active adolescent.
3. Treat with IV antibiotics.

XIV. Genetic Disorders

Inborn errors of metabolism are almost all of autosomal recessive (AR) inheritance. An exception is ornithine transcarbamylase deficiency, which is X-linked.

A. Phenylketonuria

1. Deficiency of phenylalanine hydroxylase (converts Phe to Tyr).
2. Most common inborn error of metabolism (incidence is 1 in 10,000).
3. Presents as mental retardation, hypertonicity, tremors, and behavioral problems that occur in childhood (not in infancy) due to accumulation of Phe in the brain.
4. Can be diagnosed by a Phe level greater than 20 mg/dL and tyrosine (Tyr) level less than 1 mg/dL.
5. Treat with dietary restriction of foods containing Phe for life.

B. Homocystinuria

1. Deficiency of cystathionine synthetase leading to increased homocystine and methionine levels.
2. Presents with Marfan-like body, dislocated lens, moderate mental retardation, and thromboses (can cause myocardial infarction or stroke).
3. Treat with dietary management.

C. Galactosemia

1. Deficiency of galactose-1-phosphate uridyl-transferase.
2. Causes liver problems, renal dysfunction, and cataracts in the first days of life. Ovarian failure develops later.
3. Diagnose by high AST and ALT and low levels of galactose-1-phosphate uridyl-transferase.
4. Treat through elimination of dietary galactose. Dietary galactose should be restricted in future pregnancies.

D. Glycogen Storage Disease

1. Type I (von Gierke's): Glucose-6-phosphatase deficiency. Causes hypoglycemia, lactic acidemia, liver, kidney, and platelet problems. Give supportive therapy, but patients die early.
2. Type II (Pompe's): Lysosomal α-glucosidase deficiency. Causes symmetric muscle weakness, cardiomegaly, heart failure. Recombinant therapy is promising, but patients still die early.
3. Type III (Forbes'): Debranching enzyme deficiency. Causes hypoglycemia, ketonuria, and hepatomegaly that resolves with age.

Common X-linked disorders are hemophilia A and B, glucose-6-phosphate dehydrogenase deficiency, Duchenne muscular dystrophy, ornithine transcarbamylase deficiency, and fragile X syndrome.

4. Type IV (Andersen's): Branching enzyme deficiency. Hepatic cirrhosis with early liver failure. Death by age 4.
5. Type V (McArdle): Muscle phosphorylase deficiency. Causes muscle fatigue beginning in adolescence.
6. Types VI, VII, VIII: Less important, less dangerous.

E. X-linked Disorders (Table 11-9)

TABLE 11-9 High-yield X-linked and Chromosomal Syndromes

Disorder	Description
Ornithine transcarbamylase deficiency (X-linked)	(1) Defect in a uric acid cycle enzyme that causes severe hyperammonemia upon protein challenge. (2) Newborn becomes lethargic with seizures after eating protein. Carriers may develop headaches, emesis, and learning disabilities. (3) Diagnose with urinary orotic acid level. (4) Treat with low-protein diet.
Fragile X syndrome (X-linked)	Patients have macrosomia, macroorchidism, large jaw and ears, and mental retardation.
Down syndrome (trisomy 21)	Patients have mental retardation, flat facial profile, short ears with downfolding lobes, microcephaly, sandal gap toe, simian creases. Cardiac septal defects, duodenal atresia, Hirschsprung's disease, atlantoaxial instability, and dementia after age 40 are commonly found.
Trisomy 13	Patients have midline defects and congenital heart problems and rarely live longer than 6 months.
Trisomy 18	Patients have rocker bottom feet and hip problems. Otherwise appears similar to trisomy 13. Patients rarely live past 1 year.
Turner's syndrome (45 XO)	(1) Patients have lymphedema of hands and feet at birth, webbed neck, short stature, shield chest, multiple pigmented nevi, gonadal dysgenesis, renal anomalies, coarctation of the aorta, cardiac defects, and autoimmune thyroiditis. (2) Treat with growth hormone and estrogen therapy.
Klinefelter's syndrome (47 XXY)	Patients have incomplete masculinization at puberty, mild mental retardation, and long legs and arms. Treat with testosterone.
Prader-Willi syndrome	(1) Lack of paternal copy of chromosome 15q11–13. (2) Patients have severe hypotonia, hypogonadism, and failure to thrive in infancy followed by truncal obesity in childhood. They eat constantly and have mental retardation with impulse control problems.
Angelmann's syndrome	(1) Loss of the maternal allele of the 15q11–13. (2) Patients have severe mental retardation, seizures, happy demeanor, and characteristic facies.

XV. Neonatology
  A. Prenatal Teratogens
    1. Alcohol: Fetal alcohol syndrome happens in 40% of infants whose mothers drink more than 4–6 drinks per day while pregnant. Features include microcephaly, mental retardation, intrauterine growth retardation (IUGR), facial dysmorphism (midfacial hypoplasia, micrognathia, flattened philtrum, short palpebral fissures, and a thin vermilion border), and renal/cardiac defects.
    2. Cocaine: Causes diminished placental blood flow.
      a. Associated with an increased rate of spontaneous abortion, placental abruption, fetal distress, meconium staining, preterm birth, IUGR, and low Apgar scores.
      b. Can also cause congenital anomalies (cardiac defects, skull abnormalities, GU malformations), intracranial hemorrhage, and necrotizing enterocolitis.
    3. Heroin/Methadone
      a. Maternal use of heroin causes IUGR, an increased risk of sudden infant death syndrome (SIDS), and infant narcotic withdrawal syndrome.
      b. Methadone use can cause microcephaly, an increased risk of SIDS, and infant narcotic withdrawal syndrome.
      c. Methadone maintenance is prescribed for pregnant heroin users because withdrawal places too much stress on the fetus.
      d. Narcotic withdrawal syndrome: Occurs within the first 4 days of life and presents with irritability, poor sleeping, high-pitched cry, diarrhea, sweating, sneezing, seizures, poor feeding, and poor weight gain. Symptomatic treatment includes holding, rocking and providing the neonate with frequent small feedings of hypercaloric formula. Tincture of opium, phenobarbital, and paregoric can also be used.
  B. Apgar Scoring (Mnemonic—**a**irway, **p**allor, **g**rimace, **a**ctivity, **r**eflex)
    1. Take scores at 1 and 5 minutes after birth.
    2. A score of 0–3 indicates the need for resuscitation.
    3. Most low scores are due to difficulty in establishing adequate ventilation and are not associated with cardiac pathology.
  C. Birth Trauma
    1. Cephalohematoma: Traumatic subperiosteal hemorrhage usually involving the parietal bone that does not cross the suture lines. It may not appear until hours after delivery, but usually resolves spontaneously over several weeks.
    2. Caput succedaneum: Diffuse, edematous, dark swelling of the soft scalp tissue that crosses suture lines following vaginal birth.
    3. Clavicle fracture: The right clavicle is more likely to fracture than the left (since the right shoulder must move below the pubic symphysis during delivery). A fracture presents with swelling and fullness over the fracture site, crepitus, and decreased arm movement.
    4. Erb-Duchenne palsy: Brachial plexus injury due to excessive traction on the neck, resulting in an inability to abduct the arm at the shoulder,

externally rotate the arm, or supinate the forearm. Treat with physical therapy and positioning to avoid contractures.

D. Prematurity
  1. Low-birth-weight infants (<2500 g) are 40 times more likely to die in the neonatal period than term infants.
  2. Very low birth weight infants (<1500 g) are 200 times more likely to die in the neonatal period than term infants.

E. Postmaturity (Gestation > 42 weeks)
  1. Can be associated with anencephaly, trisomy 18, and Seckel's syndrome (bird-headed dwarfism).
  2. Syndrome of postmaturity: Results in dry, peeling skin and a malnourished appearance (normal length and head circumference but decreased weight). Possible complications include meconium aspiration, perinatal depression at birth, persistent pulmonary hypertension of the newborn, hypoglycemia, hypocalcemia, and polycythemia.

The lungs usually are fully mature at 32 weeks' gestation. Surfactant production can be accelerated with maternal steroid administration, prolonged rupture of fetal membranes, maternal narcotic addiction, preeclampsia, placental insufficiency, maternal hyperthyroidism, and theophylline.

F. Neonatal Respiratory Disease
  1. Respiratory distress syndrome (RDS)
    a. Tachypnea, grunting, nasal flaring, chest wall retractions, and cyanosis in the first 3 hours of life. The patient can worsen over the first 24–48 hours of life, but symptoms should resolve by 72 hours postnatally.
    b. Occurs when the amniotic fluid lecithin/sphingomyelin ratio is less than 2.0. Chest radiograph reveals uniform reticulonodular (ground glass) appearance.
    c. Treat with respiratory support until spontaneous resolution occurs. Artificial surfactant can also be used. Continuous positive airway pressure (CPAP) and oxygen are usually used to keep the PaO_2 greater than 50 mm Hg.
    d. Complications include pulmonary hypertension, chronic lung disease, and bronchopulmonary dysplasia (BPD) (as a result of the mechanical ventilation therapy).
  2. Meconium aspiration: Caused by perinatal asphyxia and presents with tachypnea, hypoxia, and hypercapnia that may develop into pneumonia. Risk factors include postmaturity, intrauterine growth retardation, and breech presentation. Aspiration can be avoided by clearing the oropharynx in infants that are at risk, before the initiation of ventilation. If aspiration occurs, provide supportive care.

Jaundice occurs when serum bilirubin levels become higher than 5 mg/dL in neonates and higher than 2 mg/dL in children.

Jaundice is pathologic in neonates if it is evident in the first day of life, if the peak bilirubin is greater than 13 mg/dL in term infants, if the direct bilirubin fraction greater than 1.5 mg/dL, or if hepatosplenomegaly and anemia are present.

  3. Persistent pulmonary hypertension of the newborn (PPHN): A disorder of infants who have experienced hypoxia in utero that involves the failure of the pulmonary vascular resistance to fall with postnatal lung expansion and oxygenation and subsequent hypoxemia. Patients have rapidly progressive cyanosis and respiratory distress that usually resolves within 5–10 days of birth. Treat with supplemental oxygen, hyperventilation, HCO_3 administration, pulmonary vasodilators (nitric oxide), and support of systemic blood pressure.

G. Neonatal Gastrointestinal Disease
  1. Hyperbilirubinemia

a. Indirect hyperbilirubinemia

(1) Common causes (Table 11-10).

(2) Indirect bilirubin levels greater than 25 mg/dL (or lower in preterm infants) can cause kernicterus. Kernicterus presents as lethargy, hypotonia, and a high-pitched cry after 4 days of life and can progress to fever, bulging fontanelle, hypertonicity, seizures, and pulmonary hemorrhage. Avoid this complication with exchange transfusion if the child's indirect bilirubin climbs too high.

Other causes of jaundice include polycythemia, extravascular blood loss, and swallowed maternal blood.

b. Direct hyperbilirubinemia: Direct bilirubin is greater than 1.5 mg/dL.

(1) Can be caused by hyperalimentation cholestasis, perinatal infections, neonatal hepatitis, sepsis, or a variety of congenital syndromes (biliary atresia, cystic fibrosis, α_1-antitrypsin deficiency).

(2) Do not treat these patients with phototherapy or exchange transfusion. Phototherapy can cause bronzing of the skin that can last for months. Treatment depends on the specific cause of the hyperbilirubinemia.

2. Necrotizing enterocolitis (NEC): Caused by ischemic necrosis of the bowel and secondary invasion of the intestinal wall. The cause is unknown.

a. Risk factors include maternal age above 35, maternal infection requiring antibiotics, premature rupture of membranes (PROM), and cocaine exposure.

b. Patients have feeding intolerance with bilious aspirates and abdominal distention, occult blood in the stool, and dilated bowel loops on radiographs. NEC can become a surgical emergency because it can progress to sepsis, disseminated intravascular coagulation (DIC), and respiratory distress. Pneumatosis intestinalis and perforation can also occur and appears as dilated thickened bowel loops, portal air, and pneumoperitoneum on an abdominal radiograph.

c. Treat by nasogastric decompression of the GI tract, systemic antibiotics, IV fluid administration, and abdominal radiographs every 6 hours to monitor pneumatosis intestinalis. If free air is seen, then exploratory laparotomy should be done.

H. Neonatal CNS Disorders

1. Apnea of prematurity: Cessation of breathing for longer than 15–20 seconds or a shorter pause associated with cyanosis, pallor, hypotonia, or bradycardia with a heart rate less than 100 bpm.

a. Types of apnea include central (cessation of air flow and respiratory effort with no chest wall movement) and obstructive (respiratory effort and chest wall movement with no air flow). Apnea of prematurity is central apnea due to immaturity of the medullary respiratory control center.

b. Types of bradycardia include self-stimulation (infant arouses itself and stops the apneic spell), tactile stimulation (a caregiver must touch the infant to discontinue the apnea), and bradycardia requiring intervention (infant is hypotonic with pallor and bag mask ventilation is required).

TABLE 11-10
Causes of Indirect Hyperbilirubinemia

Type	Symptoms	Tests	Treatments
Physiologic	(1) Begins after 24 hours of life, peaks at levels of 12–15 mg/dL at postnatal day 3, and returns to normal by postnatal day 7. (2) Ask about family history, ABO incompatibility, TORCH infections, and gray stools. (3) In neonates, jaundice follows a cephalopedal progression.	Complete blood count (CBC) with reticulocyte count, blood typing, Coombs test, and measurements of conjugated and unconjugated bilirubin.	Phototherapy or exchange transfusion.
Hemolytic *(immune, drug, or red blood cell defects)*	Hepatosplenomegaly, anemia	Same as above.	(1) Transfuse as needed for anemia. (2) Exchange transfusion if indirect bilirubin >20 mg/dL to prevent kernicterus.
Breast milk jaundice	Presents in the second week of life. Due to dehydration or poor feeding in the first week of life.	None needed.	Increase feedings.
Disorders of bilirubin metabolism *(Gilbert, Crigler-Najjar, and Lucey-Driscoll syndromes)*	Can result in severe unconjugated (indirect) hyperbilirubinemia.	CBC with reticulocyte count, blood typing, Coombs test, and measurements of conjugated and unconjugated bilirubin.	(1) Hepatic enzyme induction by phenobarbital can help in Crigler-Najjar syndrome. (2) Exchange transfusion if bilirubin >20 mg/dL to prevent kernicterus.
Endocrine disorders *(hypothyroidism, maternal diabetes, hypopituitarism)*	See text.	(1) CBC with reticulocyte count, blood typing, Coombs test, and measurements of conjugated and unconjugated bilirubin. (2) Endocrine function tests.	(1) Treat primary endocrine disorder. (2) Exchange transfusion if bilirubin >20 mg/dL to prevent kernicterus.

c. Treatments include supplemental oxygen, tactile stimulation, and administration of respiratory stimulants (caffeine, aminophylline, doxapram). The infant can be discharged when it is 34–35 weeks of gestational age, is tolerating foods orally, and has not had an apneic or bradycardic episode for 7 days.

2. Intraventricular hemorrhage (IVH): Results from bleeding of the germinal matrix (Fig. 11-2).

a. Can present with anemia, pallor, hypotension, focal neurologic signs, seizures, apnea, or bradycardia, usually within the first 3 days of life.

b. Evaluate using ultrasonography through the fontanelle.

c. Risk of IVH can be minimized by preventing premature delivery when possible and using supportive measures to prevent hypoxemia.

d. Grades I and II often resolve without sequelae. Posthemorrhagic hydrocephalus (in more severe cases) is treated by serial lumbar punctures, external ventriculotomy, or ventriculoperitoneal shunting.

3. Neonatal seizures (see Chapter 8).

a. Causes of neonatal seizures include metabolic dysfunction, drug intoxication or withdrawal, hemorrhage in the CNS, infection (meningitis or encephalitis), and genetic syndromes (cerebral dysgenesis, chromosomal abnormalities, tuberous sclerosis).

b. Diagnostic testing should include blood and CSF cultures, urinalysis (for metabolic errors), tests for TORCH infections, and cranial ultrasonography.

c. Treatment includes bedside EEG and video tracking, anticonvulsants (usually phenobarbital), and symptomatic treatment for drug withdrawal. Toxic causes can also be treated with exchange transfusions. Status epilepticus can be managed with benzodiazepines.

Neonatal seizures can be subtle (eye deviation, mouth movements, apnea, vital sign fluctuations), focal clonic (localized jerking movements), multifocal clonic (multiple random clonic movements), tonic (extensor posturing with tonic eye deviation), myoclonic (synchronized single or multifocal rapid jerks), or tonic-clonic.

I. Neonatal Hematologic Disorders

1. Polycythemia: Can be an absolute erythrocytosis (increase in RBC mass) or a relative erythrocytosis (decrease in plasma volume).

a. Neonatal polycythemia: Absolute erythrocytosis with hematocrit (HCT) greater than 55%.

b. Infants appear ruddy and plethoric with irritability, lethargy, poor feeding, emesis, seizures, and acute renal failure. Hepatomegaly, hyperbilirubinemia, PPHN, NEC, and hypoglycemia may also occur.

c. Treat with partial exchange perfusion to remove whole blood, and replace it with normal saline or albumin. The desired HCT is 50% after dilution.

Hyperviscosity syndromes can occur when HCT is greater than 65%. Neonatal erythrocytes are less filterable or deformable than adult ones, which further contributes to hyperviscosity.

2. Anemia: Can result from blood loss, hemolysis, decreased RBC production, or decreased erythropoiesis. Inquire about familial history of anemia to assess the risk of congenital causes.

a. Anemia due to acute blood loss can present with shock, tachypnea, tachycardia, low venous pressure, weak pulses, and pallor.

b. Anemia due to chronic blood loss can present with extreme pallor, low HCT, possibly CHF or hydrops fetalis.

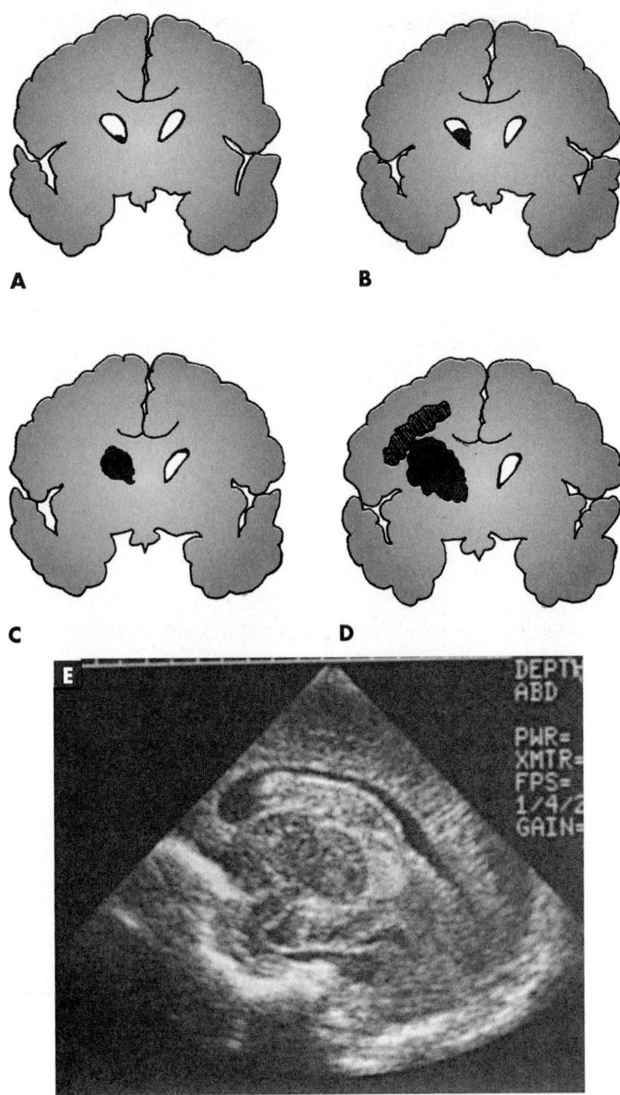

11-2: *Grading of intraventricular hemorrhage. A, Grade I: Small hemorrhage that is confined to the germinal matrix. B, Grade II: Small amount of blood in the ventricle with no ventriculomegaly. C, Grade III: Hemorrhage that extends into the ventricle with ventricular dilation. This can result in some permanent functional impairment in 50% of cases. D, Grade IV: Extension into the brain parenchyma. This can result in some permanent functional impairment in 80% of cases. E, Ultrasound of a Grade III intraventricular hemorrhage. Note that blood (white) fills and distends the ventricles but there is no evidence of extension into the brain parenchyma.*

c. Anemia due to chronic hemolysis can present with pallor, jaundice, and hepatosplenomegaly.
d. Useful diagnostic tests include reticulocyte count, bilirubin levels, Coombs test, RBC morphology, Apt test (identifies swallowed maternal blood), Kleihauer-Betke preparation (identifies fetomaternal transfusion), and ultrasound for intracranial bleeds (see Chapter 5).
e. Treatment typically depends on severity of anemia. Mild anemia will self-correct if iron intake is adequate. Hypovolemic shock can be treated with volume expander (albumin or normal saline). Anemia of prematurity can be treated with the vitamin E and iron administration present in premature formulas.

J. Neonatal Dermatology
1. Erythema toxicum neonatorum: Papules, vesicles, and pustules on an erythematous base that usually occur on the trunk and contain numerous eosinophils. This can develop within 72 hours of birth and usually resolves spontaneously over 3–5 days.
2. Milia: Pearly white or pale yellow epidermal cysts found on the nose, chin, and forehead that disappear within the first few weeks of life.
3. Seborrheic dermatitis: Erythematous dry, scaling, crusted lesions in areas rich in sebaceous glands (face, scalp, etc.) that appear between 2 and 10 weeks of age. Severe cases can be treated with baby oil and dandruff shampoo (for cradle cap) or 1% hydrocortisone cream (for dermatitis in the diaper area).
4. Mongolian spots: Found in darkly pigmented babies. The spots do not disappear but appear to fade as the surrounding skin darkens with age.

K. Neonatal Endocrine Disorders
1. Hypothyroidism: Usually caused by sporadic athyreosis or thyroid ectopy.
a. Patients may have characteristic facies (thick lips, large tongue, periorbital edema), weakness, and myxedema.
b. State law requires neonatal screening for hypothyroidism. A low T_4 and an elevated TSH indicates primary hypothyroidism.
c. If screening is positive, repeat and start levothyroxine. Adjust dose to an age-appropriate level after 4 days of treatment.
2. Hypoglycemia: Can occur with or without hyperinsulinism.
a. Presents with poor feeding, apathy, lethargy, and hypotonia with a blood glucose level less than 30 mg/dL. Severe cases can cause seizures, apnea, and cyanosis.
b. In asymptomatic infants, oral feedings or total parenteral nutrition (TPN) can be used. In symptomatic infants, infuse dextrose and give IV fluids to keep the blood glucose between 45 and 120 mg/dL.

L. Perinatal Infection (Tables 11-11 and 11-12)

M. Major Congenital Anomalies (Table 11-13)

Eighty percent of pediatric AIDS results from maternal transmission. Transmission rates of HIV from mother to child range from 30% to 50% but decrease to less than 10% with AZT treatment.

Risk factors for sepsis:
History of PROM (>24 h)
Chorioamnionitis
Maternal fever or leukocytosis
Fetal tachycardia
Preterm birth

TABLE 11-11 Antenatal Infections

Type	Symptoms	Tests	Treatment
Toxoplasmosis *(Only primary infection of the mother [asymptomatic] results in congenital infection.)*	(1) Maternal exposure to cats or cat feces. (2) Fetuses exposed early in pregnancy may get intrauterine meningoencephalitis, causing microcephaly, hydrocephalus, microphthalmia, chorioretinitis, intracranial calcifications, and seizures. They may also appear septic and have jaundice, hepatosplenomegaly, purpura, petechiae, and a maculopapular rash.	Four-fold rise in antibody titer or seroconversion.	Pyrimethamine and sulfadiazine with folic acid. Corticosteroids can be used for severe CNS or eye disease. Best prevention is avoidance and emptying of litter boxes daily by another person.
Rubella	(1) First trimester infection include heart defects, ophthalmologic defects (cataracts, microphthalmia, glaucoma, and chorioretinitis), auditory defects (sensorineural deafness), and neurologic malformations (microcephaly, meningoencephalitis, and mental retardation). (2) Chronic sequelae include growth retardation, radiolucent bone disease, hepatosplenomegaly, thrombocytopenia, jaundice, and purple skin lesions (blueberry muffin spots).	Most commonly associated with nasopharyngeal secretions. Specific rubella IgM antibody or persistence of rubella IgG in the infant is diagnostic.	Treat specific defects.
CMV	(1) CMV infections acquired during the birth process, via breast-feeding, or from blood or platelet transfusions do not produce neurologic deficits. (2) In congenital CMV: Most cases are clinically inapparent, but 5% have a syndrome of IUGR, microcephaly, intracerebral calcifications, and chorioretinitis. More commonly, the presentation involves IUGR, hepatosplenomegaly, and persistent jaundice. (3) In premature infants, severe interstitial pneumonia can be fatal.	(1) CMV present in high amounts in urine and saliva. (2) Can perform IgG CMV a ntibody testing at 6–12 weeks of age, LFTs, and imaging (CT, radiograph) to detect other abnormalities.	Evaluate for specific deficits, and test hearing using brainstem auditory evoked responses (repeated evaluations necessary because postnatal deafness can occur).

TABLE 11-11 Antenatal Infections—cont'd

Type	Symptoms	Tests	Treatment
Herpes simplex virus (HSV)	(1) Disseminated infection can involve the liver and other organs. May mimic sepsis in disease presentation. (2) Localized CNS disease presents with fever, lethargy, poor feeding, hypoglycemia, DIC, and irritability, followed by intractable focal or generalized seizures. (3) Localized infection of the skin, eye, and mouth can also occur.	(1) Viral culture or rapid assay. (2) Brain biopsy can be performed if encephalitis is suspected.	(1) Evaluate mother for active lesions prior to delivery. If active herpes lesions are present, deliver by cesarian section. (2) In cases of neonatal herpes infection, give intravenous acyclovir.
Syphilis	(1) Those symptomatic at birth exhibit nonimmune hydrops with anemia, thrombocytopenia, leukopenia, pneumonitis, hepatitis, and osteochondritis. (2) Symptoms in the first year of life include fever, osteitis, osteochondritis, hepatosplenomegaly, LAD, mucocutaneous lesions, persistent rhinitis (snuffles), jaundice, and failure to thrive. (3) Late sequelae: Bone signs (saber shins, frontal bossing), Hutchinson teeth, mulberry molars, saddle-nose deformity, rhagades, paresis, tabes, interstitial keratitis, deafness, and Clutton joints (painless joint effusions).	RPR and FTA-ABS on mother and infant.	(1) For infants without CNS disease, give penicillin G IV for 10–14 days. (2) For infants with CNS disease, give aqueous crystalline penicillin G for 3 weeks.

continued

TABLE 11-11 Antenatal Infections—cont'd

Type	Symptoms	Tests	Treatment
VZV	(1) First or second trimester exposure can cause cutaneous scars, abnormalities of the digits or limbs, eye defects, CNS anomalies, and low birth weight. (2) Third trimester exposure can cause diffusely disseminated skin lesions in varying states, which may progress to fatal pneumonia.	None.	(1) If mother has had VZV >5 days before birth: Isolate the infant for 7 days after rash onset. (2) If maternal VZV infection <5 days before birth or 2 days after birth: Give VZIG within 96 hours of birth. (3) Any infant who shows signs of neonatal infection should be given acyclovir for 10 days.
Human immunodeficiency virus	Asymptomatic at birth. Within first month, infants develop persistent thrush, hepatosplenomegaly, and LAD. This is followed by recurrent infections and failure to thrive throughout the first year of life.	HIV testing for mother and child.	(1) Treat mother with AZT, and deliver infant by cesarean section to prevent transmission. (2) For infected infants, give nutritional support, PCP prophylaxis, antiviral therapy, and anti-infective agents for specific infections. AZT therapy can be tried in an attempt to eradicate the virus from the neonate

AZT, azathioprine; CMV, cytomegalovirus; CNS, central nervous system; DIC, disseminated intravascular coagulation; FTA-ABS, fluorescent treponemal antibody absorption test; IUGR, intrauterine growth retardation; LAD, lymphadenopathy; LFTs, liver function tests; PCP, *P. carinii* pneumonia; RPR, rapid plasma reagin; VZIG, varicella-zoster immune globulin; VZV, varicella zoster virus.

TABLE 11-12
Postnatal Infections

Type	Symptoms	Tests	Treatments
Early-onset sepsis (*Presents within 1 week, and organisms include group* B Streptococcus, E. coli, Klebsiella, *and* Listeria)	(1) Overwhelming multiorgan system disease manifested by respiratory failure, shock, meningitis, DIC, acute tubular necrosis, and symmetric peripheral gangrene. (2) Patients at birth have nonspecific cardiorespiratory signs such as grunting, tachypnea, and cyanosis.	Blood, urine, and CSF culture and gram staining, cell count/differential, and protein and glucose levels. Radiograph and ABG measurements to screen for respiratory pneumonia and other problems.	Combination of ampicillin and gentamycin for 10–14 days. If meningitis is present, the treatment is extended to 21 days. If gram-negative meningitis (due to *Klebsiella* or *E. coli*) is present, use cefotaxime and amikacin synergistically.
Late-onset sepsis (*Occurs mostly in premature infants. Often caused by multidrug resistant strains in the NICU, including* S. aureus, S. epidermidis, *gram-negative bacteria, and* Candida.)	Patients have lethargy, poor feeding, hypotonia, apathy, seizures, bulging fontanelle, direct hyperbilirubinemia, and fever or hypothermia.	Same as above.	Basically the same as for neonatal sepsis. If *H. influenzae, S. pneumoniae*, or N. meningitidis is suspected, treat with ampicillin and cefotaxime for 10–14 days. For nosocomial staphylococcal infections, a combination of vancomycin and gentamycin is used. Candidal sepsis is treated with amphotericin B.
Chlamydia (Transmitted from the genital tract at a rate of 50%.)	(1) Symptomatic infection of the conjunctiva, pharynx, rectum, or vagina in the infant can persist for more than 2 years. (2) Afebrile pneumonia (with a repetitive, staccato cough) can develop between 3 and 19 weeks postnatally.	Same as above.	Oral erythromycin for 14 days. Topical therapy is not effective.

ABG, arterial blood gas; DK, disseminated intravascular coagulation; NICU, neonatal intensive care unit.

TABLE 11-13 Major Congenital Anomalies

Anomaly	Symptoms and Signs	Diagnostic Test	Treatment
Tracheoesophageal fistula (TEF)	(1) Presents with excessive drooling, inability to feed, gagging, and respiratory distress. (2) Can be associated with other abnormalities (VACTERL syndrome includes *v*ertebral, *a*nal, *c*ardiac, *t*racheal, *e*sophageal, *r*enal, and *l*imb anomalies).	Chest radiograph shows a blind pouch with air in the GI tract if the TEF is associated with esophageal atresia.	(1) Place infant in head-up 60-degree position to prevent aspiration of gastric contents. (2) Surgery.
Duodenal atresia	Bilious emesis beginning within a few hours of the first feeding after birth.	Abdominal radiographs show a "double bubble" sign.	Surgery.
Congenital diaphragmatic hernia	(1) Defect in the posterolateral diaphragm that allows abdominal contents to enter the thorax. Usually on the left side. (2) Presents as respiratory distress with decreased breath sounds on the affected side, a shift of heart sounds to the opposite side, and scaphoid abdomen. Bowel sounds may be heard in the chest.	Can often be visualized on prenatal ultrasonogram.	Intubation and mechanical ventilation followed by surgery.
Omphalocele	(1) Abdominal viscera herniated through the umbilical and supraumbilical portions of the abdominal wall into a sac covered by peritoneum and amniotic membrane. (2) Associated with polyhydramnios and premature birth.	Can often be visualized on prenatal ultrasonogram.	Do not reduce the sac. Give broad-spectrum antibiotics, and get surgical consultation.
Gastroschisis	Intestinal herniation (without a sac) through the abdominal wall 2 cm lateral to the umbilicus that is also associated with polyhydramnios and premature birth.	Can often be visualized on prenatal ultrasonogram.	Surgical closure if possible.
Cleft palate	May be associated with hypertelorism, hand defects, and cardiac anomalies.	None needed.	(1) Repair is usually done at 12–24 months. (2) Until then, feed the baby on its side, and reposition the tongue to avoid respiratory difficulties. (3) Complications include speech difficulties, dental disturbances, and recurrent otitis media.

12 CHAPTER

Psychiatry

I. General Concepts
   A. DSM-IV Axis Method of Psychiatric Assessment
      1. Axis I: Psychiatric disorders except for personality and developmental disorders
      2. Axis II: Personality or developmental disorders
      3. Axis III: Other medical issues
      4. Axis IV: Psychosocial or environmental issues
      5. Axis V: Global assessment of functioning (GAF) score
         a. 0–20: The patient is believed to be a danger to self or others.
         b. 21–50: The patient is not a danger to self or others but cannot hold a job or live independently. The patient is most likely an inpatient.
         c. 51–80: The patient has psychiatric issues that require therapy but is able to live independently and be treated as an outpatient.
         d. 81–100: There are no psychiatric issues that require treatment.
   B. Mental Status Examination
      1. A mental status examination is a process that assesses the physical appearance, arousal/attention, psychomotor activity, speech, mood, affect, memory, thought process, and thought content of the patient.
      2. The examination incorporates information from the entire encounter that is used to establish the mental state of the patient.
   C. Reasons to Admit Psychiatric Patients
      1. Danger to self
      2. Danger to others
      3. Inability to care for self
         a. Inability to give informed consent
         b. Psychosis
         c. Agitation
         d. Failure of outpatient treatment
   D. Treatment of Agitated Patients
      1. Haloperidol: Give orally (PO) or intramuscularly (IM) every 8 hours.
      2. Lorazepam: Give PO or IM.
      3. Risperidone: Preferable for elderly patients because it is not as likely to cause delirium.
   E. Suicide Assessment
      1. Risk factors
         a. Suicide plan.
         b. Previous suicide attempt: This is not true for manipulative attempts or attempts at self-mutilation. Assess the beliefs of the patient to determine his or her impression of the risk of the attempt. Attempts that seem to be low risk may actually be high risk if the patient thinks that he or she would have succeeded.

c. Voiced suicidal ideation.

d. Diagnosed psychiatric disorder: Especially major depressive disorder, bipolar disorder, schizophrenia, substance abuse, and delirium.

e. Age: Suicide rates are higher in adolescents and the elderly than in other age groups.

f. Sex: Women are more likely to attempt suicide, and men are more likely to succeed in a suicide attempt.

g. Social influences: Marital status, unemployment, personal loss, firearm ownership.

h. Hopelessness: Ask about the patient's plans for the future. Hopelessness is associated with long-term risk more than any other psychiatric symptom.

2. Treatment of the suicidal patient
   a. Treat underlying medical or psychiatric issues
   b. Psychotherapy
   c. Remove harmful objects and detain
   d. Patient can be discharged home when risk is gone and if there are good support systems in place and contacts for safety. Admit the patient with appropriate precautions if risk remains.
   e. Precautions
      (1) Suicide precaution I (SP-I): Arm's length observation (also referred to as "one-on-one" supervision).
      (2) Suicide precaution II (SP-II): Checks every 15 minutes.

II. Major Depressive Disorders (MDD)

A. Criteria for Diagnosis: Patient has depressed mood, including five or more of the following signs and symptoms (mnemonic—SIG E CAPS):
1. Decreased **s**leep
2. Decreased **i**nterest
3. **G**uilt
4. Decreased **e**nergy
5. Decreased **c**oncentration
6. Decreased **appetite**
7. **P**sychomotor retardation
8. **S**uicidal ideation

Women are twice as likely to develop MDD as are men.

The risk of MDD is three times higher in patients with a family history of depression.

B. Course
1. Episodes can last for years (usually last for 8–18 months).
2. Dysthymic disorder: Chronic low-grade depression.
3. Double depression: Dysthymia with an MDD episode interposed.

C. Subtypes of Depression
1. Melancholia: MDD with anhedonia, excessive guilt, and mood worse in the morning.
2. Atypical: Oversleeping, overeating, leaden paralysis, and mood reactivity (does not respond well to tricyclic antidepressants).
3. Psychotic: Nihilism, delusions, and hallucinations; must rule out bipolar disorder.

4. Postpartum: Begins 1 month after birth of infant.
5. Seasonal: Highest incidence is from October to February. Light therapy appears to be as effective as antidepressants.

D. Remission versus Recovery
1. Remission: Return to baseline.
2. Recovery: Remission and remaining at baseline for more than 6 months.
3. Relapse: New episode occurs less than 6 months after remission. This can be due to noncompliance associated with medications, stress, loss of medication efficacy, or absence of psychotherapy.
4. Recurrence: Another episode occurs following recovery. Risk of recurrence is 50% after one episode, 70% after two episodes, and 90% after three episodes.

E. Treatment
1. Pharmacotherapy (Table 12-1)
2. Psychotherapy: Can be beneficial.
   a. Indications for psychotherapy alone
      (1) Patient preference
      (2) Mild to moderate functional impairment
      (3) Acute onset related to adverse events
      (4) First depressive episode
   b. Types of psychotherapy
      (1) Structured (time limited): Effective as an adjunct to medication; it is not as time-consuming as other types of therapy.
      (2) Cognitive: Works on correction of the abnormal thought connections, but it requires a major time commitment and effort by both physician and patient.
      (3) Interpersonal: Effective when grief or interpersonal interaction difficulties are a cause of depression.
      (4) Behavioral: Focuses on behaviors that allow reduction of stress.
      (5) Insight oriented: Requires a major time commitment and can be costly. Goal is to effect a personality change.

III. Bipolar Disorder

A. Mania
1. Criteria for diagnosis: Patients have three of the following signs and symptoms for a period of 1 week (or less if hospitalization is required; mnemonic—DIG FAST):
   a. **D**istractibility
   b. **I**nsomnia
   c. **G**randiosity
   d. **F**light of ideas
   e. Increase in **a**ctivity/agitation
   f. Pressured **s**peech
   g. **T**houghtlessness
2. Bipolar I: Full mania and major depressive episodes.
3. Bipolar II: Hypomania with major depressive episodes.

Risk of bipolar disorder is increased by 15% if a first-degree relative has the disorder.

TABLE 12-1 Antidepressant Medications

Drug Class	Drug Name	Indication	Comments
Selective serotonin reuptake inhibitors (SSRIs)	Citalopram Fluoxetine Fluvoxamine Paroxetine Sertraline	Drugs of choice for bulimia, OCD, impulse control problems, panic disorder, generalized anxiety disorder, social anxiety, PTSD, and premature ejaculation.	Nonlethal in overdose. Serotonin syndrome can occur if an SSRI is taken in combination with an MAOI or tryptophan; this will cause sweating, mental status changes, agitation, and hyperreflexia. SSRI discontinuation syndrome occurs if SSRI is abruptly withdrawn (usually drug should be tapered over a 4-week period); symptoms include gait disturbance, sleep problems, mental status changes, and agitation.
Tricyclic antidepressants (TCAs)	Amitriptyline Clomipramine Desipramine Imipramine Nortriptyline	Reuptake inhibitors of serotonin and norepinephrine. Now used more for severe or psychotic depressions that do not respond to SSRI treatment. Amitriptyline is often used for neuropathic pain.	Fatal in overdose. Severe anticholinergic, antihistaminic, and α-adrenergic side effects; also can cause cardiac arrhythmias, orthostatic hypotension, and seizures. Use with caution in the elderly.
Monoamine oxidase inhibitors (MAOIs)	Isocarboxazid Phenelzine Selegiline (MAO-B inhibitor) Tranylcypromine	Blocks the breakdown of norepinephrine and serotonin. Best drugs used to treat atypical depression.	Orthostasis and edema. Interactions with dietary tyramine (e.g., cheese, wine, narcotics, antihistamines, pseudoephedrine) can produce a hypertensive crisis.
Serotonin and norepinephrine reuptake inhibitors	Venlafaxine	Most likely single agent used to treat depression to remission.	More adrenergic side effects than SSRIs (hypertension).
Other	Buspirone	Generalized anxiety disorder or medication-induced sexual dysfunction.	Headache, nervousness.

TABLE 12-1 Antidepressant Medications—cont'd

Drug Class	Drug Name	Indication	Comments
Other	Wellbutrin	Adjunct to SSRI therapy and help with cognitive symptoms.	Do not give to patients with bulimia or anorexia because it may cause seizures. Minimal sexual side effects.
Other	Trazodone	Patients with depression and insomnia respond well to this drug.	Sedating with minimal anticholinergic side effects. Priapism is a unique side effect of this drug.

OCD, obsessive-compulsive disorder; PTSD, post-traumatic stress disorder.

4. Course
    a. Average of one episode every 2 years.
    b. Average episode lasts 1–4 months, but patients can be ill continuously for up to 7 years.
    c. Patients who have one manic episode have an 85% chance of having another.
    d. Untreated patients will usually have about 10 episodes over a lifetime.

Among patients with bipolar disorder, 25% attempt suicide and 10% complete suicide.

B. Hypomania: Same features as mania, but the patient is not as impaired socially and symptoms need to last only 4 days to meet the criteria for diagnosis.
C. Cyclothymia
    1. A 2-year period of hypomania with periods of depressive symptoms (but not major depression).
    2. If the criteria for major depression are met, then diagnosis is changed to bipolar II disorder.
D. Mixed Episode: Manic criteria and major depressive criteria are both met for a period of 1 week.
E. Rapid Cycling: Four episodes of mood disturbance in the previous 12 months.
F. Treatment (Table 12-2)

Mania can be induced in a patient with bipolar disorder who is given antidepressants.

IV. Anxiety Disorders
  A. Generalized Anxiety Disorder (GAD)
    1. Criteria for diagnosis: Patients may appear anxious and have three of the following signs and symptoms (mnemonic—PREMIS):
        a. **P**oor concentration
        b. **R**estlessness
        c. **E**asy fatigability
        d. **M**uscle tension
        e. **I**rritability
        f. **S**leep disturbances
    2. Treatment
        a. Pharmacotherapy: Benzodiazepines, venlafaxine, and buspirone.

TABLE 12-2 Therapies Used in the Treatment of Bipolar Disorder

Treatment	Indication	Side Effects
Lithium	Onset of action is a few weeks. Better than other mood stabilizers for bipolar depression. When patients are not responsive to lithium therapy, add valproic acid or carbamazepine.	Narrow therapeutic index; maintain between 0.6 and 1.5 mEq/L. Most common side effects are gastrointestinal upset (from direct contact with lithium), tremor, and muscle weakness. Drug is not tolerated in one-third of patients. Monitor renal and thyroid function. Lithium toxicity: severe tremor, nausea, dysarthria, ataxia, and delirium.
Valproic acid	Can load rapidly, so responders show the greatest improvement within the first 3 days of treatment. Most patients will show a major decrease in symptoms, and one third will be symptom-free.	Common side effects include drowsiness, upset stomach, dizziness, and tremor. Long-term side effects can include weight gain, hair thinning, mild changes in liver function, and (rarely) liver damage and pancreatitis. Can increase the circulating levels of most other psychiatric drugs and seizure medications through binding to plasma proteins and/or inhibition of metabolism. Contraindicated during pregnancy due to teratogenicity.
Carbamazepine	Onset of action is within 1–2 weeks. May be more effective than lithium for mixed mania or rapid cyclers.	Short-term side effects include dizziness, headache, diplopia, sedation, and ataxia. Long-term side effects include leukopenia, changes in liver function, and Stevens-Johnson syndrome. Rarely can cause rash and blood dyscrasias (aplastic anemia, agranulocytosis). Perform serial complete blood counts before and during treatment. Can increase the metabolism of other drugs.
Gabapentin	Good for adjunctive use.	No drug interactions or side effects.
Lamotrigine	Good for adjunctive use and bipolar depression.	Rash that is difficult to differentiate from Stevens-Johnson syndrome.

TABLE 12-2 Therapies Used in the Treatment of Bipolar Disorder—cont'd

Treatment	Indication	Side Effects
Electroconvulsive therapy (ECT)	Indications for ECT include major depression, acute manic episode, acute psychosis, or depression or mania that is unresponsive to medication. Contraindications for ECT include increased intracranial pressure, recent myocardial infarction, coronary artery disease, heart failure, and bronchopulmonary disease.	Limited retrograde amnesia, but no lasting effects on memory or cognition.
Antidepressants	Can be used, but must discontinue within 6–12 weeks of remission of the depressive episode to prevent induction of mania.	See Table 12-1.

(1) Benzodiazepines
(a) Most commonly used: Lorazepam, diazepam, alprazolam, clonazepam, chlordiazepoxide, midazolam, triazolam.
(b) Act through the GABA receptor to decrease neuronal excitability.
(c) Used in the treatment of anxiety, agitation, insomnia, alcohol withdrawal, and seizure cessation and prophylaxis.
(d) Side effects: Respiratory depression (if taken in combination with other sedatives) and physical dependence.
(2) Tricyclic antidepressants are not effective in the treatment of GAD.

Benzodiazepines should not be used by pregnant women because they can cause floppy baby syndrome.

b. Psychotherapy can be effective.

B. Panic Disorder
1. Signs and symptoms
a. Recurrent unexpected panic attacks consisting of intense feelings of anxiety and fear of dying that may be accompanied by shortness of breath and chest pains. Attacks typically last less than 30 minutes. A workup for medical causes (such as myocardial infarction) is negative.
b. Phobic avoidance of situations in which attacks have occurred
c. Anticipatory anxiety

d. One third to one half of patients develop agoraphobia within 1 year of onset of panic disorder.
e. Women are twice as likely to have attacks as are men.

2. Neurologic disorders can cause secondary panic attacks (e.g., temporal lobe epilepsy, Parkinson's disease, postconcussion syndrome, multiple sclerosis).
3. Associated conditions include mitral valve prolapse.
4. Treatment
   a. Psychotherapy
   b. Pharmacotherapy: Tricyclic antidepressants (imipramine), selective serotonin reuptake inhibitors (SSRIs), or benzodiazepines (alprazolam). Use alprazolam cautiously owing to the increased potential for addiction. Longer-acting benzodiazepines (such as clonazepam) are less addictive and cause less severe withdrawal symptoms.

C. Phobias: Intense recurrent, unreasonable fear of an object, activity, or situation.
1. Agoraphobia: Fear of being unable to obtain help.
2. Specific phobia: Fear of an animal (e.g., spiders, snakes), the natural environment (e.g., heights, water), blood, injections, injury, or certain situations. Treatment involves systematic desensitization.
3. Social phobia: Fear of social situations in which patient is exposed to unfamiliar people or scrutiny. Treatment involves psychotherapy and/or SSRIs.

D. Post-traumatic Stress Disorder (PTSD)
1. Signs and symptoms
   a. Persistent re-experience of events (flashback) with thoughts, images, behaviors, or dreams.
   b. Decreased general responsiveness and avoidance of stimuli that bring back memories of the event.
   c. Hyperaroused state accompanied by affective lability, startle response, and difficulty concentrating and sleeping.
2. Treatment
   a. Psychotherapy.
   b. Pharmacotherapy: SSRIs, tricyclic antidepressants, monoamine oxidase inhibitors (MAOIs), or mood stabilizers; cautious use of benzodiazepines.

E. Obsessive-compulsive Disorder (OCD)
1. Obsessions: Recurrent, intrusive, unwanted thoughts and impulses that are recognized as senseless and unpleasant by the patient.
2. Compulsions: Repetitive acts that the patient recognizes as relieving the obsession but that are not always driven by obsessive thoughts.
3. There is a 10% risk of OCD in family members.
4. Comorbid conditions include Tourette's syndrome, a disorder involving tics and involuntary vocalizations that usually manifests before age 15 and lasts throughout life.

Pediatric autoimmune neuropsychiatric disorder associated with streptococcal infection (PANDAS) can occur in children with attention-deficit/hyperactivity disorder (ADHD)–like symptoms, separation anxiety, and obsessive-compulsive disorder (OCD).

5. Treatment
    a. Complete remission is uncommon.
    b. Pharmacotherapy: SSRIs, clomipramine, neuroleptics (if severe), benzodiazepines for anxiety.

V. Schizophrenia and Related Disorders
  A. Signs and Symptoms
    1. Major criteria for diagnosis of schizophrenia
      a. Symptoms usually not present in healthy patients (positive symptoms).
      b. Symptoms that involve deficiencies of traits that are present in healthy patients (negative symptoms).
    2. Positive symptoms
      a. Delusions: Strange thoughts that are out of touch with reality
      b. Hallucinations: Hypnagogic (at onset of sleep) or hypnopompic (upon awakening) hallucinations are less worrisome than those that occur at other times.
      c. Disorganized thinking: Can include tangential thought process, loose associations, word salad. This will impair effective communication.
      d. Disorganized behavior: Includes poor goal-directed behavior, inappropriate sexual behavior, and catatonic behavior.
    3. Negative symptoms: Bleuler's 4 As
      a. **A**ffective flattening
      b. **A**logia (without language)
      c. **A**volution (without motivation)
      d. **A**nhedonia (without pleasure)
  B. Prevalence
    1. Lifetime prevalence in the general population is 1%.
    2. Risk of developing schizophrenia is increased by 10% if a sibling or parent has the disorder and by 40% if both parents have it.
  C. Duration of Symptoms and Diagnosis
    1. Less than 1 month = brief psychotic episode or psychosis not otherwise specified (NOS).
    2. 1–6 months = schizophreniform disorder (one third of patients progress to schizophrenia).
    3. More than 6 months = schizophrenia.
  D. Subtypes of Schizophrenia
    1. Disorganized: The patient is disinhibited and has poor grooming habits and inappropriate emotional responses. This type has the worst prognosis of all the subtypes.
    2. Catatonic: Stupor, waxy flexibility (catalepsy).
    3. Paranoid: Delusions/hallucinations, good self-care; this type has the best prognosis.
    4. Undifferentiated: Includes characteristics of several subtypes.

Among patients with schizophrenia, 50% attempt suicide and 10% complete it.

E. Schizophrenia versus Schizoaffective Disorder: The patient must meet the criteria for schizophrenia, have mood symptoms, and show psychotic symptoms in the absence of a mood episode to be diagnosed with schizoaffective disorder.

F. Differential Diagnosis

1. Delusional disorder: The patient has nonbizarre delusions and does not meet the other criteria for schizophrenia. Delusion types include erotomanic, grandiose, jealous, persecutory, somatic, and mixed. Onset is usually in middle age or later. Treat with antipsychotics and anxiolytics.
2. Mood disorders: Psychosis occurs only during mood episodes.
3. Substance- or medication-induced psychosis.
4. Psychosis induced by a general medical condition.
5. Developmental disorder: Autism, Rett syndrome, Asperger's syndrome. Patients have poor social skills and poor communication skills but do not have delusions or hallucinations.
6. Personality disorders, especially cluster A (see section VIII.B.1).

Positive and negative symptoms of schizophrenia are differentially affected by many medications used for therapy.

G. Treatment: Antipsychotics (Table 12-3)

1. Dopamine antagonists (effective at the D_2 receptor)
2. Optimal clinical response is seen within 1–6 weeks.
3. Be alert for the development of dyskinetic symptoms when using antipsychotics (Table 12-4).

VI. Disorders of Childhood and Adolescence

A. Attention-deficit/Hyperactivity Disorder (ADHD)

1. Signs and symptoms
   a. Triad of inattention, hyperactivity, and impulsivity that occurs in multiple settings.
   b. Onset is before age 7, and symptoms have been present for more than 6 months.
   c. Physical examination and mental status examination are unremarkable.
2. Course
   a. Symptoms usually persist throughout childhood; 30% of patients retain some features of ADHD into adulthood.
   b. Some patients may develop other disorders, such as oppositional defiant disorder, conduct disorder, or antisocial personality disorder.
3. Treatment
   a. Specialized educational techniques and family psychotherapy may be useful.
   b. Stimulant medications: methylphenidate, amphetamines.
      (1) Stimulants act through an unknown mechanism to increase attention and decrease motor activity.
      (2) Side effects can include insomnia, temporary growth retardation, anorexia, and hepatotoxicity.
   c. Tricyclic antidepressants: may be useful if stimulant therapy fails. Antidepressant therapy is more effective in treating the symptoms of hyperactivity than the cognitive symptoms of ADHD.

TABLE 12-3 Antipsychotic Medications

Drug Class	Drug Name	Indication	Side Effects
Typical Antipsychotics			
High potency	Fluphenazine Haloperidol	High potency, effective for patients who have conditions or take medications that cause undesirable anticholinergic or hypotensive side effects (the elderly).	Movement disorders due to extrapyramidal effects (from nigrostriatal tract); can be treated by switching to an atypical antipsychotic. Galactorrhea, sexual dysfunction, antihistamine action, and anticholinergic action. Haloperidol has a decreased incidence of extrapyramidal symptoms if administered intravenously rather than orally; also QT prolongation, which can lead to torsades de pointes and other cardiac arrhythmias.
Medium potency	Perphenazine Loxapine Molindone	Effective in patients in whom sedative effects are desirable.	Tardive dyskinesia; anticholinergic and antihistaminic effects.
Low potency	Chlorpromazine	Effective for patients in whom extrapyramidal symptoms (EPSs) are particularly undesirable, those who can tolerate sedation, or for whom anticholinergic or hypotensive side effects would not present a danger.	Tardive dyskinesia is less severe than with other typical antipsychotics, but the anticholinergic and antihistaminic effects may be more severe.
Atypical Antipsychotics			
	Clozapine Risperidone Olanzapine Quetiapine (Geodon)	Better side effect profile (costly). More effective in treating the negative symptoms of schizophrenia than the typical antipsychotics. Olanzapine and quetiapine are first-line treatment of schizophrenia in patients who are adversely affected by extrapyramidal symptoms.	Clozapine has fewest extrapyramidal symptoms of all atypical agents, but monitor for agranulocytosis, seizures, and neuroleptic malignant syndrome. Risperidone has a minimal anticholinergic profile.

TABLE 12-4 Movement Disorders Associated with Antipsychotic Medications

Disorder	Symptoms and Treatment
Tremor	Resting and essential tremors.
Parkinsonism	Masked facies, slowed thought and movement, cogwheel rigidity.
Chorea	Dancelike movements that occur in the limbs.
Tardive dyskinesia	Abnormal oral and facial movements (tongue protrusion and lip smacking) that may be associated with abnormal limb and truncal movements.
Akathisia	Inner sense of restlessness. Treat with propranolol or benztropine.
Dystonia	Sustained abnormal posture. Types of specific dystonia can occur in the neck (torticollis), jaw (trismus), or eyes (oculogyric crisis). Treat dystonias with intramuscular anticholinergics (benztropine, trihexyphenidyl, or diphenhydramine).
Neuroleptic malignant syndrome	High fever, autonomic instability, muscle rigidity, rhabdomyolysis, renal failure. Treat with discontinuation of the antipsychotic and with supportive care. If untreated, 25% mortality rate.

B. Oppositional Defiant Disorder
   1. Signs and symptoms
      a. A pattern of defiance and hostility toward authority figures for at least 6 months that is in excess of the defiance typical of children of similar age.
      b. Behavior does not include physical hostility toward people or animals, theft, or deceit (all of which can be seen in conduct disorder).
      c. Patients frequently also have ADHD.
   2. Treatment
      a. Pharmacotherapy is not warranted unless the patient has comorbid ADHD.
      b. Psychotherapy for parents and family is useful for establishing coping skills to deal with the child's behavior.
      c. Behavioral management is necessary because the pattern of defiance might otherwise continue throughout life.

C. Conduct Disorder
   1. Signs and symptoms
      a. Consistent disregard for the rights of others and voluntarily causing others harm; may involve assault, torturing animals, or running away from home.
      b. About 40% of patients will progress to antisocial personality disorder as adults. ADHD may be a comorbid diagnosis in these patients.
   2. Treatment
      a. Family and parental psychotherapy is useful in establishing a home environment that does not reward tantrums and that appropriately responds to the patient's behavior. These therapies are more effective if they are started at an earlier age.

b. Pharmacotherapy for ADHD or mood disorders (if present); also, medications such as SSRIs, lithium, and antipsychotics can be used to manage excessive emotional lability, impulsiveness, and hallucinations.

D. Pervasive Developmental Disorders (Autism)

1. Subtypes

a. Asperger's syndrome: Patients have intact language and cognitive functioning.

b. Rett syndrome: Caused by a defective gene on the X chromosome that primarily affects girls and causes severe retardation and hand-wringing.

2. Signs and symptoms

a. Impairment of social interaction, communication, and restricted, repetitive, stereotyped patterns of behavior.

b. The first indicators of autism are the failure to reach language milestones, but the full diagnosis is usually made after 3 years of age.

3. Treatment: Consists mainly of behavioral therapy, which can increase the level of social functioning in mild cases if it is started at an early age.

E. Mental Retardation

1. Mental functioning below average, as measured by an intelligence quotient (IQ) score of less than 70, with onset before 18 years of age, and accompanied by impaired functioning.

Criteria for diagnosis of mental retardation: IQ less than 70, age under 18, impaired functioning.

a. Fragile X syndrome: Most common inherited cause of mental retardation (Fig. 12-1A).

b. Fetal alcohol syndrome: Most common preventable cause of mental retardation (Fig. 12-1B).

c. Trisomy 21 (Down syndrome): Chromosomal anomaly frequently associated with mental retardation (Fig. 12-1C).

2. Patients with mild mental retardation may not be recognized until schooling starts. Syndromes associated with severe mental retardation can often be recognized at birth owing to other congenital anomalies.

3. Treatment: Involves mainly behavioral therapy, with a goal of allowing the person to function as independently as possible.

VII. Eating Disorders

A. Types

1. Anorexia nervosa

a. Person is about 15% below ideal body weight with distorted body image and morbid fear of feeling fat or of being fat.

b. Amenorrhea is present for at least 3 months.

c. Presenting signs: Amenorrhea, lanugo, cold intolerance, lethargy, excess energy, emaciation, hypotension, hypothermia, skin dryness, bradycardia, and hypocarotenemia.

d. Death can occur as a result of cardiac arrest or suicide; 5% of patients die within 4 years of onset of the disorder.

2. Bulimia nervosa

a. Weight fluctuation with self-evaluation unduly affected by weight.

Some patients with bulimia nervosa may have normal body weight.

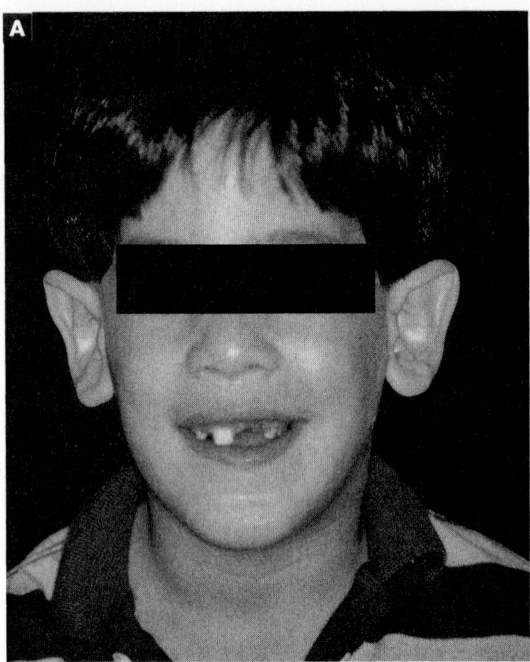

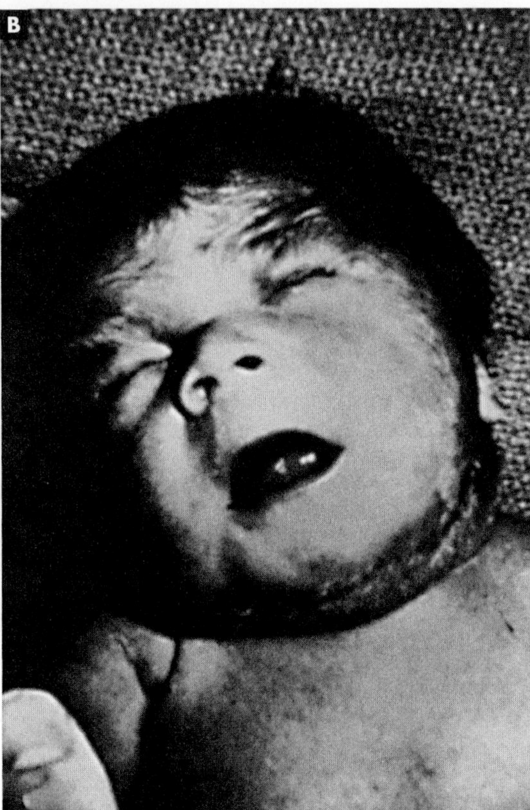

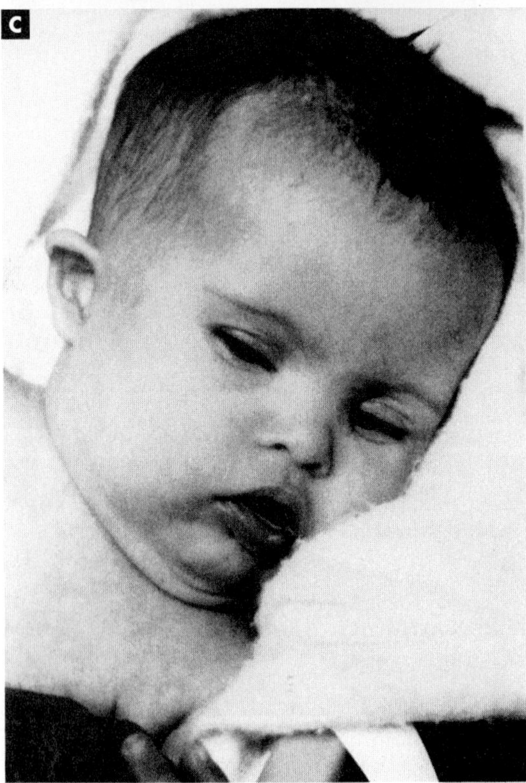

12-1: A, *Patients with fragile X syndrome have flat faces, protrusion of the tongue, and small ears.* B, *Patients with fetal alcohol syndrome have short palpebral fissures, a flat philtrum, facial hirsutism, and ptosis.* C, *Patients with Down syndrome have epicanthal folds, a depressed nasal bridge, and a simian crease on the hands.*

b. Episodes of bingeing and purging twice a week for 3 months. Purging can involve vomiting, laxative abuse, diuretics, enemas, fasting, or excessive exercise.

c. Presenting signs: Dental enamel erosion, enlarged parotid glands, scars on the dorsal surfaces of the hands, menstrual irregularities, and laxative dependence.

d. About 1% of patients die within 6 years of onset of the disorder.

B. Complications

1. Central nervous system (CNS): Irreversible gray matter changes.
2. Bone: Stunted growth, osteopenia, osteoporosis.
3. Gynecologic: Reduced fertility, higher risk of prematurity and perinatal complications.

C. Treatment

1. Restoration of nutrition and electrolytes: Refeeding at 30–40 kcal/kg per day is gradually increased to 40–60 kcal/kg per day.
2. Psychotherapy: To reevaluate and treat underlying psychiatric and environmental issues.
3. Pharmacotherapy: Antianxiety medications (SSRIs such as fluoxetine) can decrease premeal anxiety; atypical neuroleptics may decrease compulsivity.
4. Prognosis: About 70% of patients respond to treatment, but relapse rates are high.

VIII. Personality Disorders

A. Diagnosis

1. Persistent behavior that deviates markedly from the patient's culture.
2. Pattern manifests itself in two or more of the following areas:
   a. Cognition (perceptions or interpretations)
   b. Affectivity
   c. Interpersonal function
   d. Impulse control
3. Pattern is inflexible.
4. Behavior is not due to another psychiatric, medical, or substance-induced disorder.

B. Types of Personality Disorders (Clusters)

1. Cluster A (weird): Includes paranoid, schizoid, and schizotypal personality disorders. Patients often benefit most from cognitive behavioral therapy and supportive therapy and typically reject group psychotherapeutic approaches.
2. Cluster B (wild): Includes antisocial, borderline, histrionic, and narcissistic personality disorders. Patients often benefit from cognitive behavioral therapy and group psychotherapy.
3. Cluster C (worried): Includes avoidant, dependent, and obsessive-compulsive personality disorders. Patients often benefit from cognitive behavioral therapy and group psychotherapy.

3 Ws of personality disorders: Cluster A = "weird"; cluster B = "wild"; cluster C = "worried."

C. Defense Mechanisms (Table 12-5)

1. Just as individual personality disorders have characteristic dysfunctional behaviors and attitudes, the physician may also encounter characteristic defense mechanisms that can complicate communication with the patient.

TABLE 12-5 Common Defense Mechanisms Encountered in Personality Disorders

Defense Mechanism	Characteristics
Acting out	The patient deals with stressors with actions rather than feelings.
Controlling	The patient manipulates events and people.
Denial	The patient refuses to accept reality.
Devaluation	The patient sees attributes of self or others as worthless.
Dissociation	Alteration of consciousness, identity, or behavior to avoid emotional distress.
Distortion	The patient reshapes reality to meet inner needs.
Idealization	Exceedingly positive qualities are ascribed to self and others.
Identification	The patient adopts characteristics of people he or she admires to increase self-esteem.
Isolation of affect (intellectualization)	Separation of thought from associated feelings (intellectualization).
Projection	Attribution of unacceptable internal feelings to external sources.
Reaction formation	The patient rejects an impulse by embracing its opposite.
Regression	A return to a previous level of functioning.
Repression	The patient withholds a feeling from his or her conscious awareness.
Somatization	Manifestation of internal feelings through physical complaints.
Splitting	Compartmentalizing of opposite affective states.

2. Recognition of these defense mechanisms can be important in the establishment and maintenance of trust between the doctor and the patient.

D. Transference/Countertransference
   1. Transference occurs when something about the physician reminds the patient of someone else.
   2. Countertransference occurs when something about the patient reminds the physician of someone else.
   3. Both reactions can interfere with effective communication between physician and patient.

E. Cluster A

Paranoid = suspicious

   1. Paranoid personality disorder
      a. Criteria for diagnosis: Mistrust and suspicion of others, including four of the following:
         (1) Suspects others of deceiving or harming him or her without sufficient basis.
         (2) Preoccupied with doubts of trustworthiness.
         (3) Reluctant to confide in others.

(4) Reads threatening meanings into benign remarks.
(5) Bears grudges.
(6) Perceives attacks on character not apparent to others.
(7) Has recurrent suspicions about fidelity of partners.

b. Capsule snapshot: The patient with paranoid personality disorder believes the world is against him or her, is constantly on the defense against perceived outside threats (which are not present), and may hold a variety of conspiracy theories.

Schizoid = solitary

2. Schizoid personality disorder

a. Criteria for diagnosis: Detachment from social relationships and emotional expression, including four or more of the following:
(1) No interest or enjoyment in close relationships.
(2) Chooses solitary activities.
(3) No interest in sex.
(4) Anhedonia.
(5) Lacks close friends.
(6) Indifferent to the praise or criticism of others.
(7) Emotional coldness or flat affect.

b. Capsule snapshot: The patient with schizoid personality disorder is solitary by choice, with no interest in friendships, and may have a job that incorporates enjoyment of solitude, such as tending a lighthouse.

Schizotypal = strange

3. Schizotypal personality disorder

a. Criteria for diagnosis: Unusual perceptual experiences (including body illusions); odd thinking, speech, and behavior patterns; paranoia and suspicion.

b. Other features: Excessive social anxiety that does not lessen with familiarity, lack of close friends.

c. Capsule snapshot: The patient with schizotypal personality disorder has a bizarre impression of the world that may manifest as belief in bizarre abilities or powers. These individuals can be suspicious and solitary, but the strange beliefs and behavior are what classify them as schizotypal.

F. Cluster B

Antisocial = disregards others

1. Antisocial personality disorder

a. Criteria for diagnosis: Disregard for the rights of others since age 15, including three of the following:
(1) Repeated crimes
(2) Deceitfulness (including use of aliases)
(3) Impulsivity
(4) Aggressiveness
(5) Disregard for safety of others
(6) Financial and job irresponsibility
(7) Lack of remorse

b. Behaviors do not occur exclusively during a manic or psychotic episode but instead are present in the patient's daily behavior.

c. Capsule snapshot: The patient with antisocial personality disorder has the characteristics of a career criminal and is 18 years of age or older.

Younger patients with similar symptoms are assigned the diagnosis of conduct disorder, which may or may not progress to antisocial personality disorder when they become adults.

d. Treatment

(1) Valproic acid, lithium, or clozapine may be useful in controlling impulsivity.

(2) Antisocial patients frequently have substance abuse issues, which should also be addressed.

Borderline = impulsive

2. Borderline personality disorder

a. Criteria for diagnosis: Impulsivity and instability of relationships, affects, and image, including five of the following:

(1) Frantic efforts to avoid abandonment
(2) Unstable relationships
(3) Identity disturbance
(4) Impulsivity in several areas
(5) Recurrent suicidal ideation or attempts or self-mutilation
(6) Affective instability
(7) Chronic feelings of emptiness
(8) Inappropriate intense anger
(9) Stress-related paranoia

b. Capsule snapshot: The patient with borderline personality disorder shows significant emotional instability and frequently is on the verge of self-mutilation or suicide.

c. Treatment: Valproate and clozapine can be used to diminish aggression and impulse control issues.

Histrionic = exaggerated

3. Histrionic personality disorder

a. Criteria for diagnosis: Excessive emotionality and attention seeking, including five of the following:

(1) Seeks to be center of attention.
(2) Inappropriate seductive or provocative behavior.
(3) Rapidly shifting, shallow emotional experiences.
(4) Uses physical appearance to draw attention.
(5) Speech lacks detail.
(6) Theatrical and exaggerated emotion.
(7) Easily influenced by others.
(8) Considers relationships more intimate than others do.

b. Capsule snapshot: The patient with histrionic personality disorder craves attention and seeks to obtain it through any means necessary (e.g., clothing, inappropriate language, emotional outbursts).

c. Histrionic versus borderline personality disorder: Symptoms may appear similar, but patients with histrionic personality disorder are not as prone to self-mutilation or suicide as are those with borderline personality.

Narcissistic = grandiose

4. Narcissistic personality disorder

a. Criteria for diagnosis: Grandiosity and lack of empathy, including five of the following:

(1) Grandiose self-importance, but low sense of self-worth.

(2) Preoccupied with fantasies of success.
(3) Believes he or she can only be understood by other high-functioning people.
(4) Requires admiration.
(5) Sense of entitlement.
(6) Interpersonally exploitative.
(7) Lacks empathy (e.g., believes others must somehow have earned whatever misfortunes they are experiencing).
(8) Envious of others.
(9) Arrogant (e.g., believes he or she deserves promotion to the highest levels).

b. Capsule snapshot: The patient with narcissistic personality disorder is "out" for himself or herself and, regardless of actual position in life, acts as if he or she is the most important person around.

G. Cluster C

1. Avoidant personality disorder

Avoidant = inhibited

a. Criteria for diagnosis: Social inhibition and feelings of inadequacy, as indicated by four of the following:
(1) Avoids occupations with interpersonal contact.
(2) Unwilling to become involved with people unless acceptance is ensured.
(3) Fear of being ridiculed.
(4) Preoccupied with being criticized.
(5) Inhibited in new situations.
(6) Sees self as inferior.
(7) Reluctant to take personal risks.

b. Capsule snapshot: The patient with avoidant personality disorder is terrified of criticism and tries to be as invisible as possible.

c. Treatment: SSRIs can be used to decrease the anxiety these patients feel in social situations.

2. Dependent personality disorder

Dependent = helpless

a. Criteria for diagnosis: Submissive and clingy person with separation anxiety and five of the following:
(1) Needs others to assume responsibility for major areas of their life.
(2) Difficulty expressing disagreement.
(3) Difficulty initiating projects.
(4) Goes to excessive lengths to obtain nurturance.
(5) Feels helpless when alone.
(6) Urgently seeks another relationship when one ends.
(7) Unrealistically preoccupied with fears of being left to care for self.

b. Capsule snapshot: The patient with dependent personality disorder is extremely preoccupied with his or her primary interpersonal relationship and may tolerate a very poor relationship (e.g., abuse, adultery) because of fear of being alone.

3. Obsessive-compulsive personality disorder (OCPD)

Obsessive-compulsive = perfectionistic

a. Criteria for diagnosis: Preoccupation with orderliness at the expense of flexibility and efficiency, as indicated by four of the following:
   (1) Preoccupation with details, rules, order, or schedules to the point that the major point of the activity is lost.
   (2) Perfectionism that interferes with task completion.
   (3) Devoted to work at the expense of personal life.
   (4) Overly conscientious about morality.
   (5) Unable to discard worthless objects.
   (6) Reluctant to delegate tasks.
   (7) Miserly spending style.
   (8) Rigidity and stubbornness.

b. Capsule snapshot: The patient with OCPD is someone who "dots the i's and crosses the t's," but his or her actual job performance suffers from this fixation on perfection. This patient sees the work of others as inferior and is convinced that his or her attitude is the only one that will allow successful completion of the job.

c. OCPD versus OCD
   (1) OCPD is ego syntonic: The patient does not know that his or her behaviors are odd.
   (2) OCD is ego dystonic: The patient knows that the compulsions are odd but is unable to stop.

d. Treatment: SSRIs can be used to decrease the anxiety involved with the need for perfection and control.

IX. Somatoform Disorders

A. Somatization Disorder

1. Symptoms: Multiple complaints concerning various organ systems over time for which no physical basis can be found.

2. Treatment
   a. Chart diagnosis and inform physicians.
   b. Maintain contact with family members.
   c. Set limits on patient demands.

B. Conversion Disorder

1. Symptoms: Patients experience sensory or motor deficits that are thought to be caused by psychological factors (e.g., a woman loses her vision shortly after the death of her son). The deficit is not intentionally produced or feigned, but it causes clinically significant distress.

2. Treatment: Social learning, mimicry, and suggestion. Use amobarbital or methylamphetamine to strengthen suggestion if necessary.

C. Psychogenic Pain

1. Symptoms: These patients often have pain in the absence of identifiable physical causes, or they experience pain to a much more severe degree when a physical cause is present.

2. Treatment: Medications for acute pain syndromes (such as opioids) should not be given. Instead, patients should be managed with psychotherapy and medications for chronic pain disorders (including tricyclic antidepressants or gabapentin).

D. Hypochondriasis
   1. Preoccupation with the idea that a person has a disease owing to misinterpretation of bodily symptoms.
   2. Belief persists despite medical assurance.
   3. Belief is not strong enough to be delusional.
E. Factitious Disorder
   1. Intentional production or feigning of physical signs.
   2. Motivation is to assume the sick role.
   3. No external motives are present.
F. Malingering (Munchausen Syndrome)
   1. The intentional production of false symptoms for the acquisition of external incentives.
   2. When a dependent is harmed with the intention of acquiring such incentives, the condition is called Munchausen syndrome by proxy.

X. Substance Abuse
A. Abuse versus Dependence
   1. Abuse: Irresponsible use without the development of tolerance and without the induction of withdrawal symptoms on abstinence.
   2. Dependence or addiction: Tolerance has developed and the patient will show signs of withdrawal on abstinence. The patient will also continue use despite knowledge of the harmful consequences of continued substance abuse.
B. Commonly Abused Substances (Table 12-6)

TABLE 12-6 Commonly Abused Substances

Drug	Abuse Symptoms	Withdrawal Symptoms	Treatment
Alcohol	Alcohol-induced mood disorders: The patient will only associate the mood symptoms with periods of substance use, and the symptoms should resolve within days to weeks of drinking cessation. Complications of chronic use include: Wernicke's encephalopathy (ataxia, memory loss, and delirium), which can be reversed with administration of thiamine and vitamin B intramuscularly.	Common symptoms include anxiety and hypertension. Symptoms peak in about 3 days and diminish by day 5. Delirium tremens (DTs): gross cognitive disturbances (delirium) with agitation and tactile and visual hallucinations.	Use chlordiazepoxide to minimize withdrawal symptoms and gradually taper dosage. Group psychotherapy and support groups (e.g., Alcoholics Anonymous). Relapse can be prevented with disulfiram.

continued

TABLE 12-6 Commonly Abused Substances—cont'd

Drug	Abuse Symptoms	Withdrawal Symptoms	Treatment
	Korsakoff's syndrome: pronounced anterograde and retrograde amnesia along with other cognitive deficits. Can also be due to thiamine deficiency. Usually reversible. Alcohol-induced dementia: broader deficits than Korsakoff's syndrome, with evidence of cortical atrophy. Peripheral neuropathy: can also be due to vitamin B_{12} deficiency.	Seizures can occur. If untreated, DTs will cause death in 20% of cases.	
Opioids	Intoxication causes euphoria, followed by dysphoria, apathy, psychomotor problems, impaired judgment. Pupillary constriction, slurred speech, and impaired attention and memory can also occur. Mood disorders and psychotic disorders can occur as a result of opioid use. Overdose (OD) will present with depressed respiration, coma and pinpoint pupils with pulmonary edema and frothing at the mouth. Treat meperidine OD more aggressively because, in addition to respiratory depression, it can also cause seizures.	Patient becomes irritated and anxious, with dilated pupils, hypertension, tearing, and rhinorrhea; may also complain of insomnia and myalgias. Not life-threatening.	Methadone: used as a long-acting opioid to minimize withdrawal symptoms. Clonidine: can be used alone or in combination with methadone to treat the constitutional withdrawal symptoms. Naltrexone: can be used with clonidine to displace opioids from receptors. Buprenorphine: partial opioid agonist
Cocaine or amphetamines	Intoxication produces intense euphoria and self-confidence with hypervigilance. Psychosis can develop that usually clears up within 48 hours.	Anxiety, depression, anorexia, craving, and hypersomnia.	Can give lorazepam for agitation or haloperidol for psychosis.

TABLE 12-6 Commonly Abused Substances—cont'd

Drug	Abuse Symptoms	Withdrawal Symptoms	Treatment
	Complications of intoxication (not withdrawal) include cardiovascular problems (e.g., cardiac arrhythmias, myocardial infarction, myocarditis) and seizures. Example: in cocaine use, patients may hallucinate that bugs are crawling under their skin (formication).	Extended vulnerability to relapse.	Can give bromocriptine, or nothing at all, for withdrawal. Behavioral therapy can be useful to prevent relapses.
Cannabis	Euphoria; conjunctival injection; reduced concentration, motivation, and new learning; impaired coordination and increased appetite; can also produce anxiety, persecutory delusions, and psychosis. Complications of long-term use include delirium, decreased heart rate, infertility, and gynecomastia.	Irritability and restlessness.	—
Phencyclidine (PCP)	Intoxication can produce behavioral disinhibition and aggression with disruption of sensory input. Seizures, psychosis, and anticholinergic symptoms can also occur. Hypertension is also present, and there is a risk of hypertensive crisis with increasing doses. Ketamine (Special K) is a related compound that acts through NMDA receptor antagonism.	Not typically encountered.	Give lorazepam for agitation and haloperidol for psychosis. Minimize sensory input.

continued

TABLE 12-6 Commonly Abused Substances—cont'd

Drug	Abuse Symptoms	Withdrawal Symptoms	Treatment
Benzodiazepines	Effects of intoxication appear similar to those of alcohol intoxication.	Anxiety, insomnia, tachycardia, tremor, hallucinations, and seizures. Withdrawal will be most severe in patients who are dependent on short-acting benzodiazepines, such as alprazolam.	Dangerous withdrawal effects can be avoided by switching to a long-acting benzodiazepine (chlordiazepoxide) and gradually tapering over several days.
Hallucinogens	Intoxication can produce perceptual changes (usually not full hallucinations), psychosis, pupillary dilation, and tachycardia.	No physical addiction; no withdrawal.	Reassurance and prevention of patient from self-injury.
Nicotine	Intoxication produces symptoms of malaise; usually happens only to people who smoke while using the nicotine patch.	Irritability, anxiety, depression, insomnia, hunger and weight gain.	Smoking cessation may be facilitated with nicotine gum or patches. Wellbutrin may be useful in decreasing nicotine craving during withdrawal.
Caffeine	Intoxication produces anxiety, nervousness, gastrointestinal disturbances, tremors, and tachycardia.	Headache, malaise.	—

13 CHAPTER

Pulmonology

Risk factors for pulmonary embolism consist of Virchow's triad of venous stasis, injury to the endothelium, and a hypercoagulable state.

I. Pulmonary Embolism (PE)
   A. Symptoms and Signs
      1. Patients have dyspnea, chest pain, cough, anxiety, and sometimes hemoptysis.
      2. Physical examination findings include tachycardia, increased pulmonary component of S_2, tachypnea, and low-grade fever (high-grade fever suggests pneumonia rather than a pulmonary embolism).
      3. A deep vein thrombosis (DVT) may be present as an embolic source. DVT can present with calf pain, edema, and venous distention.
   B. Evaluation
      1. ECG usually displays sinus tachycardia, but the ECG also helps rule out myocardial infarction (MI) as a cause of chest pain.
      2. Chest radiograph is usually normal, but a wedge-shaped infarct (Hampton's hump) may be present. Spiral CT scanning with contrast is becoming the imaging modality of choice for visualization of pulmonary emboli.
      3. Arterial blood gas (ABG) measurement shows a respiratory alkalosis with a pO_2 greater than 80 mm Hg.
      4. D-dimer is elevated. This is not a specific test for PE, but a negative D-dimer helps rule out PE.
      5. Ventilation/perfusion (V/Q) scan: A normal result can rule out PE. A high-probability result gives a 90% chance of PE, and a low-probability result a 30% chance of PE.
      6. Doppler ultrasonography: Can be used to check for DVT.
      7. MRI, ultrafast CT scans, and pulmonary angiography are alternative imaging modalities for detection of PE.
   C. Treatment
      1. Anticoagulate with heparin, and start warfarin to build up therapeutic levels, as indicated by an international normalized ratio (INR) of 2–3. Anticoagulation should be continued for 6 months following discharge.
      2. Consider an inferior vena cava (Greenfield) filter if the patient has repeated PEs from the legs or if anticoagulation is contraindicated. Even with a filter, anticoagulation should be continued, if possible, because of the possibility of thrombosis of the filter.
      3. Thrombolysis is indicated if the DVT or PE is causing hemodynamic compromise.

II. Asthma
   A. Signs and Symptoms
      1. Patients have cough, dyspnea, wheezing, and chest tightness.
      2. Physical examination findings include decreased breath sounds, wheezing, hyperresonance, and use of accessory respiratory muscles.

Variant presentations of asthma include cough variant asthma (in which cough is the major presenting symptom) and exercise-induced asthma (in which attacks occur several minutes after stopping exercise). Exercise-induced asthma can be avoided by the use of pre-exercise β-agonist inhalers, by exercising in a humid environment, or by wearing a mask during exercise.

3. Some patients may have Sampter's triad of asthma, nasal polyps, and aspirin sensitivity.
4. Precipitants for asthma attacks can include allergens, irritants, infection, reflux disease, cold air, and drugs (aspirin, beta-blockers).

B. Evaluation

1. Peak flowmeter: Measurements vary with age and size but peak flow is typically greater than 400 L/min. Admit the patient if the peak flow is less than 60 L/min or does not improve to 50% of the predicted value after 1 hour of treatment.
2. ABG: Will show respiratory alkalosis (decreased $PaCO_2$) early, followed by pseudonormalization and eventual respiratory acidosis as the patient's blood oxygen falls. An increased $PaCO_2$ indicates respiratory failure, and the patient should be admitted.
3. Chest radiograph: In an acute exacerbation, it may reveal hyperinflation, flat diaphragms, and a vertical heart. It also may display attack precipitants such as pneumonia or mimics such as pulmonary edema.
4. Pulmonary function tests (PFTs): Patients have low FEV_1, and a low FEV_1/FVC ratio indicates obstruction during an attack. There should be a 10% to 15% improvement in FEV_1 in response to a bronchodilator.
5. Airway hyperreactivity can be tested using a methacholine or cold air challenge.

C. Treatment

1. Usually incorporates an inhaled corticosteroid on a regular basis for long-term control and a β-agonist inhaler as needed.
2. Short-term therapies for asthma attacks include albuterol (inhaled or nebulized) and anticholinergics (ipratropium).
3. Long-term therapy includes the following:
   a. Corticosteroids (methylprednisolone) for prevention of airway inflammation.
   b. Long-acting β_2-agonists (salmeterol).
   c. Cromolyn, nedocromil, and theophylline can be used.
   d. Antileukotriene agents (zileuton and zafirlukast) are particularly useful in exercise-induced asthma or aspirin sensitivity.

III. Chronic Obstructive Pulmonary Disease (COPD): The two main forms of COPD are chronic bronchitis and emphysema.

A. Symptoms and Signs

1. Chronic bronchitis: Sometimes referred to as "blue bloaters," these patients are overweight and have mild dyspnea and copious sputum production. ABGs can show high pCO_2 with marked hypoxemia, and PFTs show normal elastic recoil with markedly increased airway resistance.
2. Emphysema: Sometimes referred to as "pink puffers," these patients are often thin with complaints of severe dyspnea, pursed lip breathing, and minimal sputum production. ABGs show normal pCO_2 with mild hypoxemia. PFTs show severely reduced elastic recoil with mildly increased resistance.

3. Symptomatic exacerbations can be triggered by infection, irritation, or congestive heart failure.
4. General physical findings include increased anteroposterior chest diameter, hyperresonant lung fields, decreased breath sounds, increased length of expiratory phase, rhonchi, and wheezing. Diaphragmatic flattening can cause Hoover's sign (inward movement of the lower rib cage during inspiration) and thoraco-abdominal paradox (simultaneous inward movement of the abdominal wall and outward movement of the chest during inspiration).

B. Evaluation
1. Chest radiograph shows clear lung fields with flattened diaphragms and hyperinflated lungs (Fig. 13-1A).
2. CBC: Patients have high HCO_3 and high hemoglobin as compensation for chronic hypoxia.
3. PFTs: Patients have decreased FEV_1, FVC, and FEV_1/FVC due to obstruction. Total lung capacity (TLC) and residual volume (RV) are increased due to hyperinflation. See Table 13-1 for a comparison to restrictive lung disease.
4. ABG: Patients have varying degrees of hypoxemia and hypercapnia depending on the type of COPD, as described previously.

C. Treatment
1. Supplemental O_2.
a. Home O_2 therapy is indicated if the patient's resting pO_2 is less than 55 mm Hg or oxygen saturation is less than 88%.
b. CO_2 retainers (patients with chronic high pCO_2) may do worse with supplemental O_2 because they are accustomed to high HCO_3 levels and are predominantly using hypoxemia for their respiratory drive. Acutely increasing their O_2 saturation may cause them to lose their respiratory drive altogether.
c. The reactive airway component can be managed similarly to asthma. Albuterol inhalers or nebulizers are used for bronchodilation, along with corticosteroids and anticholinergic agents.
d. Patients should receive the pneumococcal vaccine, and chronic bronchitis can be treated with trimethoprim/sulfamethoxazole (TMP-SMX).

TABLE 13-1 Comparison of Pulmonary Function Test Measurements in the Evaluation of Obstructive and Restrictive Lung Disease

Type	Obstructive Lung Disease	Restrictive Lung Disease
FVC	Decreased	Decreased
FEV_1/FVC	Decreased	Normal or increased
TLC	Normal or increased	Decreased

FEV_1, forced expiratory volume in 1 second; FVC, forced vital capacity; TLC, total lung capacity.

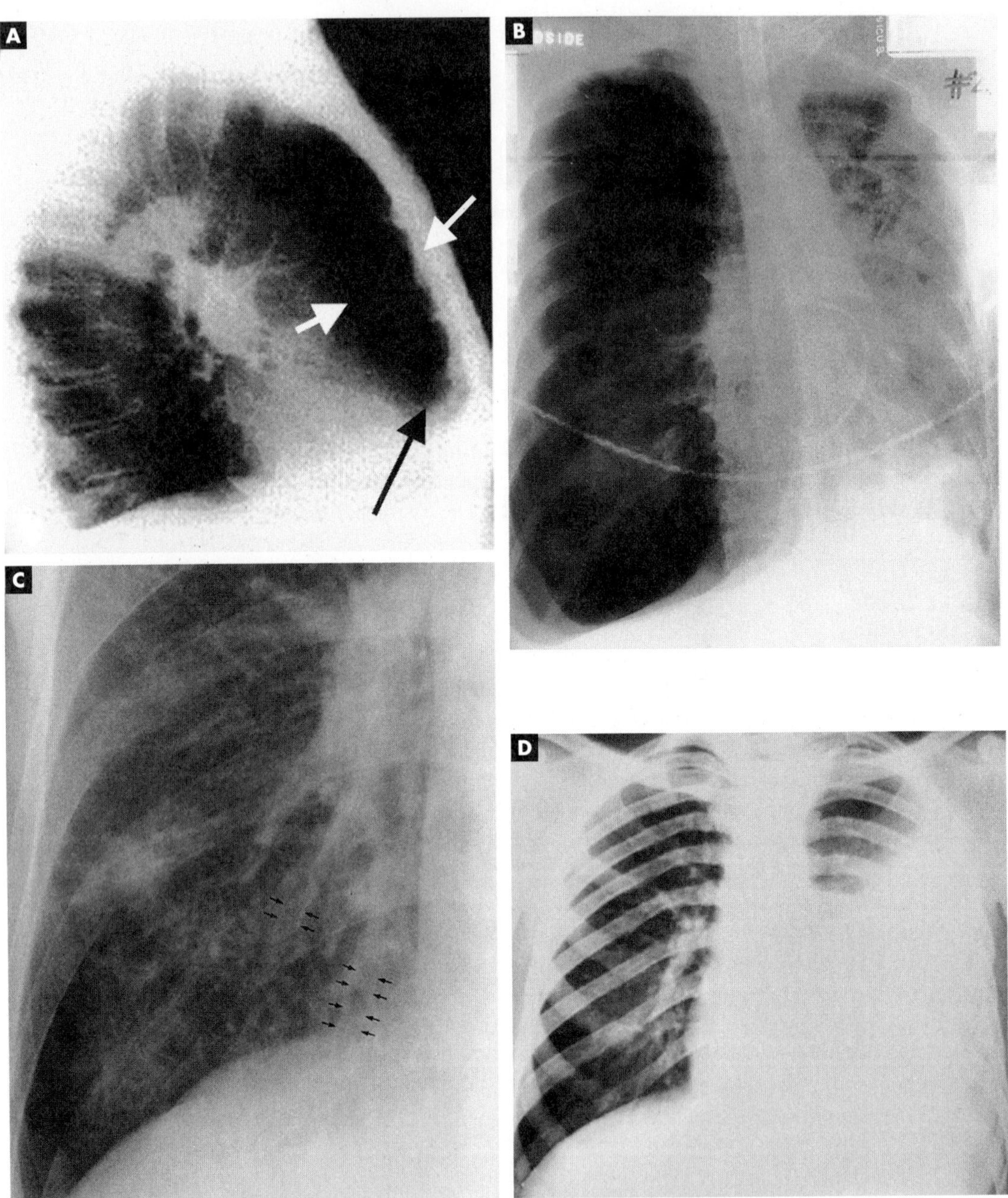

13-1: *Representative chest radiographs of common pulmonary disorders.* A, *In chronic obstructive pulmonary disease (COPD), patients have clear lung fields with hyperinflated lungs* (white arrows) *and clear diaphragms* (black arrow). B, *Tension pneumothorax displays hyperlucency and diaphragmatic flattening on the affected side, with deviation of the trachea away from the affected lung.* C, *Bronchiectasis displays a "tram track" appearance* (arrows) *with thickening of the bronchial walls.* D, *Pleural effusion displays a fluid collection with a visible meniscus denoting the air-fluid level.*

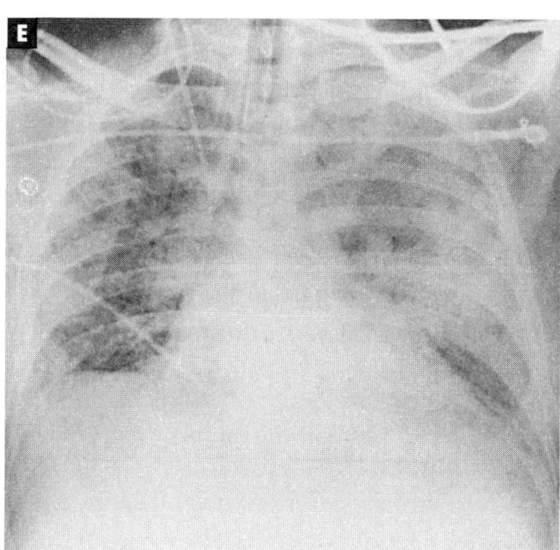

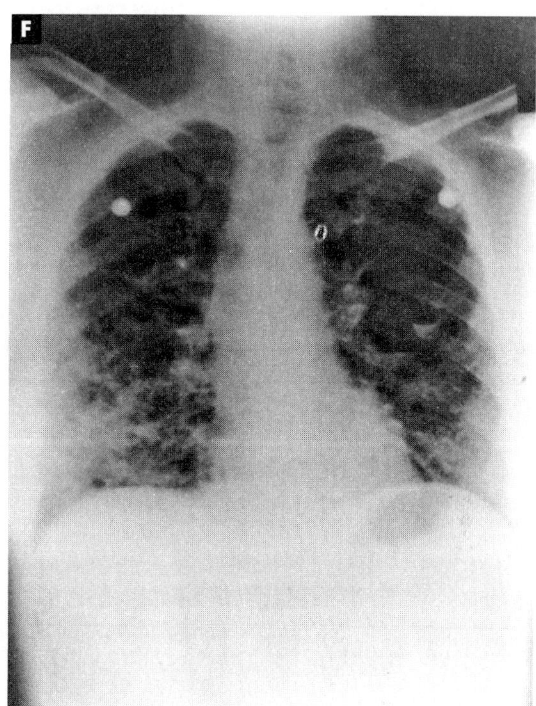

13-1: cont'd. E, *Acute respiratory distress syndrome (ARDS) presents with pulmonary infiltrates diffusely throughout the lung fields that develop within 24 hours.* F, *Sarcoidosis can produce hilar lymphadenopathy and diffuse interstitial lung disease.*

IV. Pneumothorax

A. Causes

1. Primary: Due to subpleural apical blebs or Marfan's syndrome.
2. Secondary: Due to COPD, asthma, tuberculosis (TB), trauma, or *Pneumocystis carinii* pneumonia.
3. Iatrogenic: Due to thoracentesis, subclavian lines, positive pressure ventilation, or bronchoscopy.

B. Symptoms and Signs

1. Patients complain of acute-onset of pleuritic chest pain and dyspnea.
2. Physical findings include diminished breath sounds, hyperresonance to percussion, and decreased tactile fremitus.
3. Tension pneumothorax presents with respiratory distress, falling O_2 saturation, hypotension, and tracheal deviation.

C. Evaluation (see Fig. 13-1B): Chest radiograph displays hyperlucency in the affected lung field, deviation of the trachea away from the affected lung, and flattening of the diaphragm on the affected side.

D. Treatment

1. Small pneumothoraces can resolve spontaneously.
2. Large or severely symptomatic pneumothoraces can be treated with chest tube insertion and supplemental O_2. Recurrent pneumothorax can be treated surgically with pleurodesis (fusion of the pleural membranes).

3. Tension pneumothorax can be treated with immediate needle thoracostomy with a 14-gauge needle in the second or third intercostal space at the midclavicular line.
4. Any patient with a pneumothorax on mechanical ventilation should have a chest tube inserted owing to the high risk of tension pneumothorax development.

V. Pneumonia (see Chapter 6)

VI. Bronchiectasis (Abnormal dilation of the bronchi due to smooth muscle destruction)
A. Causes
1. Allergic bronchopulmonary aspergillosis.
2. Chronic respiratory infections associated with immunodeficiency.
3. Abnormal airway clearance (Kartagener's syndrome is a ciliary defect causing sinusitis, situs inversus, and infertility in which bronchiectasis frequently occurs).
4. Cystic fibrosis.
B. Symptoms and Signs: Patients have a chronic cough that may be productive of large amounts of sputum (which may be blood tinged).
C. Evaluation (see Fig. 13-1C): Chest radiograph shows a "tram track" appearance due to thickening of the bronchial walls.
D. Treatment: Regimens vary but often involve bronchodilators, mucolytic agents, and anti-inflammatories, with the addition of TMP-SMX or amoxicillin for acute exacerbations.

VII. Interstitial Lung Disease
A. Symptoms and Signs: Patients have cough and progressive dyspnea, but the diagnosis is usually made only after lung biopsy.
B. Causes (Table 13-2)
C. Evaluation
1. PFTs show a decreased TLC with decreased diffusing capacity. See Table 13-1 for a comparison to obstructive lung disease.
2. Lung biopsy is usually necessary for diagnosis.
3. Antigen challenge tests can be used in hypersensitivity.
D. Treatment (see Table 13-2)

VIII. Pleural Effusion
A. Symptoms and Signs
1. Patients are asymptomatic or have complaints of dyspnea or chest pain.
2. Physical examination findings include decreased breath sounds, dullness to percussion, and decreased tactile fremitus.
B. Types of Effusion (Table 13-3)
1. Transudative effusions: Occur as a result of fluid movement out of the vasculature owing to high hydrostatic pressure or low oncotic pressure in the intravascular compartment.

TABLE 13-2
Major Causes of Pulmonary Fibrosis

Condition	Description
Idiopathic pulmonary fibrosis	(1) Patients usually have gradual onset of dyspnea with nonproductive cough for years. More rapidly progressive disease can be seen in Hamman-Rich syndrome. (2) CT scan shows a ground-glass appearance with linear opacities. (3) Treatment includes oral prednisone and lung transplantation.
Pneumoconioses	(1) Result from inhaling and retaining dusts in the workplace that result in inflammation and fibrosis. (2) Asbestosis: Associated with 6× risk of mesothelioma formation, 60× risk increase if the patient also smokes. Biopsy shows ferruginous bodies. (3) Silicosis: Biopsy shows birefringent crystals and alveolar proteinosis. (4) Coal: Biopsy shows anthracotic pigment accumulation. (5) Berylliosis: Biopsy shows granulomas. Can confirm the diagnosis with a lymphocyte transformation test. (6) The only treatments available are oxygen and supportive measures.
Hypersensitivity pneumonitis	(1) Similar in pathogenesis to pneumoconioses but the dust elicits a hypersensitivity reaction rather than simple inflammation and fibrosis. (2) Subtypes include farmer's lung, humidifier-associated pneumonitis, and pigeon breeder's lung. (3) Biopsy shows obliterative bronchiolitis without granulomas. (4) Avoid antigens. Give systemic corticosteroids for acute attacks.
Medication-induced	(1) Patients are taking a causative medication and have fever and cough. Many cases are mistaken for bacterial pneumonia. (2) Chemotherapeutics including bleomycin (if >450 U cumulative dose, irradiation lowers threshold), busulfan, cyclophosphamide, methotrexate, and nitrosoureas can cause disease. (3) Other drugs that cause pulmonary fibrosis include (mnemonic—HIT SNAG): **h**ydralazine, **I**NH, **t**hiazides, **s**ulfonamides, **n**itrofurantoin, **a**miodarone (especially if the patient is taking ≥400 mg/day), and **g**old. (4) Most drug-induced interstitial lung disease is reversible if the drug is discontinued early in the course of the disease.
Infection	Viral infections, *Pneumocystis carinii* pneumonia, fungal infections, and HIV can cause fibrosis.
Malignancy	Fibrosis can occur due to carcinomatosis, bronchoalveolar carcinoma, and lymphoproliferative disorders.
Collagen vascular disease	See Chapter 14.
Vasculitis (Wegener's granulomatosis)	See Chapter 14.

TABLE 13-3 Exudative and Transudative Pleural Effusions

Type	Transudative Effusion	Exudative Effusion
Causes	(1) Major causes include CHF, nephrotic syndrome, cirrhosis, protein malnutrition, or ascites. (2) Capillaries are intact.	(1) Major causes include **i**nfections, **n**eoplasm, **p**ulmonary emboli, **u**remia, **t**raumatic pleural taps, **c**ollagen vascular disease, **p**ancreatitis, and **c**hylothorax (mnemonic—INPUT CPC). (2) Capillaries are leaky due to inflammation.
Pleural fluid protein	Low protein (<0.5 pleural/serum ratio).	High protein (>0.5 pleural/serum ratio).
Pleural fluid lactate dehydrogenase (LDH)	Low LDH (<0.6 pleural/serum ratio).	High LDH (>0.6 pleural/serum ratio).
Other pleurocentesis results	Transudative effusions are similar to filtered serum and so should not contain any abnormal cells or components that are not found in serum.	(1) Lymphocytic taps indicate viral infection, TB, or malignancy. (2) Triglyceride-rich (milky) taps indicate chylothorax. (3) Pus in the pleural space (empyema) or organisms detected on Gram staining suggest infection as a cause of effusion. (4) Tumor cells may be present on cytologic examination in malignant effusions.

CHF, congestive heart failure; TB, tuberculosis.

2. Exudative effusions: Occur as a result of an increase in the permeability of the pleural compartment caused by one of several disease processes.

C. Evaluation

1. Chest radiograph shows fluid accumulation with a visible meniscus (see Fig. 13-1D).
2. Diagnostic thoracentesis can be performed and pleural fluid sent for evaluation. Protein and lactate dehydrogenase (LDH) levels in both serum and pleural fluid are useful for determining whether the effusion is exudative or transudative (see Table 13-3).

D. Treatment

1. Therapeutic thoracentesis can be performed for exudative effusions. Serial thoracentesis can be performed for malignant effusions.
2. Tube thoracostomy should be used if empyema is present.
3. Treat underlying diseases.

IX. Pulmonary Hypertension (Mean pulmonary artery pressure >25 mm Hg at rest or >30 mm Hg with exertion)

A. Causes

1. Increased pulmonary blood flow (cardiac septal defects or patent ductus arteriosus).
2. Increased pulmonary venous pressure (left heart failure or mitral valve disease).
3. Occlusion of the pulmonary arteries (pulmonary embolism, vasculitis, stenosis).
4. Pulmonary arterial vasoconstriction (due to hypoxia or acidosis).

B. Symptoms and Signs
1. Patients have dyspnea, exertional syncope, and exertional chest pain. Hoarseness may occur owing to recurrent laryngeal nerve compression by the left pulmonary artery.
2. Physical examination findings include a prominent pulmonary component of the second heart sounds, a right ventricular heave, a fourth heart sound, and murmurs from the pulmonary and tricuspid valves.

Cor pulmonale is a condition in which pulmonary hypertension or lung disease causes hypertrophy and/or failure of the right ventricle owing to increased pulmonary pressures.

C. Evaluation
1. ECG is consistent with right atrial enlargement, right ventricular hypertrophy, and right bundle branch block.
2. Echocardiogram shows right-sided pressure overload.
3. Chest radiograph, PFTs, and ABGs will rule out infection and COPD.

D. Treatment
1. Supplemental oxygen.
2. Gentle diuresis: The right ventricle is preload dependent, so a dramatic decrease in blood volume will send the patient into heart failure.
3. Vasodilators.
   a. Vasodilator challenge with nitric oxide will predict the usefulness of long-term vasodilator therapy.
   b. Nifedipine and prostacyclin can both be beneficial to the majority of patients with primary pulmonary hypertension. This has not been shown in secondary pulmonary hypertension.
   c. Consider anticoagulation because decreased cardiac output can lead to increased thrombosis.
4. Lung transplantation.

X. Acute Respiratory Distress Syndrome (Noncardiogenic pulmonary edema due to lung injury)

A. Cause: Most cases are caused by infection (systemic or pulmonary), severe trauma, or aspiration of gastric contents.

B. Symptoms and Signs
1. Patients have an acute onset of severe hypoxemia that is not responsive to supplemental oxygen.
2. These patients have no evidence of volume overload.

C. Evaluation
1. Chest radiograph shows diffuse bilateral pulmonary infiltrates that develop within 24 hours.
2. Infiltrates may give a "whiteout" appearance (see Fig. 13-1E).

D. Treatment

1. Mechanical ventilation: Use a high positive end expiratory pressure (PEEP) of 10–12 mm Hg and inspiratory time and maintain the plateau pressure at less than 35 cm H_2O.
2. Nitric oxide and prone ventilation can also be used to maximize the PaO_2.
3. Corticosteroids: Attempt IV methylprednisolone if the patient does not improve after 1 week.

E. Prognosis: Poor; 40% mortality in isolated acute respiratory distress syndrome (ARDS) and 90% mortality if the patient has multiorgan disease.

XI. Sarcoidosis

A. Symptoms and Signs (Mnemonic—LUNG RING)

1. **L**ymphadenopathy
2. **U**veitis
3. **N**egative TB test
4. **G**ranulomas
5. **R**heumatoid arthritis
6. **I**nterstitial fibrosis
7. Erythema **n**odosum
8. **G**ammaglobulinemia

B. Evaluation

1. Nodule may be visible on chest radiograph (see Fig. 13-1F).
2. Biopsy of the nodule shows noncaseating granulomas.
3. Angiotensin-converting enzyme (ACE) levels are elevated.
4. Hypercalcemia.
5. Alkaline phosphatase are elevated if the liver is involved.

C. Treatment

1. Treat with systemic corticosteroids.
2. Eye disease should be evaluated and followed by an ophthalmologist.

D. Prognosis: After 3 years, one third of cases are in remission, one third are unchanged, and one third have worsened.

XII. Solitary Pulmonary Nodule

A. Patients have a pulmonary nodule identified on chest radiograph in the absence of any symptoms suggesting a specific pulmonary diagnosis.

B. There is an increasing chance of malignancy with increasing age, smoking history, or history of other malignancies.

C. Types

1. Benign (70%)
   - a. Granuloma (90%)
   - b. Hamartoma (5%)
   - c. Cyst
   - d. Arteriovenous (AV) malformation
   - e. Various infectious, ischemic, or inflammatory foci
2. Malignant (30%)
   - a. Bronchogenic carcinoma (75%)
   - b. Metastasis (20%)

c. Carcinoid
d. Sarcoma

D. Evaluation
1. Serial chest radiographs to document changes in the nodule. Nodules of stable size for 2 years are likely to be benign.
2. Infectious workup, including PPD for TB and fungal serologies.
3. Lung biopsy usually is not indicated owing to the high probability of sampling error.

E. Management
1. Active observation.
2. Repeat chest radiograph every 3 months to monitor for changes.
3. If the patient has a significant risk for lung cancer, the mass can be removed surgically.

XIII. Lung Cancer (see Chapter 10)

CHAPTER 14

Rheumatology

I. Arthritis (Fig. 14-1 and Table 14-1)

II. Spondyloarthropathies
   A. Ankylosing Spondylitis
      1. Symptoms and signs
         a. Patients have a gradual onset of intermittent bouts of lower back pain and stiffness. This stiffness is worst in the morning and improves with a hot shower and exercise.
         b. Patients may have tenderness at the costochondral junctions, spinous processes, scapulae, iliac crests, and heels, which are indicative of sacroiliitis and spondylitis.
         c. Acute anterior uveitis can cause blurred vision, lacrimation, and photophobia. Aortic insufficiency is another potential complication.
      2. Evaluation
         a. Radiograph of the hip will show sacroiliac joint erosions and sclerosis.
         b. Radiograph of the spine shows calcification of the spinal ligaments and "bamboo spine" (Fig. 14-2).
         c. Strongly associated with the HLA-B27 genotype.
      3. Treatment includes NSAIDs, physical therapy, and sulfasalazine. Consult an ophthalmologist if uveitis is present.
   B. Reiter's Syndrome
      1. Symptoms and signs
         a. Patients have a triad of arthritis, nongonococcal urethritis, and conjunctivitis ("Can't see, can't pee, can't climb a tree"). This often occurs 1 month following a chlamydial infection.
         b. Patients can have arthritis of the large joints (they can develop sausage digits), hyperkeratotic lesions of the skin, diarrhea, and aortic insufficiency.
      2. Evaluation
         a. Radiograph shows soft tissue swelling and sacroiliitis.
         b. Test for *Chlamydia* by ELISA or DNA probe.
      3. Treatment includes NSAIDs for arthritis, topical corticosteroids for hyperkeratotic skin lesions, and azithromycin or doxycycline if the patient remains infected with *Chlamydia.*
   C. Psoriatic Arthritis
      1. Patients usually have asymmetric arthritis with sausage digits, spinal involvement, conjunctivitis, and psoriatic skin disease (Fig. 14-3A).
      2. Radiograph of the hand shows the "pencil in cup" deformity (Fig. 14-4).
      3. Treat with NSAIDs, physical therapy, local corticosteroid injections, intramuscular gold injection, hydroxychloroquine, and methotrexate.

Text continued on p. 290

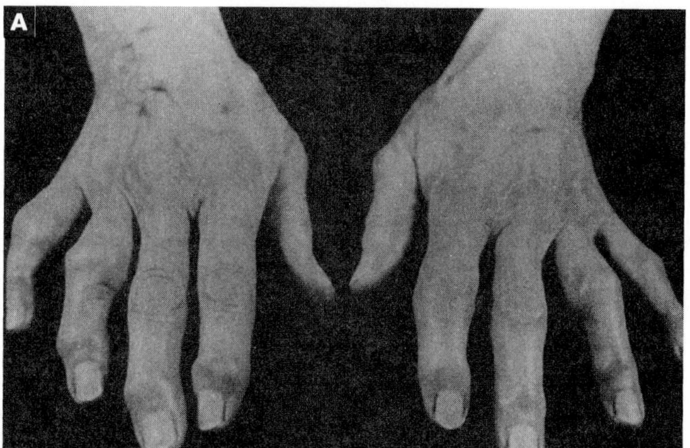

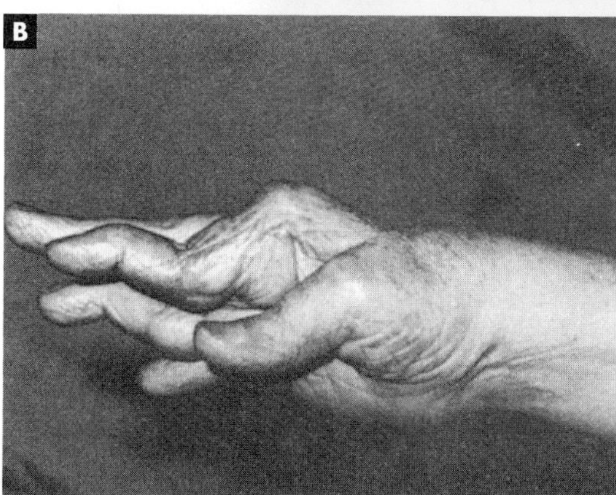

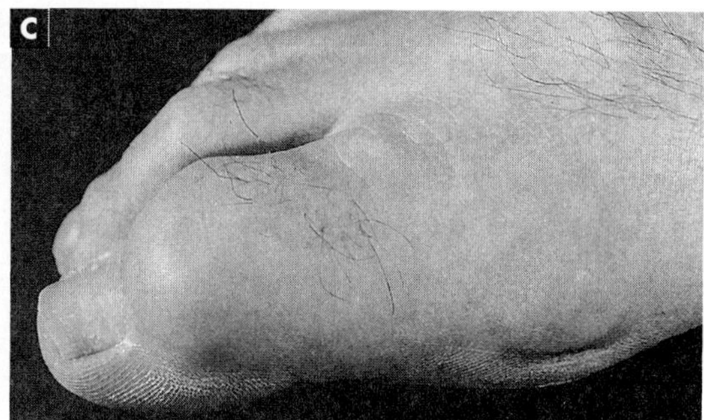

14-1: *Joint abnormalities that occur in rheumatologic disease. A, Heberden's and Bouchard's nodes in osteoarthritis. Bouchard's nodes occur at the proximal interphalangeal joints, while Heberden's nodes occur at the distal interphalangeal joints. B, Swan neck deformity in rheumatoid arthritis. C, Tophus in gout.*

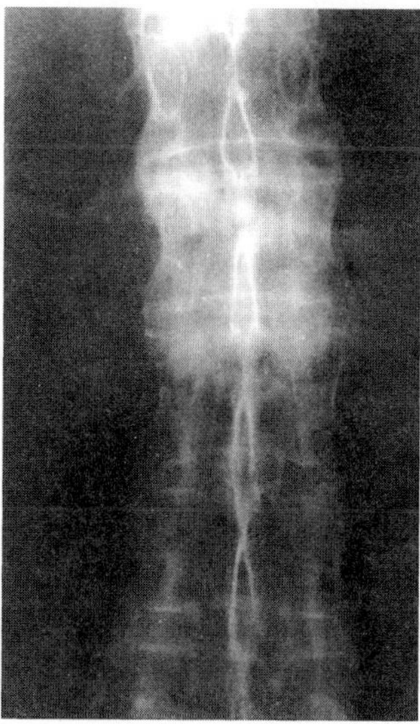

14-2: *"Bamboo spine" seen in ankylosing spondylitis.*

TABLE 14-1
Types of Arthritis

Condition	Symptoms and Signs	Diagnostic Tests	Treatment
Osteoarthritis	(1) Polyarticular degeneration of the large joints. (2) Pain worsens as the day progresses. (3) Characteristic hand deformities include Heberden's and Bouchard's nodes in the interphalangeal joints of the hand (see Fig. 14-1A).	Osteophytes may be seen on the radiograph.	NSAIDs, acetaminophen, or joint replacement surgery.
Rheumatoid arthritis	(1) Polyarticular arthritis of the small joints (especially the metacarpophalangeal and wrist joints). (2) Characteristic hand deformities include swan neck deformity (see Fig. 14-1B) and boutonnière deformity (proximal interphalangeal flexion, distal interphalangeal extension). (3) Symptoms include four of the following for >6 weeks (mnemonic—RRR SHAM): **R**heumatoid nodules on extensor tendons **R**heumatoid factor **R**adiographic changes of joint erosion **S**ymmetric joint involvement **H**and joint arthritis **A**rthritis >3 joints **M**orning stiffness (4) Also associated with interstitial lung disease with pleural effusions, pericarditis with effusion, and splenomegaly.	(1) Joint fluid shows >10,000 WBCs and a predominance of neutrophils. (2) Rheumatoid factor is present, and ESR is elevated.	(1) High-dose NSAIDs: Watch for GI irritation. (2) Glucocorticoids: Use sparingly and for a short term because of osteoporosis risk. (3) Slow-acting antirheumatoid drugs: drugs of choice are hydroxychloroquine, sulfasalazine, and methotrexate.

TABLE 14-1
Types of Arthritis—cont'd

Condition	Symptoms and Signs	Diagnostic Tests	Treatment
Gout	(1) Acute monoarticular pain due to the deposition of urate crystals. (2) Associated with a tophus of the metatarsophalangeal joint of the toe (see Figure 14-1C) and olecranon and patellar bursitis. (3) The patient may also have renal stones made of uric acid. (4) Acute attacks may be precipitated by alcohol consumption and/or high-protein meals. (5) Risk factors include obesity, diabetes mellitus, and hypertriglyceridemia.	(1) Joint fluid has >10,000 WBCs and >90% neutrophils. (2) Needle-shaped, negatively birefringent crystals are present in the joint aspirate.	(1) Can use intra-articular or oral corticosteroids. Oral corticosteroids may trigger hyperglycemia in diabetics. (2) NSAIDs (indomethacin is the drug of choice). (3) Avoid alcohol ingestion. (4) Colchicine: Good when given early in an attack. (5) Long-term treatment: Use colchicine and allopurinol.
Pseudogout	(1) Associated with deposition of calcium pyrophosphate dihydrate crystals. (2) Usually presents on a radiograph as an incidental finding, or the patient may have acute attacks of arthritis. (3) Common sites are menisci of the knee, cartilage of the wrist, or the symphysis pubis.	Joint aspirate shows rhomboid, positively birefringent intracellular crystals.	NSAIDs or intra-articular corticosteroids.

When starting allopurinol or probenecid for gout, give colchicines to prevent initiation of an attack. Do not give probenecid or allopurinol during an acute attack of gout.

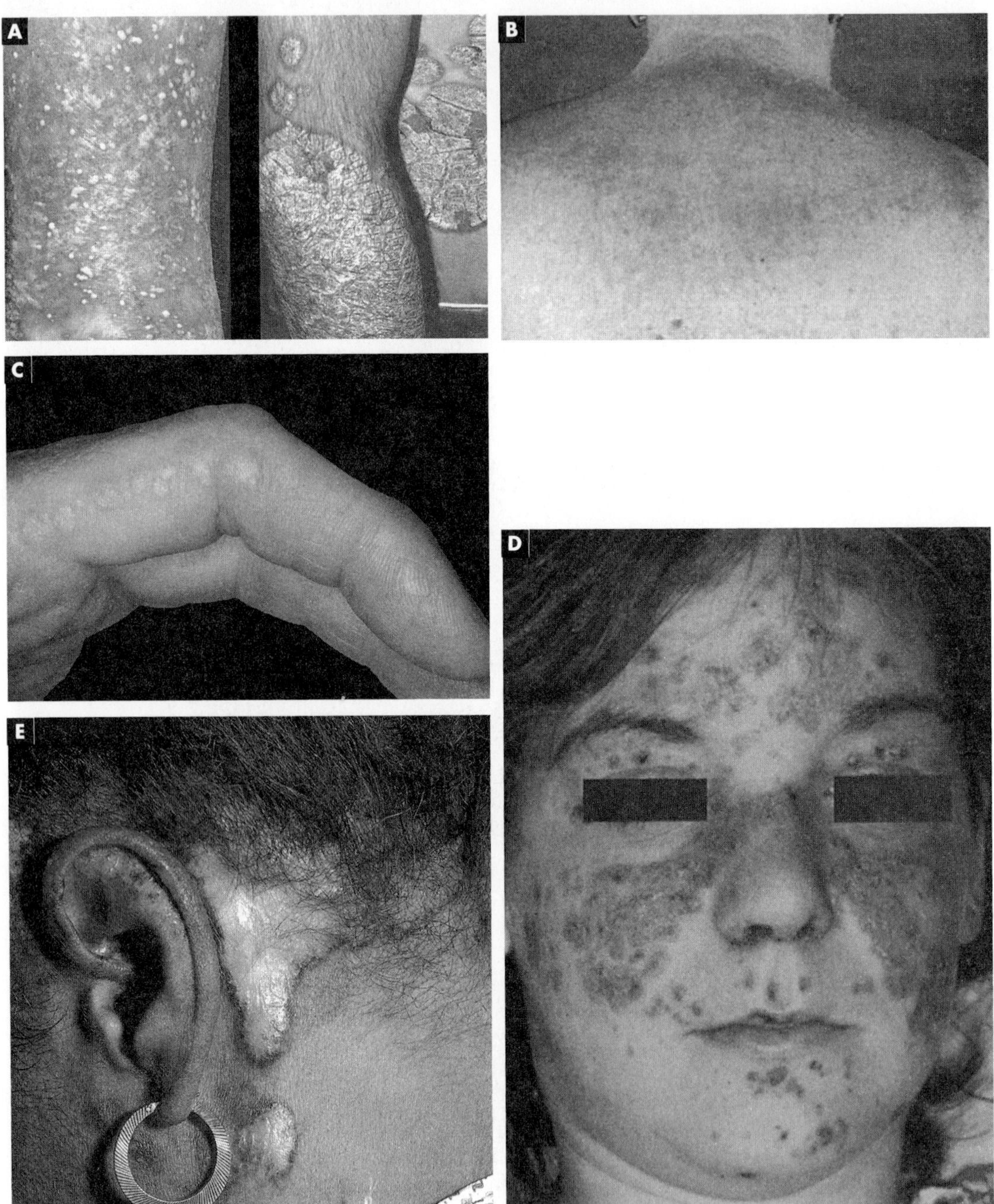

14-3: *Skin abnormalities that occur in rheumatologic disease. A, Skin changes in psoriasis. B and C, Skin findings in dermatomyositis. D, Malar rash in SLE. E, Discoid rash in SLE.*

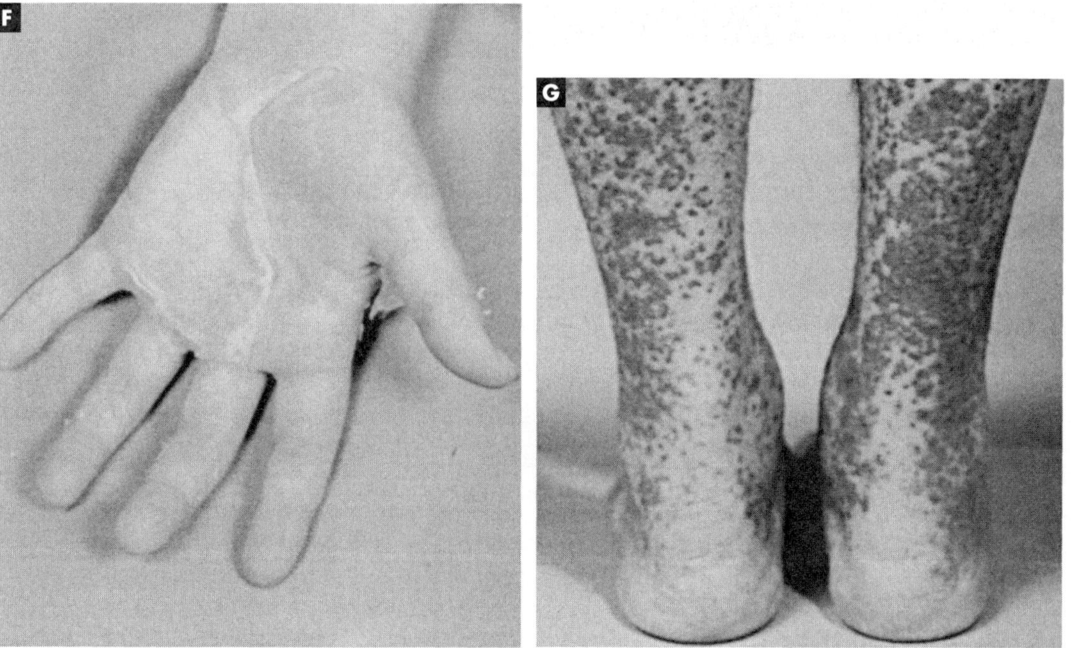

14-3: cont'd F, *Skin changes in Kawasaki disease.* G, *Skin changes in Henoch-Schönlein purpura.*

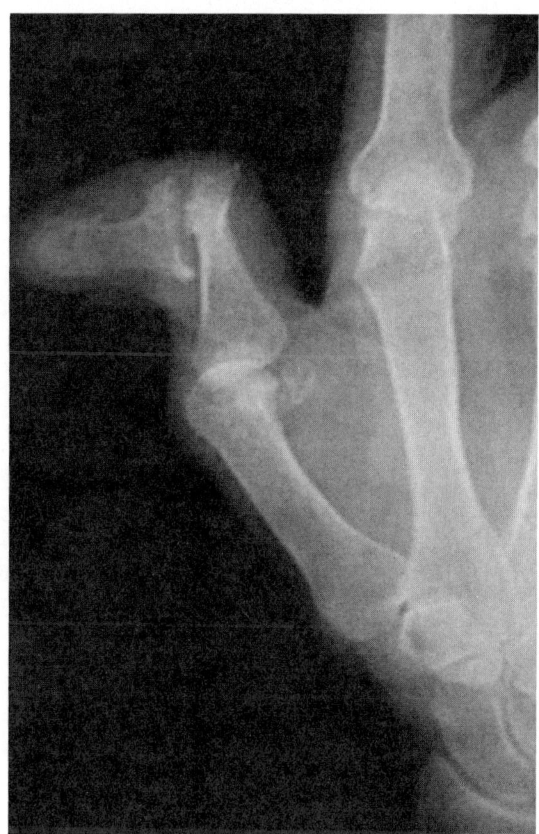

14-4: *"Pencil in cup" abnormality found in psoriatic arthritis. In this case, the joint developed instability and is shown here following subluxation.*

D. Arthritis Associated with Inflammatory Bowel Disease (Nonerosive oligoarticular arthritis; see Chapter 4)

III. Connective Tissue Disease

A. Scleroderma

1. Symptoms and signs (mnemonic—SIT FAR).

a. **S**kin thickening of the extremities, face, and trunk.

b. **I**nfertility and amenorrhea are common.

c. **T**elangiectatic skin rash.

d. **F**ibrosis: Myocardial and pulmonary.

e. Poly**a**rthralgia and joint stiffness.

f. Sclerodermal **r**enal crisis: Sudden onset of severe hypertension and rapidly progressive glomerulonephritis.

The CREST syndrome associated with some cases of scleroderma includes **c**alcinosis, **R**aynaud's phenomenon, **e**sophageal dysmotility, **s**clerodactyly, and **t**elangiectasias.

2. Evaluation

a. Anti–Scl 70, anticentromere, and antinuclear antibodies can all be seen.

b. Elevated ESR and anemia of chronic disease also are present.

3. Treatment

a. Calcium channel blockers and smoking cessation for Raynaud's phenomenon.

b. Proton pump inhibitors for GERD, if present.

c. ACE inhibitors for hypertensive renal crisis.

d. D-Penicillamine for visceral disease.

e. Corticosteroids for pulmonary fibrosis or cyclophosphamide for inflammatory lung disease.

B. Polymyositis and Dermatomyositis

1. Symptoms and signs

a. Polymyositis causes proximal muscle inflammation and weakness, particularly in the shoulder and pelvic girdle.

b. Dermatomyositis presents with skin findings in addition to the symptoms of polymyositis (see Figs. 14-3B and 14-3C).

(1) An erythematous rash may be present on sun exposed areas.

(2) Butterfly (red) and heliotrope (purple) rashes may be present on the face and eyelids.

(3) Scaling and cracking of the skin on the hands may occur.

2. Evaluation

a. Elevated CPK, aldolase, LDH, and AST.

b. Anti-Jo, anti-Mi, and antinuclear antibodies can be found.

c. Muscle involvement can be documented by abnormal EMG and muscle biopsy.

3. Treat with high-dose corticosteroids.

C. Sjögren's Syndrome

1. Symptoms and signs

a. Patients have dry eyes, dry mouth, and chronic arthritis.

b. They may also have type 1 renal tubular acidosis or nephritis (see Chapter 7).

2. Evaluation
   a. Anti-SSA/Ro, anti-SSB/La, RF, and antinuclear antibodies can be found.
   b. Biopsy of the salivary glands shows plasma cell infiltration.
3. Treatment is symptomatic.
   a. Replacement of tears, gum to promote salivation.
   b. NSAIDs or corticosteroids for arthritis.
   c. Hydroxychloroquine, azathioprine, methotrexate, or cyclosporine can be used if there are symptoms of rheumatic disease.

IV. Systemic Lupus Erythematosus (SLE)
   A. Symptoms and Signs (Mnemonic—SOAP BRAIN MD)
      1. **S**erositis.
      2. **O**ral ulcers.
      3. **A**rthritis.
      4. **P**hotosensitivity.
      5. **B**lood: Hemolytic anemia, leukopenia, or thrombocytopenia.
      6. **R**enal: proteinuria.
      7. **A**ntinuclear antibodies.
      8. **I**mmunologic: Anti-dsDNA, anti-Sm, false-positive VDRL.
      9. **N**eurologic: Psychosis, seizures.
      10. **M**alar rash: Mostly in sun-exposed areas (see Fig. 14-3D).
      11. **D**iscoid rash: Erythematous papules with keratosis and plugging.
   B. Association with Certain Drugs
      1. **Q**uinidine, **c**hlorpromazine, **h**ydralazine, **I**NH (isoniazid), **m**ethyldopa, **p**rocainamide (mnemonic—Q CHIMP).
      2. Drug-induced lupus is usually a milder disease and reversible within 4–6 weeks (see Fig. 14-3E).
   C. Treatment
      1. NSAIDs
      2. For mild disease, the following agents can be used:
         (1) Hydroxychloroquine: Screen regularly for retinal toxicity.
         (2) Methotrexate.
         (3) Azathioprine: Causes leukopenia and anemia.
      3. Corticosteroids for acute exacerbations.
      4. Cyclophosphamide for severe exacerbations and CNS disease. Toxicities include pancytopenia, alopecia, and hemorrhagic cystitis.
      5. Avoid sun exposure.

V. Vasculitis (Table 14-2)

VI. Amyloidosis
   A. Amyloidosis
      1. Causes multisystem deposition of protein.
      2. Commonly involved systems include:
         a. Renal: Nephropathy.
         b. Cardiac: Restrictive cardiomyopathy.

TABLE 14-2
Types of Vasculitis

Condition	Symptoms and Signs	Diagnostic Tests	Treatment
Wegener's granulomatosis (small vessel)	(1) Pulmonary involvement causes cough, pulmonary hemorrhage, or hemoptysis. (2) Other symptoms can include hematuria, rapidly progressive glomerulonephritis, proptosis, uveitis, and neuropathy.	(1) cANCA. (2) Biopsy shows necrotizing granulomatous inflammation of the arterioles. (3) Hematuria with RBC casts on urinalysis.	(1) Mortality if untreated is 100%. (2) Cyclophosphamide and methylprednisolone.
Microscopic polyangiitis (small vessel)	Presents in same way as Wegener's granulomatosis without the granulomas.	(1) HBV-negative. (2) Biopsy does not show granulomas in the arterioles.	Methylprednisolone and cyclophosphamide.
Churg-Strauss syndrome (small vessel)	Patients have asthma, eosinophilic pneumonia, and systemic small vessel vasculitis.	(1) Eosinophilia on CBC with differential. (2) pANCA. (3) Biopsy shows vasculitis with granulomas.	High-dose corticosteroids.
Polyarteritis nodosa (medium vessel)	(1) Associated with hepatitis B virus. (2) Patients can have constitutional symptoms, abdominal bleeding and pain, and mononeuritis multiplex. (3) There is no pulmonary involvement, but renal involvement can cause hypertension and focal segmental glomerulonephritis.	(1) Angiogram shows irregular vessels. (2) Biopsy shows vasculitis without granulomas. (3) Elevated ESR and WBC. (4) Positive HBV serology.	(1) Glucocorticoids. (2) Antiviral therapy can be used in hepatitis B– or C–positive patients.
Kawasaki disease (medium vessel)	(1) Stage I: high fever, conjunctival infection, strawberry tongue, and rash with desquamation of the palms and soles (see Figure 14-3F). (2) Stage 2: coronary vasculitis with possible thrombosis. Coronary artery aneurysms can also occur. (3) Stage 3: regression of disease with fibrosis of affected vessels.	(1) Elevated ESR. (2) Coronary aneurysms on echocardiography or coronary angiography.	High-dose IVIg with aspirin (one of the only indications for aspirin use in children).

TABLE 14-2
Types of Vasculitis—cont'd

Condition	Symptoms and Signs	Diagnostic Tests	Treatment
Takayasu's arteritis (large vessel)	(1) Phase I: inflammatory period with fever, arthralgias, and weight loss. (2) Phase II: vessel pain and tenderness. Unequal pulses in the extremities. (3) Phase III: burnt-out fibrotic period.	(1) Elevated ESR. (2) Arteriography shows arterial stenosis and irregularity. (3) Biopsy shows panarteritis with granulomas.	Corticosteroids, cyclophosphamide
Temporal arteritis (large vessel)	(1) Patients have constitutional symptoms, headache, jaw claudication, and tender temporal arteries. (2) Visual changes may occur, including amaurosis fugax, blurred vision, eye pain, and blindness.	(1) Elevated ESR. (2) Temporal artery biopsy shows vasculitis and granulomas.	High-dose glucocorticoids for 6–12 months.
Polymyalgia rheumatica (large vessel)	(1) Patients have pain and stiffness of the hip and shoulder girdles. (2) Can be found in patients with temporal arteritis, and vice versa.	Associated with elevated ESR and anemia.	Glucocorticoids at a much lower dose than that needed for temporal arteritis.
Henoch-Schönlein purpura (immunocomplex)	(1) Purpuric rash on the extensor surfaces and buttocks (see Figure 14-3G) in children. (2) Arthralgias may be present in the lower extremities. (3) Colicky abdominal pain may be present, which can be associated with intussusception.	(1) Elevated serum IgA and IgM. (2) Biopsy shows vasculitis with IgA and complement deposition.	Corticosteroids.

continued

TABLE 14-2 Types of Vasculitis—cont'd

Condition	Symptoms and Signs	Diagnostic Tests	Treatment
Hypersensitivity vasculitis (cutaneous leukocytoclastic angiitis) (immunocomplex)	(1) Abrupt onset of purpura, cutaneous ulceration, and transient arthralgias. (2) Symptoms are a response to exposure to drugs (penicillin, ASA, amphetamines, thiazides, immunizations), infections (streptococcal throat infection, endocarditis, tuberculosis, hepatitis, staphylococcal infection), or tumor antigens.	(1) Elevated ESR and low complement levels. (2) Skin biopsy shows vasculitis with eosinophils and neutrophils.	Withdraw offending agent, and treat with prednisone.
Behçet's syndrome (immunocomplex)	Patients have recurrent oral and genital ulcers, conjunctivitis, arthritis, and focal neurologic deficits.	(1) Elevated ESR. (2) Biopsy shows only nonspecific changes.	Corticosteroids, dapsone, colchicines, azathioprine, cyclosporine, chlorambucil.

cANCA, circulating antineutrophil cytoplasmic antibodies; ESR, erythrocyte sedimentation rate; HBV, hepatitis B virus; IVIg, intravenous immunoglobulin; pANCA, perinuclear antineutrophil cytoplasmic antibodies.

c. Skin: Nonpruritic papules and easy bruising.
d. GI tract: Diarrhea and macroglossia.
e. Nerve: Peripheral neuropathy with pain and autonomic neuropathy.
f. Musculoskeletal: Arthritis.
g. Pulmonary: Airway obstruction.

B. Diagnosis
   1. Can be made with subcutaneous biopsy.
   2. Amyloid deposits have apple-green birefringence on Congo-red staining.

C. Treatment: Includes melphalan and prednisone.

APPENDIX I

appendix I

Medical Ethics

I. Confidentiality

A. Situations in which confidentiality can be broken:

1. Permission from the patient.
2. Suspicion of child abuse.
3. Court order.
4. The patient is a danger to himself/herself or others. This includes patients with reportable diseases.
5. Specific legal situations, including gunshot wounds, knife wounds, and intoxicated drivers.

B. Do not hide the diagnosis from the patient if the family requests it. However, refrain from telling the patient the diagnosis if the patient requests it.

C. Cases in which patients under 18 years of age do not need parental consent:

1. Emancipation.
2. Marriage.
3. Parents of children: Teenage parents have autonomy when it comes to the care of their children, but they may not have autonomy when it comes to their own medical care.
4. Serving in the armed forces.
5. Issues involving sexually transmitted disease, birth control, or pregnancy.
6. Drug treatment or counseling. However, it should be noted that a competent minor can not be given involuntary urine testing without receiving informed consent.

D. Physicians are obligated to tell patients if a mistake has been made during the course of their care.

II. Consent

A. Informed Consent: Tells the patient about the diagnosis, prognosis, proposed treatments, alternative treatments, and the risks and benefits of treatment. The patient should then be free to accept or decline the treatment. A written form is not required, so long as the consent is documented in some way.

B. Consent is implied in emergency (life-threatening) situation in which the patient cannot communicate and no family is available. Do what must be done to stabilize the patient.

C. Patients are allowed to withdraw their consent for an intervention at any time.

III. Refusal of Care

A. Jehovah's Witness: Has the right to refuse blood products for himself/herself. If a child desires a transfusion in a Jehovah's Witness family and the parents are against the transfusion, then the transfusion should be given (because it is within both the medical and the stated interest of the patient).

B. Refusal by parents to administer a straightforward, life-saving treatment for their child:

1. Try to convince them.
2. Court order.

C. A doctor can refuse to perform an intervention when he/she believes such an intervention would be futile. This can occur when there is no rationale for the treatment, the treatment has been unsuccessful in a previous trial, or the maximum degree of care for the disorder is currently being performed.

IV. Advance Directives and the Dying Patient

A. Durable Power of Attorney: Designates that a single individual will be responsible for health care decisions if the patient becomes incompetent or incapacitated.

B. Living Will: Written document that addresses the patient's wishes for specific health care situations. These usually involve whether they patient desires cardiopulmonary resuscitation, intubation, or other extraordinary measures that might be available in the intensive care unit. Even when the patient does not want to be resuscitated or intubated, he/she should be treated by all medical means possible that do not involve these measures.

C. Surrogate Decision Makers: Incapacitated or incompetent patients with no advance directives can have decisions made by one of several parties (in this order):

1. Family members: Heed the wishes of the family if they are in agreement. Consult the hospital ethics committee if the family does not agree on an issue. Court intervention may be necessary if the family can not decide with the hospital's intervention.
2. Friend.
3. Personal physician.

D. Allow competent adult patients to die if they want to. This includes the discontinuation of life-sustaining therapy. There is no distinction between withholding and withdrawing life-sustaining therapy.

E. Pain control for the terminally ill should focus on relief of the pain. Addictive potential is not an issue in these cases.

APPENDIX II

Statistics and Preventive Medicine

I. Statistical Equations and Terminology Used in Medical Literature (Fig. A2-1)

A. Sensitivity: Ability to detect disease. This is desirable for a screening test.

Sensitivity = True positives/number of people with disease

B. Specificity: Ability to detect healthy nondiseased individuals. This is desirable for a confirmatory test.

Raising the sensitivity of a test lowers its specificity.

Specificity = True negatives/number of people without the disease

C. Positive Predictive Value (PPV): Given a positive test, it expresses the likelihood that the patient has the disease. The positive predictive value will be higher for diseases that have a high prevalence.

PPV = True positives/number of people with a positive test

D. Negative Predictive Value (NPV): Given a negative test, it expresses the likelihood that the patient does not have the disease. The negative predictive value will be higher for diseases that have a low prevalence.

NPV = True negatives/number of people with a negative test

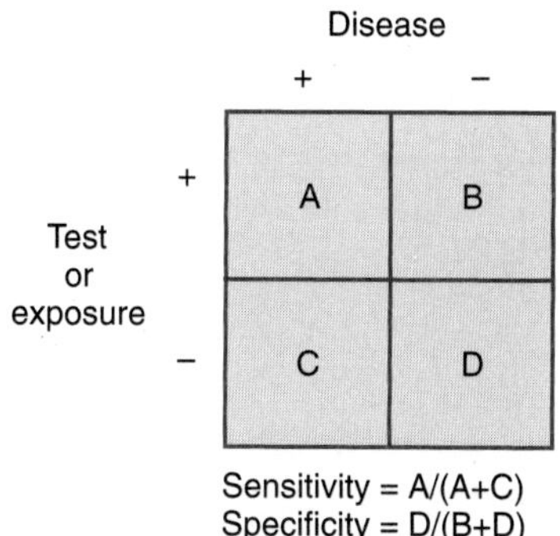

Sensitivity = A/(A+C)
Specificity = D/(B+D)
PPV = A/(A+B)
NPV = D/(C+D)
OR = (A*D)/(B*C)
RR = (A/(A+B))/(C/(C+D))

A2-1: *Use of a 2 × 2 table to determine statistical values. This format is used to organize the data from a study into true positives (A), false positives (B), false negatives (C), and true negatives (D).*

E. Odds Ratio (OR): Describes the odds of having been exposed to a certain factor in diseased individuals compared to healthy individuals.

F. Relative Risk (RR): Compares the disease risk in a population exposed to a factor or treatment to the disease risk in a population that has not been exposed to this factor or treatment. Relative risk greater than 1 suggests that the factor contributes to the disease, whereas relative risk less than 1 suggests that the factor may protect against the disease. Relative risks with 95% confidence intervals (see later discussion) that include values both above and below 1 are not statistically significant.

G. Relative Risk Reduction: This is calculated by subtracting the relative risk from 1. In cases where an intervention decreases the relative risk to 0.8, the relative risk reduction would be 0.2 (or 20%).

H. Number Needed to Treat (NNT): NNT = 1/(Pc–Pi), where Pc is the proportion of people with disease in the control group and Pi is the proportion of people with the disease in the intervention group. Basically, the NNT tells you how many times you would have to perform the intervention in order to have one success. For instance, if the intervention decreased the proportion of people with the disease by 50%, then the NNT would be 2.

I. Standard Deviation: Assuming a bell-shaped distribution curve of the data, 68% of the values will be within 1 standard deviation (SD) of the mean, 95% of values will be within 2 SD of the mean, and 99.7% of values will be within 3 SD of the mean.

J. Confidence Interval (CI): This is usually presented as a 95% CI and is an indication of the distribution of the data. This measurement states the range of values within which 95% of the population values can be found in the data. It is possible to generate a 95% CI if you know the mean and SD and you know that the data have a bell-shaped distribution. Because 95% of the data is within 2 SD of the mean, the low end of the 95% confidence interval will be the mean − 2 SD, and the high end of the 95% confidence interval will be the mean + 2 SD.

K. Incidence: Number of new cases of a disease that are diagnosed in a unit of time (usually 1 year).

L. Prevalence: Total number of cases of a disease that exist in a population (this incorporates both the patients who have survived with the disease and the new cases that have been diagnosed within a unit of time).

II. Research Terminology

A. Blinding: Refers to whether the participants in a study were aware of the experimental group to which they belonged. In terms of therapeutic trials, single blinding is present when the patient does not know whether he or she is in the treatment or the placebo group. Double blinding is present when both the patient and the physician do not know whether the patient is in the treatment or the placebo group.

B. Prospective (Cohort) Trial: Trials in which the experimental group is exposed to a factor after the start of the trial, and the results are compared to an equivalent placebo group. Ideally, both the experimental group and the placebo group should be selected from the same population (people with the same disorder and health status) so that the only variable is exposure to the factor being tested. The trial is stopped if the study reaches an acceptable end-point or the factor (or lack of exposure to the factor, in the case of the placebo group) has a significant and clear positive or negative impact on the study participants' health.

C. Retrospective (Case-control) Trial: A common paradigm for studies evaluating the risk factors for a disease. In this case, the study is performed after exposure to the variables in question, and the study is divided into two populations—patients with or without a certain disease. The two populations should be as similar as possible except for the presence of the disease. A drawback of this design is that it can be heavily biased, given that the healthy people will not remember as much about their hazardous exposures as the diseased people will.

D. Meta-analysis: Pooling together of data regarding a particular topic into a single study. This allows the pooling of several small studies (where the findings may not have been statistically significant owing to low numbers) to determine whether statistical differences would be present with larger sample numbers.

E. Case Study: Basically, reports of low numbers of cases in which a specific condition is present. The study is not controlled. This can be useful for rare diseases, or for inclusion in a meta-analysis to incorporate greater numbers. However, the low numbers and lack of controlled conditions limit the usefulness of these studies beyond that point.

III. Selection of Appropriate Statistical Tests

A. *t* Test: For the comparison of two means.

B. Analysis of Variance (ANOVA): For the comparison of three or more means.

C. Chi-Squared: For comparison of percentages or proportions.

D. *P* Value: Each statistical test gives you a *P* value, which tells you the probability that the data could have occurred by chance. In most studies, the threshold for statistical significance is $P < 0.05$, which means that there is a less than 5% chance that these observations would have occurred by chance. Using *P* values, several types of error can be made:

1. Type I error: Claiming a significant event is occurring when (in reality) it is not.
2. Type II error: Claiming that no significant event is occurring when (in reality) an event is occurring.

IV. Types of Bias

A. Confounding Variables: Variables that are present, but not accounted for, that will affect the outcome of a trial and make the two groups appear different from each other.

B. Nonrandom Sampling: Differences between the inclusion criteria for the experimental and control groups are likely to introduce confounding factors.

C. Lead Time Bias: This can occur when an intervention or study allows the earlier diagnosis of a particular disorder. If a terminal condition is diagnosed at an earlier age but the patient dies at the same age as he or she would have without the intervention, it may appear that the patient survived for a longer period because he or she was aware of the disease for a longer period of time.

D. Recall Bias: Patients with a disease are more cognizant of their exposure to risk factors than healthy patients.

E. Interviewer Bias: When the investigator (consciously or subconsciously) treats the patients in the experimental and control groups differently from one another. This bias can be minimized by double-blinded studies.

V. Preventive Medicine

A. Types of Screening

1. Primary prevention: Measures to prevent the acquisition of the disease in patients who do not have the disease. Examples of primary prevention include immunizations and safety measures (bicycle helmets, seat belts).
2. Secondary prevention: Measures to prevent the development of symptomatic disease in patients who have significant risk factors or preclinical disease. Secondary screening is performed for conditions such as hypertension, hyperlipidemia, breast cancer, and prostate cancer.
3. Tertiary prevention: Measures to restore or maximize function in patients who have established disease.

B. Guidelines for Preventive Screening (Table A2-1)

C. Guidelines for Immunization (Tables A2-2 and A2-3)

TABLE A2-1
Routine Preventive Testing

Condition	Age	Procedure
Congenital hypothyroidism	Birth	Thyroid-stimulating hormone (TSH) and T_4 levels
Phenylketonuria	Birth	Phenylalanine level
Hypertension	25 years of age and older	Routine blood pressure measurements over multiple visits
Hyperlipidemia	25 years of age and older	Routine cholesterol and blood lipid testing
Colorectal cancer	>50 years of age	(1) Sigmoidoscopy every 5 yr (2) Stool occult blood yearly
Prostate cancer	>40 years of age	Digital rectal examinations yearly
Cervical cancer	(1) Start at 18 years of age or when the patient becomes sexually active (2) Stop screening at 65 years of age	Pap smear yearly until two consecutive normal examinations occur; then Pap smear every 3 yr
Breast cancer	(1) Clinical examinations should start after 20 years of age (2) Mammography start date is variable but usually begins at 40–50 years of age	(1) Clinical breast examinations by a physician every 3 yr (2) Mammography
Endometrial cancer	Menopause	Endometrial biopsy

TABLE A2-2
Commonly Used Pediatric Vaccinations and Their Recommended Dosing Schedules

Immunization	Disease Covered	Time of Administration
Hepatitis B	Hepatitis B	Birth, 1 mo, 6 mo
Hib	*Haemophilus influenzae* type b	2, 4, 6, and 12 mo
PCV	Pneumococcal	2, 4, 6, and 12 mo
IPV	Inactivated poliovirus	2, 4, and 6 mo and then at 4 yr
DTaP	Diphtheria, tetanus, pertussis	2, 4, 6, and 15 mo and then at 4 yr
Td	Tetanus	Every 10 yr after 4 years of age
Varicella	Varicella zoster virus	12 mo
MMR	Measles, mumps, rubella	12 mo, then at 4 yr
Influenza	Influenza viruses	Yearly, especially for patients with lung disease
Hepatitis A	Hepatitis A	As needed for foreign travel

TABLE A2-3 Routine Vaccinations That Are Administered to Adults

Vaccination	Comments
Rubella	Also give to all women of childbearing age who do not have a record of immunization for rubella (but do not immunize if already pregnant)
Hepatitis B	Indicated for people who are likely to be exposed to blood (including health care workers)
Influenza	All adults over 50 years of age and all patients with chronic respiratory, cardiac, or renal conditions
Pneumococcus	All adults over 65 years of age, immunocompromised patients, diabetics, and patients with chronic respiratory, cardiac, or renal conditions
Tetanus	(1) Maintenance boosters should be given every 10 years (2) Give a booster to patients with dirty wounds if they have not received a tetanus shot in >5 years

QUESTIONS

questions

CARDIOLOGY

A 65-year-old man with a history of smoking and asthma presents to his primary care physician's office with complaints of decreased exercise tolerance and an irregular thumping in his chest. His blood pressure is 160/90, and his pulse is irregularly irregular at 125 beats per minute (bpm). His lungs are clear to auscultation, and there is minimal edema in his extremities. No other abnormalities are noted on physical examination. An electrocardiogram (ECG) displays the following:

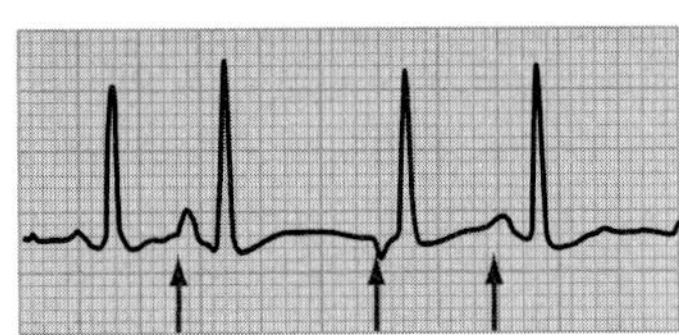

1. Which of the following is the most appropriate pharmacotherapy for this patient?
   A. Propranolol
   B. Verapamil
   C. Quinidine
   D. Sotalol
   E. Ibutilide

2. Which of the following is an indication for cardiac stress testing?
   A. Assessment of a patient who has had a myocardial infarction 1 week ago
   B. Assessment of a patient who has had a myocardial infarction 1 day ago
   C. Assessment of a patient with a history of untreated atrial fibrillation
   D. Assessment of a patient with unstable angina
   E. Assessment of a patient with severe aortic stenosis

A 75-year-old patient with a history of angina, hypertension, and diabetes comes to the emergency room with acute onset of crushing substernal chest pain that radiates to the left jaw. The pain began 30 minutes ago while he was walking in the grocery store and was not relieved by use of sublingual nitroglycerin. The patient's blood pressure is 150/90, and his heart rate is 120. The patient appears diaphoretic and in distress.

3. Which of the following tests is most likely to be abnormal at this time?
   A. Chest radiograph
   B. CK-MB
   C. CT scan of the chest
   D. Electrocardiogram
   E. Troponin

A 30-year-old woman with no significant past medical history presents to her primary care physician with frequent headaches and persistent high blood pressure readings measured at her local pharmacy. Her blood pressure in the office was 155/105 and 160/110 on two measurements taken 25 minutes apart. The pressure was symmetric in both arms. The only abnormality detected on physical examination is a bruit in her left flank.

4. Which of the following medications is contraindicated?
   A. Verapamil
   B. Metoprolol
   C. Penicillin
   D. Captopril
   E. Novocain

A 77-year-old man with a history of myocardial infarction presents with fatigue, shortness of breath, and the inability to sleep while lying flat. On physical examination, crackles are audible in the lungs and the point of maximal impulse of the heart is laterally displaced. 2+ pitting edema is present up to the level of the mid-shin.

5. Medications that are contraindicated in this condition include which of the following?
A. Verapamil
B. Captopril
C. Nitroglycerin
D. Spironolactone
E. Morphine

A 40-year-old man visits you for the first time because of concern about his cholesterol level. He had been told by his previous physician that his LDL level was high on his previous tests, and since then he has tried to change his diet to prevent taking any more medications.

6. At the outset of the interview, the patient insinuates that he already takes several medications. Which of the following medications can increase this patient's LDL?
A. Aspirin
B. Albuterol
C. Hydrochlorothiazide
D. Antacids
E. Captopril

A 29-year-old man with a history of IV heroin use presents to the emergency room with weight loss, fever, chest pain, and hemoptysis for several days. Physical examination findings include a heart murmur at the left lower sternal border and red spots on the palms of his hands and under the nail beds.

7. Which of the following is the most appropriate initial pharmacotherapy?
A. Penicillin and gentamycin
B. Nafcillin and gentamycin
C. Intravenous ceftriaxone
D. Vancomycin and rifampin
E. Amoxicillin

A patient with a history of unstable angina visits his primary care physician for a routine evaluation. No abnormalities are noted on physical examination, but the patient does have a significant abnormality on lead aVF of his ECG (see top of next column), with similar changes seen in leads II and III.

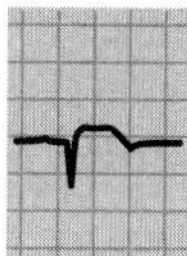

8. Which of the following diagnoses can adequately explain this abnormality?
A. Unstable angina
B. Prinzmetal's angina
C. Acute myocardial infarction
D. Old myocardial infarction
E. Left bundle branch block

9. The patient undergoes surgical correction for his problem, and encounters postoperative complications including hypovolemia, metabolic acidosis, and electrolyte abnormalities on the day of surgery. Which of the following is the probable cause for these complications?
A. Cross-clamping of the aorta
B. Withdrawal from hormones secreted by the tumor
C. Strangulation of the bowel
D. Postoperative atelectasis
E. Postoperative infection

A 50-year-old woman with a previous history of breast cancer and radiation therapy presents to her primary care physician with fatigue and decreased exercise tolerance over the past several months. Peripheral edema, hepatomegaly, and ascites are noted on physical examination. The point of maximal impulse of the heart displays a strong beat. Previous attempts at treatment of these symptoms with furosemide were unsuccessful. Bedside ECG shows diffusely low-voltage QRS complexes.

10. Which of the following is the most likely diagnosis?
A. Hypertrophic cardiomyopathy
B. Dilated cardiomyopathy
C. Restrictive cardiomyopathy
D. Constrictive pericarditis
E. Pericardial tamponade

EMERGENCY MEDICINE TOPICS

A 70-kg, 42-year-old patient presents to the emergency room with a scalding injury. On physical examination, you note that the burn extends throughout one arm and across the front of his torso. The burn appears superficial, but blisters are beginning to form.

11. How would you describe the severity and the time course for healing this injury?
A. First-degree burn, and it will take days to heal
B. First-degree burn, and it will take weeks to heal
C. Second-degree burn, and it will take weeks to heal
D. Second-degree burn, and it will not heal without skin grafting
E. Third-degree burn, and it will not heal without skin grafting

A 25-year-old man arrives in an ambulance after a rescue from a burning office. The patient is unconscious and in respiratory distress at presentation, and subsequently undergoes intubation in the emergency department. On physical examination, minor burns are present on the patient's face and arms, and the patient's skin is a bright red color. Wheezes are heard on auscultation of the lungs. When the patient's blood is drawn, it is bright red in color.

12. Which of the following is the most effective management?
A. Bronchoscopy to evaluate the patient for inhalation injury
B. Immediate treatment with 100% humidified O_2
C. Chest radiograph to assess for consolidation in the lungs
D. Transfusion with packed red blood cells
E. Volume resuscitation and topical wound treatment

A 22-year-old female is brought by ambulance to the emergency department following involvement in a motor vehicle crash as an unrestrained passenger. Her blood pressure is 90/40. On physical examination, she is minimally responsive, with a bruise and palpable mass in the left upper quadrant of her abdomen and pale, cool, clammy skin. She opens her eyes and moves (withdrawal movements) only in response to painful stimuli, and her only speech is composed of incomprehensible sounds.

13. The patient is showing signs of shock. Which type of shock is most likely present?
A. Hypovolemic
B. Distributive
C. Cardiogenic
D. Extracardiac obstructive shock
E. Neurogenic shock

A 64-year-old woman is delivered by ambulance to the emergency room after experiencing severe chest pain and syncope at home 30 minutes ago. The patient's blood pressure is 90/40 and her heart rate is 100 bpm. The patient appears pale and diaphoretic and has been unconscious since the onset of syncope.

14. Which of the following is the most effective management?
A. Surgical intervention
B. Aggressive volume resuscitation with IV fluids
C. Typing and cross-matching, followed by transfusion
D. Antibiotic therapy
E. Ventilation/perfusion (V/Q) scan of the chest

Items 15–20:
Match the following symptoms of poisoning or drug toxicity with the appropriate antidotes.
A. Calcium chloride
B. N-acetylcysteine
C. Deferoxamine
D. Vitamin K
E. Physostigmine
F. Pralidoxime chloride

15. Nausea, vomiting, delayed jaundice, and hepatic failure within 96 hours.

16. Mania, delirium, dry mouth and eyes, and tachycardia.

17. Miosis, salivation, urination, bronchospasm, weakness, and confusion.

18. Hematemesis, diarrhea, hypotension, and hepatic failure, with pills that can be seen on the radiograph.

19. Hypotension and dizziness in a patient who has a history of hypertension.

20. Bruising and bleeding in a patient with chronic atrial fibrillation.

ENDOCRINOLOGY

A 10-year-old boy presents to his pediatrician because of his parents' concern over his height and weight. He has always been shorter than his peers and unable to tolerate exercise to the same extent. On physical examination, he appears symmetrically small with excess adiposity of his abdomen. His height is in the third percentile for his age. He has two older siblings who were consistently in the 70th percentile during their growth, and his parents appear to be of average height.

21. Insufficiency of which hormone is the most likely cause of the short stature?
A. Prolactin
B. Growth hormone
C. Gonadotropin-releasing hormone (GnRH)
D. Thyroid-stimulating hormone (TSH)
E. Adrenocorticotrophic hormone (ACTH)

A 25-year-old woman with a history of schizophrenia visits the primary care clinic with complaints of amenorrhea and galactorrhea for the past several years. She was diagnosed with schizophrenia 5 years ago, and her symptoms are currently well controlled with haloperidol. On physical examination, the only abnormality is a small amount of white discharge from the left nipple.

22. Which of the following is the most appropriate therapy?
A. Bromocriptine
B. Oral contraceptive pills
C. Estrogen replacement therapy
D. Surgical removal of the ovaries
E. Craniectomy

A 45-year-old woman presents to the primary care clinic with complaints of weakness, fatigue, constipation, and irregular menses over the past year. She has no pertinent past medical history. Her blood pressure is 110/70, and her heart rate is 55 bpm. On physical examination, the thyroid is enlarged and tender. The extremities are dry and cold and exhibit nonpitting edema. The deep tendon reflexes are 1+ in all limbs. Subsequent testing reveals antithyroid antibodies.

23. Which of the following is the most appropriate therapy?
A. Levothyroxine
B. Total thyroidectomy
C. Thyroid lobectomy
D. Aspirin
E. Ibuprofen

A 50-year-old woman presents to the primary care clinic with complaints of weakness, fatigue, constipation, and irregular menses over the past year. She has a history of breast cancer that was treated with lumpectomy and irradiation 5 years ago. Her blood pressure is 110/70, and her heart rate is 55 bpm. On physical examination, the thyroid gland is enlarged and has an irregular, firm, nontender mass in the right lobe. Her deep tendon reflexes are 1+ in all limbs.

24. Which of the following is the most likely diagnosis?
A. Toxic adenoma
B. Toxic multinodular goiter
C. Papillary thyroid cancer
D. Medullary thyroid cancer
E. Hashimoto's thyroiditis

A 34-year-old woman presents to the primary care clinic with increased appetite, weight loss, insomnia, and diarrhea for the past 2 months. Her heart rate is 110 bpm. Abnormalities on physical examination include exophthalmos, an enlarged thyroid, and a thyroid bruit. Subsequent testing detects antithyroid antibodies.

25. Which therapy for this disorder is most likely to allow resolution of the exophthalmos?
A. Thyroid surgery
B. Propylthiouracil
C. Radioiodine
D. Ibuprofen
E. Plasmapheresis

A 40-year-old woman presents to the primary care clinic with increased appetite, weight loss, insomnia, and diarrhea for the past 6 months. Her heart rate is 120. Abnormalities on physical examination include an enlarged thyroid and a single palpable nodule extending from the surface of the thyroid. Subsequent testing did not detect antithyroid antibodies in the patient's blood.

26. Which of the following is the most effective management?
A. Treatment with propylthiouracil and iodine followed by subtotal thyroidectomy surgery
B. Treatment with aspirin and prednisone followed by subtotal thyroidectomy surgery
C. Treatment with propylthiouracil and iodine followed by thyroid lobectomy surgery
D. Treatment with aspirin and prednisone followed by thyroid lobectomy surgery
E. Subtotal thyroidectomy surgery alone

A 45-year-old woman with a history of toxic multinodular goiter and subtotal thyroidectomy presents 1 month after surgery with perioral numbness, tingling of the fingers, and muscle spasms. Physical examination findings include facial muscle contraction after the cheek is tapped and carpopedal spasms.

27. Which of the following sets of laboratory abnormalities is most likely present?
A. Low serum calcium, high serum phosphorus, low serum parathyroid hormone
B. Low serum calcium, low serum phosphorus, low serum parathyroid hormone
C. Low serum calcium, high serum phosphorus, high serum parathyroid hormone
D. High serum calcium, low serum phosphorus, low serum parathyroid hormone
E. High serum calcium, low serum phosphorus, high serum parathyroid hormone

A 50-year-old man with a history of chronic renal failure, currently on dialysis, presents to his primary care physician with bone pain and progressive muscle pain and weakness over the past few months, which is most severe in his legs. Physical examination is normal except for pain in several muscles and bones in all of his limbs. A radiograph of the patient's arm displayed several extraskeletal calcifications at the location of the patient's muscle pain.

28. Which of the following is the most effective management?
A. Subtotal thyroidectomy
B. Radioiodine
C. Removal of parathyroid tissue
D. Renal transplantation
E. Local radiation therapy

A 60-year-old man presents to the primary care clinic for a routine annual examination with complaints of recent headaches. His blood pressure is 160/90 mm Hg with a heart rate of 70 bpm. On physical examination, the lungs are clear to auscultation, and there are no abnormalities on cardiac examination. No bruits are heard in the carotid canal or the flank. Serum electrolytes reveal a sodium of 150 mEq/L (normal 136–146 mEq/L) and a serum potassium of 2.8 mEq/L (normal 3.5–5.0 mEq/L). Plasma renin levels are decreased.

29. Which medication is most useful prior to surgical correction of this disorder?
A. Metoprolol
B. Diltiazem
C. Captopril
D. Furosemide
E. Spironolactone

A 35-year-old woman presents to the primary care clinic with complaints of poor appetite, dizziness upon standing, weakness, and a gradual darkening of her skin despite a lack of sun exposure. Her family history is significant for Graves' disease in her mother and multiple sclerosis in her sister. Her blood pressure is 110/70 while sitting and 90/50 after standing. The heart and lung examination is unremarkable, and no bruits or peripheral edema is noted.

30. Which of the following medications can produce these symptoms?
A. Ketoconazole
B. Streptomycin
C. Metoprolol
D. Niacin
E. Losartan

GASTROENTEROLOGY

A 35-year-old man presents to the emergency room with protracted vomiting several hours after eating at a Chinese food buffet. During his initial evaluation, the patient experiences sudden postemetic pain in his chest and neck, and there is a small amount of blood present in his emesis. On physical examination, the patient's blood pressure is 160/100 mm Hg and his heart rate is 115 bpm. Breath sounds in the left lung are decreased. Auscultation of the heart detects a crunching sound.

31. Which of the following is the most effective management?
A. Drainage and repair surgery with antibiotics within 24 hours
B. Stopping the bleeding with electrocautery during endoscopy
C. Pneumatic dilation
D. Surgical section of the cricopharyngeus muscle
E. Antibiotic and antiemetic pharmacologic treatment alone

A 55-year-old woman with a history of mild asthma presents with substernal chest pain and an increase in wheezing for the past 6 months. The pain usually lasts less than 5 minutes and is often associated with a sour taste in her mouth. She more frequently experiences this pain when she is in a horizontal or recumbent position. There is no history of heart disease, and her only medication is an albuterol inhaler that she takes on an as-needed basis.

32. Which of the following is the most effective management?
A. Cimetidine
B. Omeprazole
C. Aluminum hydroxide
D. Pneumatic dilation
E. Graham patch procedure

A 50-year-old man with a history of smoking presents to the primary care clinic with complaints of epigastric pain and anorexia for the past few months. The pain has a burning quality and is worsened by eating and relieved by over-the-counter antacids. On physical examination, the patient has slight tenderness to deep palpation of the epigastric region. The heart and lung examination is unremarkable.

33. Which of the following is the most effective management?
A. Short-term treatment with omeprazole along with antibiotic therapy including clarithromycin and metronidazole
B. Short-term treatment with sucralfate along with antibiotic therapy including clarithromycin and metronidazole
C. Short-term treatment with omeprazole followed by surgical correction with Nissen fundoplication
D. Short-term treatment with metoclopramide followed by antibiotic therapy with tetracycline and metronidazole
E. Short-term treatment with omeprazole and sucralfate followed by antibiotic therapy with tetracycline and metronidazole

A 45-year-old man with a history of alcoholism presents to the emergency department with severe abdominal pain, nausea, vomiting, and fever. The pain is stabbing in nature and is located in the epigastric area with radiation to the back. The patient also describes foul-smelling diarrhea for the past several days. He has never experienced these symptoms in the past. On physical examination, the patient has abdominal tenderness in the epigastric region and ecchymosis in his flank and periumbilical regions. Laboratory test results on his admission to the hospital reveal the following:

Serum glucose: 275 mg/dL
Serum lactate dehydrogenase: 400 units/L
Serum AST: 2500 units/L
WBC count: 18,000 mm^3
Hematocrit: 40%

34. Which of the following factors are more favorable in terms of this patient's prognosis?
A. The blood glucose level
B. The lactate dehydrogenase level
C. The white blood cell count
D. The hematocrit
(E.) The patient's age

A 15-year-old boy presents to the emergency department with periumbilical pain for the past 4 hours and nausea and vomiting that started 1 hour ago. The patient's temperature is 39°C, his heart rate is 90 bpm, and his blood pressure is 120/70 mm Hg. The patient's periumbilical region is acutely tender even to light palpation, and pain is elicited upon flexion of the hip against resistance. During the course of the examination, the patient's pain shifts from the epigastric region to the right lower quadrant.

35. Which of the following is the most effective management?
A. Aggressive intravenous rehydration, cessation of oral feedings, and observation
B. Débridement with drain and jejunostomy tube placement
C. Pharmacologic therapy with clarithromycin, omeprazole, and metronidazole
(D) Surgical removal of the appendix followed by 1 day of antibiotic therapy
E. Surgical removal of the appendix followed by 7 days of antibiotic therapy

A 67-year-old female with a history of uterine fibroids, status post–abdominal hysterectomy, presents to the emergency department with epigastric abdominal pain, nausea, and vomiting that have been increasing over the past few days. The patient says that she has intervals without pain and the pain is relieved by vomiting. She has not had a bowel movement for 1 week, which is much less frequent than her normal bowel function. The patient's temperature is 37°C, her heart rate is 95 bpm, and her blood pressure is 100/60 mm Hg. Findings on physical examination include dry mucous membranes and hyperactive bowel sounds, with no focal pain or tenderness since she last vomited 10 minutes ago.

36. Which type of acid-base abnormality would you expect to encounter in this patient?
A. Hypochloremic, hyponatremic metabolic acidosis
B. Hypochloremic, hyponatremic metabolic alkalosis
C. Hypochloremic, hyperkalemic metabolic acidosis
(D) Hypochloremic, hypokalemic metabolic alkalosis
E. Hypochloremic, hyperkalemic metabolic alkalosis

A 70-year-old patient with a history of alcoholism presents to the emergency department with melena and hematemesis over the past day. His heart rate is 120 bpm, and his blood pressure is 100/60 mm Hg. The patient was not vomiting prior to the hematemesis. On physical examination, the patient has jaundiced skin with caput medusae in the periumbilical region. He has a positive fluid-wave sign on abdominal examination, and hemorrhoids and guaiac-positive stools are noted on rectal examination. No oral lesions are noted. During the course of the examination, he has one episode of bright-red hematemesis.

37. Which of the following could have prevented the development of bleeding?
A. A protein-rich diet
B. Omeprazole
C. Cimetidine
(D) Metoprolol
E. Metoclopramide

A 55-year-old man with a history of alcoholism presents to the primary care clinic with nausea, malaise, fever, and fatigue. He has no history of foreign travel, IV drug abuse, blood transfusion, or unprotected sexual intercourse. Tender hepatomegaly and scleral icterus are present on physical examination. The serum AST is 450 units/L and the serum ALT is 200 units/L.

38. Which of the following is the most effective management?
A. Interferon alpha
B. Corticosteroids and cessation of drinking
C. Liver transplantation
D. N-acetylcysteine
E. Azathioprine

A 74-year-old man with a history of alcoholism returns to the primary care clinic with complaints of weight gain and indigestion. He continues to drink a liter of vodka per day despite repeated attempts by his physician and family to convince him to quit drinking. On physical examination, you note jaundice, palmar erythema, gynecomastia, and fluid in his abdomen. Splenomegaly is present, and the patient's liver is small and nodular.

39. You notice over time that this patient has developed cognitive decline, hyperreflexia, and insomnia. Which of the following medications will most likely stop or slow the development of neurologic symptoms?
A. Levodopa
B. Bromocriptine
C. Lactulose
D. Acetaminophen
E. Sucralfate

A 42-year-old obese woman presents to the emergency department with complaints of nausea, vomiting, and abdominal pain in the right upper quadrant that started several days ago. Her temperature is 39°C, her heart rate is 110 bpm, and the blood pressure is 130/90 mm Hg. The pain radiates to the right subscapular area, and it can be elicited by palpation of the right upper quadrant during inspiration. No abdominal masses are palpable.

40. What is the most likely diagnosis?
A. Acute cholecystitis
B. Chronic cholecystitis
C. Cholelithiasis
D. Choledocholithiasis
E. Klatskin's tumor

HEMATOLOGY

A 35-year-old woman presents to the primary care clinic with fatigue and dyspnea on exertion that have worsened progressively over the past week. She also says that she has been feeling lightheaded when standing over the past few days. She has no pertinent previous medical history and takes no medications or supplements. Her last menstrual period ended 4 days ago, and menses was heavier than usual. Her temperature is 37°C, her heart rate is 110 bpm, and her blood pressure is 110/70 mm Hg, which dropped to 90/45 after standing.

41. Which of the following is the most likely diagnosis?
A. Thalassemia
B. Iron deficiency anemia
C. Sideroblastic anemia
D. Autoimmune hemolytic anemia
E. Microangiopathic hemolytic anemia

A 75-year-old woman developed a stroke following an elective hysterectomy for uterine fibroids, and was admitted to the inpatient service 1 week ago. Prior to surgery, she had been on warfarin because of a history of recurrent deep vein thromboses, and she is currently receiving heparin as an inpatient. She restarted warfarin 1 day ago. Her blood pressure is 120/80 mm Hg, and her heart rate is 75 bpm. On physical examination, she has weakness in her right arm and fingers, which has been present since the stroke but has improved slightly over the past several days. Her abdominal incision is clean, dry, and intact. Her heart, lung, and abdominal examination is otherwise normal.

42. Which coagulation test findings are most likely present?
A. Increased PT and bleeding time
B. Increased PTT and bleeding time

C. Increased PT, PTT, and bleeding time
D. Increased bleeding time alone
E. Coagulation lab tests should be normal

The same patient is anticoagulated pharmacologically. The following day, this patient experiences leg pain and localized edema and tenderness. A Doppler scan of the limb confirms the presence of a deep vein thrombosis. The most recent complete blood count displayed a drop in the platelet count from 125,000/μL yesterday to 60,000/μL this morning (normal platelet count = 150,000–450,000/μL). The patient's coagulation lab tests from this morning showed a PT of 25 seconds and a PTT of 35 seconds.

43. Which of the following is the most effective management?
A. Increasing doses of both heparin and warfarin
B. Discontinuation of heparin and increased warfarin dosing
C. Discontinuation of both heparin and warfarin and starting lepirudin therapy
D. Local thrombolysis of the deep vein thrombosis
E. Plasmapheresis and prednisone with no change in the anticoagulant regimen

Match the appropriate type of bleeding disorder with the features that best describe it.
A. Von Willebrand's disease
B. Vitamin K deficiency
C. Disseminated intravascular coagulation
D. Hemophilia A
E. Coagulation factor inhibitors

44. The PT is normal. The PTT is prolonged and does not correct in a mixing study.
E

45. The PT is normal. The PTT is prolonged and corrects to normal in a mixing study.
D

46. Usually associated with trauma, malignancy, or obstetric complications. PT, fibrin degradation products, and D-dimer are increased.
C

47. This bleeding disorder may develop owing to hemorrhagic disease of the newborn, warfarin therapy, fat malabsorption, or antibiotic therapy.
B

48. The PT is normal, PTT is prolonged, bleeding time is prolonged, and factor VIII activity is decreased.
A

A 55-year-old woman presents to the emergency room with headache, monocular blindness, and mental status changes that started 2 hours ago. She has a previous history of myocardial infarction 1 year ago. The patient's heart rate is 90 bpm, and her blood pressure is 120/80 mm Hg at admission. During the course of the examination, the patient's mental status gradually improves and her vision returns to normal over the next several hours. CT scan performed at the time of admission shows no acute infarctions. A complete blood count (CBC) reveals the following results:

WBC: 13,000 mm^3
Hemoglobin: 17.0 g/dL
Hematocrit: 51%
Platelets: 450,000/μL

49. Which disorder is the most likely cause of the patient's recurrent thromboses?
A. Polycythemia vera
B. Essential thrombocytosis
C. Myelofibrosis
D. Leukostasis
E. Atrial fibrillation

A 65-year-old man presents to the primary care clinic with complaints of fatigue, dyspnea on exertion, pain in his ribs, and constipation. These symptoms have been gradually worsening over the past several months, and now impair his daily functioning. His temperature is 37°C, heart rate is 75 bpm, and blood pressure is 120/75 mm Hg. On physical examination, he is pale and his ribs are tender to palpation at several locations. No other abnormalities are noted on his heart, lung, or abdominal examination. Urinalysis reveals 2+ protein. Other laboratory tests reveal the following information.

WBC count: 11,000 mm^3
Hemoglobin: 8.0 g/dL
Hematocrit: 24%
Platelets: 150,000/µL
Serum protein 11 g/dL
Serum albumin 2.7 g/dL

50. What is the most likely diagnosis?
A. Systemic amyloidosis
B. Monoclonal gammopathy of undetermined significance (MGUS)
C. Multiple myeloma
D. Waldenström's macroglobulinemia
E. Myelofibrosis

INFECTIOUS DISEASE

A 6-year-old girl with a history of rash and wheezing following penicillin therapy presents with a sore throat for the past week. Her temperature is 101°F. On physical examination, she has an erythematous pharynx with white exudates. A sandpapery rash is present on her trunk and extremities.

51. Which complication can be prevented by antibiotic therapy?
A. Colitis
B. Glomerulonephritis
C. Rheumatic heart disease
D. Toxic epidermal necrolysis
E. Scalded skin syndrome

An 8-year-old boy is brought to the emergency department with complaints of sore throat for the past week. He had been taken to the primary care clinic 4 days ago and given empiric penicillin therapy, and has since developed a rash. His temperature is 101°F. On physical examination, he has an inflamed, erythematous pharynx and a mildly erythematous maculopapular rash on his trunk. Hepatomegaly is present.

52. Which antibiotic was used in the empiric treatment of this patient's illness?
A. Amoxicillin
B. Ampicillin
C. Clavulanic acid
D. Doxycycline
E. Tetracycline

A 5-year-old girl presents to the emergency department with a 2-day history of sore throat and fever. Her mother has also noted that she has become progressively hoarse. Her temperature is 102°F. On physical examination, the patient appears pale, ill, and drooling. Stridor is present on auscultation of the lung fields. A lateral radiograph of the neck reveals swelling of the epiglottis.

53. What is the most appropriate treatment?
A. Intubation and empiric therapy with intravenous cefuroxime
B. Fluid resuscitation and laryngoscopic exploration
C. Oral penicillin
D. Intubation with oral penicillin therapy, pending throat culture results
E. Ribavirin

A 30-year-old Chinese immigrant presents to the primary care clinic for a health insurance screening with no acute medical complaints. He received adequate health care and vaccinations in China, and has never had a serious illness requiring hospitalization. The physical examination is unremarkable, but he has a positive PPD test when he returns to the office 3 days later. Subsequent workup of this finding resulted in a clear chest radiograph and two sputum samples that were negative for acid-fast bacilli.

54. What is the most appropriate treatment?
A. No treatment is needed
B. Isoniazid therapy for 6 months
C. Isoniazid therapy for 9 months
D. Acid-fast staining of bronchial washings
E. Combination therapy with pyrazinamide, isoniazid, rifampin, and ethambutol

A 30-year-old woman with a history of HIV infection has given birth to a healthy baby boy 1 month ago. She had frequent prenatal visits and received zidovudine in the third trimester of her pregnancy. Thus far, the child has no symptoms or signs of HIV infection, and testing has been negative.

55. What test results are sufficient to determine that the child is HIV negative?
A. Negative ELISA test at 1 year of age
B. Negative PCR test at 1 year of age
C. Negative PCR and ELISA tests consistently over the first year of life
D. Negative PCR and ELISA tests consistently over the first 2 years of life
E. Negative PCR and ELISA tests consistently over the first 5 years of life

A 35-year-old man with a 7-year history of HIV infection is currently on combination antiretroviral therapy with zidovudine, zalcitabine, and indinavir, but his CD4 counts have been steadily dropping to the current level of 90 cells/mm^3. The present physical examination is unremarkable except for an oral thrush infection. He has no history of tuberculosis infection, and the PPD has consistently been negative.

56. Which of the following is the most appropriate prophylactic therapy for this patient?
A. Trimethoprim-sulfamethoxazole
B. Trimethoprim-sulfamethoxazole with isoniazid
C. Clarithromycin with trimethoprim-sulfamethoxazole
D. Clarithromycin with trimethoprim-sulfamethoxazole and isoniazid
E. Clarithromycin with isoniazid

A 27-year-old patient with a history of genital herpes develops genital ulcers consistent with herpes simplex lesions at week 34 of pregnancy.

57. What is the appropriate management to protect the child from contracting herpes perinatally?
A. Immediate cesarean section
B. Acyclovir therapy with delivery at term using either normal spontaneous vaginal delivery (NSVD) or cesarean section (depending on the presence of active lesions at the time)
C. Acyclovir with cesarean section regardless of the patient's symptoms at delivery
D. Ganciclovir therapy with delivery at term using either NSVD or cesarean section (depending on the presence of active lesions at the time)
E. No antiviral therapy with cesarean section at the time of delivery

A 26-year-old female presents to the primary care clinic with symptoms of dysuria and abdominal pain over the past week. She has been sexually active with several partners over the past year, and her use of protection has been inconsistent. On physical examination, she displays adnexal and cervical motion tenderness, and a mucopurulent discharge is noted on the cervix. Gram staining of the discharge shows the following results:

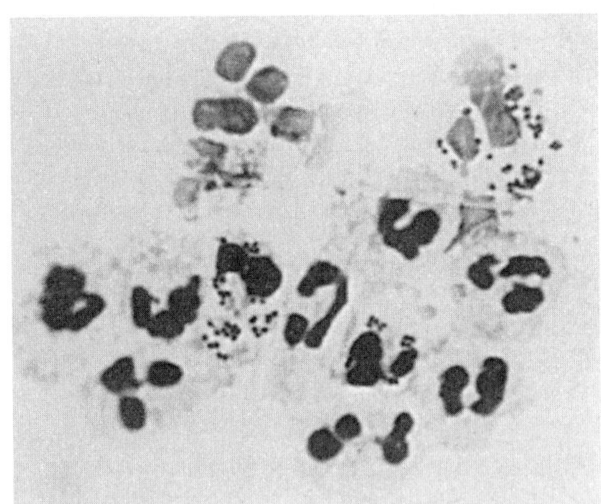

58. What is the most appropriate treatment?
A. Ceftriaxone
B. Azithromycin
C. Ceftriaxone with azithromycin
D. Metronidazole
E. Over-the-counter antifungal cream

A 10-year-old boy is brought to the primary care clinic with a recent history of rash and current symptoms of joint pain. He first developed the rash, which started on his lower back, 1 month ago. Additional foci of the rash subsequently appeared at other locations of his trunk, as the initial lesion was fading. His parents found a tick on the initial rash site shortly before he developed symptoms. Over the past week, the rash disappeared and he started to develop pain and tenderness in his knees and hips. On physical examination, the patient's vital signs are normal and his heart and lung examinations are unremarkable. No rash is present. Minor tenderness and pain are elicited on the active and passive movement of the knee and hip.

59. What is the most appropriate treatment?
A. Doxycycline
B. Amoxicillin
C. Ganciclovir
D. Chloramphenicol
E. Penicillamine

A 47-year-old man presents to the emergency room complaining of a skin infection on his arm that has markedly worsened over the past day. He had injured himself with a large splinter of wood 2 days previously and admits that he may not have gotten the entire splinter out. Today he has noted fevers, malaise, dizziness, and he has vomited once. On physical examination, his temperature is 101°F, his blood pressure is 100/70 mm Hg, and his heart rate is 90 bpm. His right arm shows a bluish discoloration of the skin and subcutaneous tissue extending from the site of the splinter, with formation of bullae. The margins of the lesion are poorly defined.

60. What is the most likely diagnosis?
A. Necrotizing fasciitis
B. Clostridial myonecrosis
C. Toxic epidermal necrolysis
D. Stevens-Johnson syndrome
E. Scalded skin syndrome

NEPHROLOGY

A 45-year-old man with a history of right knee pain presents to the primary care clinic for a routine life insurance screening examination. His knee pain has occurred consistently since an athletic injury 10 years ago, but his symptoms are well controlled with the daily use of ibuprofen. He has noted a weight gain of 10 pounds over the past year despite a consistent diet and exercise regimen. On physical examination, his blood pressure is 125/80 mm Hg with a heart rate of 80 bpm. His cardiac and lung examinations are unremarkable. Passive movement of his right knee elicits crepitus and minor tenderness. Pitting edema (2+) is noted bilaterally to mid-shin. The results of a complete blood count, basic metabolic panel, and serum cholesterol are pending. A dipstick urinalysis shows 3+ protein, trace blood, and no glucose. The urine contains fatty casts on microscopic examination.

61. Which of the following routine blood tests is most likely to be abnormal in this patient?
A. Serum cholesterol
B. Serum glucose
C. Serum sodium
D. Serum potassium
E. Serum calcium

A 30-year-old man arrives at the emergency room following a motor vehicle accident as an unrestrained driver. The patient is conscious and states that he has no major medical illnesses and takes no medications. On physical examination, the blood pressure is 110/75 mm Hg with a heart rate of 95 bpm. The cranial nerves are intact, and muscle tone is normal. Cardiac and lung examinations are unremarkable. However, numerous contusions are located on the chest and arms. He is admitted to the surgical intensive care unit, and oliguria develops over the next 24 hours. His plasma creatinine rises to 3.5 g/dL, and the bedside urine dipstick testing detects blood (4+). However, red blood cells are not seen on microscopic examination of the urine.

62. What is the most likely diagnosis?
A. Acute renal failure due to hypovolemia
B. Acute renal failure due to rhabdomyolysis
C. Acute renal failure due to kidney trauma
D. Rapidly progressive glomerulonephritis
E. IgA nephropathy

63. What is the most appropriate therapy?
A. Hemodialysis
B. Removal of the injured kidney
C. Blood transfusion
D. Cyclophosphamide and prednisone
E. Plasmapheresis

For each of the following scenarios, select the acid-base disorder that is most likely responsible for the patient's arterial blood gas (ABG) values.

A. Acute respiratory acidosis with compensation
B. Chronic respiratory acidosis with compensation
C. Acute respiratory acidosis without compensation
D. Metabolic acidosis without compensation
E. Metabolic acidosis with compensation

64. A patient with an ABG pH of 7.30, a pCO_2 of 50 mm Hg, and an HCO_3 of 25 mEq/L.

65. A patient with an ABG pH of 7.33, a pCO_2 of 60 mm Hg, and an HCO_3 of 31 mEq/L.

66. A patient with an ABG pH of 7.30, a pCO_2 of 30 mm Hg, and an HCO_3 of 14 mEq/L.

A 65-year-old man is brought to the emergency room by his wife with symptoms of confusion and poor appetite that have worsened over the past few days. He is responsive to questioning, but does not recall his medical history and is not oriented to time or place. According to his wife, he has a history of hypertension and hypercholesterolemia, for which he takes losartan, metoprolol, hydrochlorothiazide, multivitamin, and lovastatin. He has no recent history of trauma. The blood pressure is currently 140/85 mm Hg with a heart rate of 80 bpm. The heart and lung examinations are unremarkable, and there are no signs of orthostatic hypotension. The ECG shows no abnormalities, and laboratory tests show the following results:

Serum Na^+: 125 mEq/L
Serum K^+: 4 mEq/L
Serum Cl^-: 100 mEq/L
Serum HCO_3^-: 24 mEq/L
Serum glucose: 100 mg/dL
Blood urea nitrogen: 7 mg/dL
Serum osmolality: 258 mOsm/kg
Urine osmolality: 125 mOsm/kg

67. Which of the patient's medications could be causing these symptoms?
A. Losartan
B. Metoprolol
C. Hydrochlorothiazide
D. Lovastatin
E. Multivitamin

A 55-year-old man with a history of recent craniectomy for a frontal lobe oligodendroglioma presents for a postoperative visit with complaints of fatigue and increased thirst. His surgery was 2 months ago, and his recovery was unremarkable. He has no history of renal disease. The blood pressure is 145/85 mm Hg with a heart rate of 75 bpm. On physical examination, he has a healed surgical scar in the left temporal region without focal neurologic deficits. The heart and lung examinations are unremarkable. Laboratory tests show the following results:

Serum Na^+: 150 mEq/L
Serum K^+: 5 mEq/L
Serum Cl^-: 100 mEq/L
Serum HCO_3^-: 23 mEq/L
Serum creatinine: 0.8 mg/dL
Serum osmolality: 680 mOsm/kg
Urine osmolality: 100 mOsm/kg

68. Which of the following treatments is most likely to be effective in this patient?
A. DDAVP (a.k.a. desmopressin) with gradual correction of the electrolyte abnormalities
B. Correction of the electrolyte abnormalities over the ensuing 8 hours
C. Sodium restriction and hydrochlorothiazide
D. Hemodialysis
E. Calcium gluconate, insulin, and bicarbonate

A 45-year-old woman presents to the emergency room with weakness, nausea, diarrhea, vomiting, and muscle cramps over the past few days. She has no history of renal or neurologic disease and is not taking any medications. The blood pressure is 125/80 mm Hg with a heart rate of 85 bpm. The heart, lung, and abdominal examinations are unremarkable. Laboratory studies show the following results:

Serum Na^+: 135 mEq/L
Serum K^+: 2.7 mEq/L
Serum Cl^-: 114 mEq/L
Serum HCO_3^-: 14 mEq/L
Serum Ca^{++} (ionized): 5 mg/dL
Serum Mg^{++}: 0.7 mg/dL
Serum phosphorus: 3.0 mg/dL

69. Which of the following would be the most appropriate first step in the patient's treatment?
A. Potassium supplementation
B. Magnesium supplementation
C. Calcium supplementation
D. Supplementation with potassium and magnesium
E. Supplementation with potassium and calcium

A 60-year-old woman with a history of hypertension and diabetes mellitus presents to the emergency department with complaints of weakness and abdominal pain for the past week. Her medications include metoprolol, simvastatin, and glipizide. The blood pressure is 145/90 mm Hg with a heart rate of 80 bpm. The heart and lung examination is unremarkable, but there is diffuse abdominal tenderness to deep palpation. A bedside ECG shows peaked T waves in all leads with an increased PR interval. Serum laboratory test results are pending.

70. Which of the following electrolyte abnormalities is most likely to be responsible for the patient's symptoms?
A. Hypokalemia
B. Hyperkalemia
C. Hyponatremia
D. Hypercalcemia
E. Hypomagnesemia

NEUROLOGY

A 75-year-old woman with a history of hypertension and type 2 diabetes mellitus presents with weakness and sensory loss in her right leg since awakening this morning. She has not experienced nausea or vomiting and has had no changes in her vision. She has no prior history of these symptoms and no recent injuries. Her diabetes has been well controlled with metformin and glyburide since the diagnosis 3 years ago. Her hypertension has not been well controlled, and she is currently taking metoprolol and captopril. On physical examination, the temperature is 37°C, the heart rate is 90 bpm, the respiratory rate is 22, and the blood pressure is 150/90 mm Hg. The pulmonary, cardiac, and abdominal examinations are unremarkable. Visual fields are intact, and the optic discs are sharp. In the right leg, strength is 0/5 and sensation to pinprick and vibration are absent. Strength and all sensory modalities are intact in the right arm and in the left arm and leg.

71. What is the most appropriate management for the hypertension during this incident?
A. Increase the patient's dose of metoprolol
B. Increase the frequency with which the patient receives metoprolol
C. Change the patient from oral metoprolol to intravenous metoprolol
D. Change the patient's antihypertensive medication to hydralazine
E. Do not treat the patient's hypertension during the first few days after her stroke

A 70-year-old man with a history of diabetes, hypertension, and atrial fibrillation is brought to the emergency department by ambulance 1 hour after collapsing in the supermarket. He was shopping when he suddenly collapsed, and has regained consciousness since the incident. His diabetes is well controlled with glyburide and metformin, and the hypertension is well controlled with captopril and metoprolol. He has a history of chronic atrial fibrillation, for which he takes daily warfarin. On physical examination, the temperature is 37°C, the heart rate is 110 bpm, the respiratory rate is 20, and the blood pressure is 130/80 mm Hg. The heart rate is irregularly irregular and tachycardic. The pulmonary and abdominal examinations are unremarkable. Visual fields are intact with sharp optic discs. The patient is not moving his left arm, and the left side of his face is flaccid with sparing of the forehead. Vibration, proprioception, and nociception are absent over the left face and arm but are present over the left lower leg and the entire right side of the face and body. Strength is 0/5 throughout the left arm, 2/5 in the left hip flexors, and 4/5 in the left plantar flexors. Strength is 5/5 throughout the right side.

72. What is the most likely diagnosis?
   A. Ischemic stroke of the anterior cerebral artery
   (B.) Ischemic stroke of the middle cerebral artery
   C. Ischemic stroke of the posterior cerebral artery
   D. Hemorrhagic stroke of the anterior cerebral artery
   E. Hemorrhagic stroke of the middle cerebral artery

A 23-year-old woman is brought to the emergency department after having an episode of unresponsiveness at the dinner table. According to her parents, the patient stopped talking in mid-sentence and stared off into space for approximately 2 minutes. During this period, she continued to move her lips in a repetitive pattern without producing noises. She then became responsive again with no recollection of the event, but was oriented to person, place, and situation. She has no prior history of these symptoms and has not recently been injured or ill. On physical examination, the temperature is 38°C, the heart rate is 70 bpm, the respiratory rate is 20, and the blood pressure is 115/70 mm Hg. The cardiac, pulmonary, and abdominal examinations are unremarkable. She is alert and oriented to person, time, and place, and her cranial nerves, strength, and sensation are intact throughout the body.

73. What is the most appropriate diagnosis?
   A. Simple partial seizure
   (B.) Complex partial seizure
   C. Tonic-clonic generalized seizure
   D. Febrile seizure
   E. Myoclonic seizure

An 80-year-old man with a history of hypertension and diabetes mellitus is brought to the emergency department because of gradually increasing confusion over the past 2 weeks. His symptoms began with mild forgetfulness, but he has gradually become more disoriented and has begun giving inappropriate responses to questions over the past day. According to his wife, he fell in the bathroom and hit his head about two and a half weeks ago. He is currently taking captopril, glyburide, metformin, and metoprolol and has not recently changed his medications. On physical examination, the temperature is 37°C, the heart rate is 80 bpm, the respiratory rate is 20, and the blood pressure is 140/80 mm Hg. There is a healing bruise on his right parietal scalp. The cardiac, pulmonary, and abdominal examinations are unremarkable. Cranial nerve function is intact. There is 3/5 strength in the left arm and hand with decreased sensation to pinprick and vibration. Strength and sensation are normal in all other limbs.

74. What is the most likely diagnosis?
   A. Epidural hematoma
   (B.) Subdural hematoma
   C. Subarachnoid hemorrhage
   D. Ruptured berry aneurysm
   E. Pituitary apoplexy

A 70-year-old man is brought to the emergency department with symptoms of slow movement, tremor, and confusion. He appears disoriented and is uncooperative with commands and questioning. When he is brought into the room, he has a stooped posture and shuffling gait. On physical examination, the temperature is 37°C, the heart rate is 80 bpm, the respiratory rate is 20, and the blood pressure is 120/85 mm Hg. The pulmonary, cardiac, and abdominal examinations are unremarkable. There is a resting tremor in both hands, and the patient only moves minimally during the examination. The limbs exhibit cogwheel rigidity to passive movement. Reflexes are 2+ bilaterally, and strength cannot be judged owing to poor cooperation with the examination.

75. What type of toxic exposure could have caused these symptoms?
   A. Cyanide
   B. Tetrodotoxin

C. Carbon monoxide
D. Botulinum toxin
E. Mercury

A 38-year-old man comes to the primary care clinic with complaints of depression and involuntary movements. He also has had difficulty remembering names and locations over the past 6 months. His depressed mood has become increasingly severe during the same period, and he admits to thoughts of suicide. His father committed suicide at the age of 35. On physical examination, the temperature is 38°C, the heart rate is 70 bpm, the respiratory rate is 18, and the blood pressure is 120/80 mm Hg. Throughout the examination, the patient makes writhing movements with his arms, hands, and neck that he attempts to conceal by combining them with other movements. The cardiac, pulmonary, and abdominal examinations are unremarkable. Cranial nerves, strength, and sensation are intact. He has difficulty performing a tandem walk because of sudden movements of his arms and neck.

76. What is the most appropriate treatment for the patient's movement symptoms?
A. Fluoxetine
B. Haloperidol
C. Metoprolol
D. Levodopa
E. Amantadine

A 50-year-old man presents to the primary care clinic with complaints of progressive weakness, fatigability, and difficulty swallowing over the past 3 months. During this period, he noticed gradually decreasing exercise tolerance, muscle cramps, and the development of spontaneous twitching in his muscles. There is no prior history of these symptoms, and he had no severe illnesses over the past year. On physical examination, the temperature is 38°C, the heart rate is 80 bpm, the respiratory rate is 22, and the blood pressure is 130/80 mm Hg. The cardiac, pulmonary, and abdominal examinations are unremarkable. The arms and legs all show some degree of atrophy, and fasciculations are also noted in these muscles. Reflexes are 3+ bilaterally, and there is a hyperactive jaw-jerk reflex.

77. What is the most appropriate treatment for the patient's spasticity?
A. Ibuprofen
B. Levodopa
C. Baclofen
D. Amantidine
E. Metoprolol

A 40-year-old woman presents to the emergency department with eye pain and blurred vision in her right eye for the past week. Her sharp eye pain and blurred vision are improved by decreasing the intensity of light in the room. She is noticeably photosensitive. She has not had these symptoms in the past, but she did have an episode of trigeminal neuralgia last year and an episode of arm weakness 3 years ago. Both incidents lasted several months but eventually resolved completely with no residual deficits. There is no history of trauma to the eye and no recent illnesses. On physical examination, the temperature is 38°C, the heart rate is 90 bpm, the respiratory rate is 20, and the blood pressure is 130/75 mm Hg. The cardiac, pulmonary, and abdominal examinations are unremarkable. A diffuse monocular visual field deficit is present in her right eye, which she states is due to blurry vision. Mild papilledema is present in the right eye. Cranial nerves, strength, and sensory function are otherwise intact.

78. Which result would most likely be found on analysis of this patient's cerebrospinal fluid?
A. Oligoclonal IgG bands
B. Prion proteins
C. Greater than 10,000 leukocytes per mm^3
D. Tau protein
E. Gram-negative diplococci

A 50-year-old construction worker presents to the primary care clinic with complaints of neck and shoulder pain and right arm weakness since falling off a ladder 1 month ago. Since his injury, he has noticed shock-like pain in his right shoulder and difficulty lifting moderately heavy objects. On physical examination, the temperature is 37°C, the heart rate is 70 bpm, the respiratory rate is 20, and the blood pressure is 120/80 mm Hg. The cardiac, pulmonary, and abdominal examinations are unremarkable. There is mild restriction of motion of the neck, and flexion with rotation of the neck produces a shock-like pain in his deltoid region. Strength is 3/5 on arm flexion and abduction. The biceps reflex is 1+ on the right. Neurologic examination is otherwise intact.

79. What is the most likely cause of the symptoms?
  A. Compression of the nerve root by a herniated intervertebral disk
  B. Demyelination in the spinal cord
  C. Demyelination in the peripheral nerve
  D. Selective degeneration of neurons in the anterior horn
  E. Degeneration of myelin due to dysmyelination

A 40-year-old woman with a history of smoking presents to the primary care clinic with complaints of weakness and drooping eyelids for the past week. During this period, she has noticed that her general exercise tolerance has decreased and that her muscles tire soon after she starts even routine tasks. The first symptom she noticed was difficulty keeping her eyes open, despite a lack of drowsiness. She has no prior history of these symptoms and has had no recent infections or injuries. On physical examination, the temperature is 37°C, the heart rate is 80 bpm, the respiratory rate is 20, and the blood pressure is 120/80 mm Hg. Moderate ptosis of the eyelids is present. The pupils are directly and consensually reactive to light bilaterally. The cardiac, pulmonary, and abdominal examinations are unremarkable. Strength of the proximal muscles of all limbs is 4/5, and strength to the distal muscles is 5/5. No sensory deficits are noted, and reflexes are 2+ in all limbs. Subsequent electromyography detects impaired neuromuscular transmission. Supramaximal repetitive stimulation shows initially normal neuromuscular responses that decrease with successive stimuli.

80. What type of tumor is associated with this disorder?
  A. Small cell lung carcinoma
  B. Colon carcinoma
  C. Papillary thyroid carcinoma
  D. Thymoma
  E. Hepatocellular carcinoma

OBSTETRICS AND GYNECOLOGY

A 26-year-old G1P0 woman presents to the obstetrics clinic with concerns about possible fetal loss during her current pregnancy. She has a sister who lost her second pregnancy due to erythroblastosis fetalis, and the patient is aware that her blood type is A−. The father of the child has an A+ blood type. A rosette screening test identifies the fetal blood type as A+, and a follow-up Kleihauer-Betke test cannot detect fetal red blood cells in the maternal circulation.

81. Which complications are likely to occur in the patient's current pregnancy?
  A. Intraventricular hemorrhage
  B. Hydrops fetalis
  C. Autoimmune hemolytic anemia
  D. Cleft palate
  E. No complications

A 30-year-old G0 woman presents to the gynecology clinic with complaints of amenorrhea and difficulty conceiving for the past 6 months. She discontinued her oral contraceptive medications 8 months ago but has not had a menstrual cycle since then. She has taken monthly over-the-counter pregnancy tests since then, which have all been negative. She also complains of mood swings, insomnia, and dyspareunia. The physical examination is unremarkable, and she is told to take progesterone supplementation for 1 week. Two weeks later, she returns and states that she began menstruating the day before.

82. What is the cause of the amenorrhea?
  A. Endometriosis
  B. Adhesions
  C. Ovulatory failure
  D. Abnormal cervical mucus
  E. Endocrine abnormalities

A 35-year-old G0 woman presents to the gynecology clinic for a routine examination and is found to have atypical cells on a Papanicolaou (Pap) smear with changes suggestive of human papillomavirus infection.

83. Which of the following is the most appropriate next step in the evaluation of this patient?
A. Hysterectomy
B. Laser therapy
C. Radiation therapy
D. Neoadjuvant chemotherapy
E. Cone biopsy of the cervix

A 32-year-old G1P0 woman presents to the obstetrics clinic at 15 weeks' gestation with lower abdominal discomfort. Prior ultrasounds have shown a focal enlargement of the myometrium consistent with a uterine fibroid, which appears to be enlarging on more recent scans. Currently, the fibroid is not interfering with fetal growth, and the fetus is in no distress.

84. What is the most appropriate management for this patient?
A. Immediate myomectomy
B. Immediate medical therapy using mifepristone
C. Monitor the pregnancy for complications, with a cesarean section and removal of fibroids at the time of delivery
D. Monitor the pregnancy for complications, with delivery by NSVD and subsequent treatment of the fibroids by embolization
E. Monitor the pregnancy for complications, with delivery by NSVD and subsequent treatment of the fibroids medically using mifepristone

A 25-year-old G1P0 pregnant woman at 28 weeks' gestational age presents to the obstetrics clinic with headaches for the past 2 weeks. Her pregnancy has been uncomplicated thus far, and she has no pertinent medical history. During the past 2 weeks, she has experienced frontal pounding headaches several times per day. In addition, she complains of notable swelling in her arms and legs during this period. On physical examination, the temperature is 37°C, the heart rate is 80 bpm, the respiratory rate is 20, and the blood pressure is 150/95 mm Hg. Mild edema is present diffusely. The pulmonary, cardiac, and gastrointestinal examinations are unremarkable. Deep tendon reflexes are normal. Dipstick urine testing detects 3+ protein present in the urine, with no blood or glucose present.

85. What is the most appropriate treatment for this patient?
A. $MgSO_4$ and hydralazine
B. $MgSO_4$ and metoprolol
C. $ZnSO_4$ and hydralazine
D. $ZnSO_4$ and metoprolol
E. Immediate delivery of the fetus

A 33-year-old woman with a history of hypertension presents to the obstetrics clinic with a positive pregnancy test. Her last menstrual period was 8 weeks ago. Her blood pressure has previously been well controlled using metoprolol, and she has continued taking her medications. On physical examination, the temperature is 38°C, the heart rate is 75 bpm, the respiratory rate is 20, and the blood pressure is 145/85 mm Hg. The pulmonary, cardiac, and abdominal examinations are unremarkable. Gynecologic examination is consistent with early gestation.

86. Which of the following is the best treatment for the hypertension?
A. Increase the dose of metoprolol
B. Continue metoprolol at the current dose
C. Change from metoprolol to hydralazine
D. Change from metoprolol to captopril
E. Discontinue all antihypertensive medications until delivery

A 35-year-old G4P4004 woman at 30 weeks' gestation with a 20-pack-year history of smoking presents to the obstetrics clinic with complaints of painless vaginal bleeding for the past 2 days. Her pregnancy has been uncomplicated until this point, and she has not experienced any contractions. On physical examination, the temperature is 38°C, the heart rate is 90 bpm, the respiratory rate is 22, and the blood pressure is 120/80 mm Hg. The cardiac, pulmonary, and abdominal examinations are unremarkable. The fetal heart rate is 150 bpm with no decelerations. Pelvic examination is significant only for a small amount of blood oozing from the cervical os. Bedside ultrasonography displays the edge of the placenta extending over the internal os. The hemoglobin is 12 g/dL, and the hematocrit is 38%.

87. What is the most appropriate management?
   A. Betamethasone treatment followed by emergent delivery of the fetus
   B. Immediate blood transfusion
   C. Surgical ablation of the placental edge through the cervix
   D. Observation with method of delivery dependent on the placement of the placenta at term
   E. Observation with cesarean section at term, regardless of placental placement

A 35-year-old G4P4004 woman at 36 weeks' gestation with a 20-pack-year history of cigarette smoking is taken to the emergency department with contractions and abdominal pain following an automobile accident. The patient was a restrained driver when she was hit from behind, and she recalls hitting her abdomen against the steering wheel of the car. Her pregnancy has been uncomplicated until this point. On physical examination, the temperature is 38°C, the heart rate is 110 bpm, the respiratory rate is 22, and the blood pressure is 110/60 mm Hg. The fetal heart rate is 160 bpm with occasional late decelerations. Her cardiac and pulmonary examinations are otherwise unremarkable. Pelvic examination is significant only for a moderate amount of blood oozing from the cervical os. Bedside ultrasonography displays a posteriorly located placenta with no visible abnormalities. The hemoglobin is 9 g/dL and the hematocrit is 26%.

88. What is the most appropriate treatment?
   A. Stabilize the patient, and deliver when the patient reaches term
   B. Betamethasone followed by delivery of the fetus after 2 days
   C. Observation with follow-up ultrasonography in 1 week
   D. Immediate vaginal delivery
   E. Immediate delivery by cesarean section

A 20-year-old woman presents to the gynecologic clinic with complaints of amenorrhea for the past 5 months. She has taken several pregnancy tests during this period, all of which have been negative. She also expresses concern over a 25-pound weight gain over the past year, and an increased growth of hair on her facE. She is not taking oral contraceptive pills. On physical examination, the temperature is 37°C, the heart rate is 80 bpm, the respiratory rate is 20, and the blood pressure is 120/80 mm Hg. Hair is present on the face and shoulders that is thicker than on previous visits. The heart, lung, and abdominal examinations are remarkable only for mild obesity. Pelvic examination detects mild enlargement of the clitoris and enlarged and tender ovaries.

89. What is the most likely diagnosis?
   A. Adult polycystic kidney disease
   B. Serous cystadenoma of the ovary
   C. Polycystic ovary syndrome
   D. Acromegaly
   E. 21α-Hydroxylase deficiency

A 24-year-old G1P0 woman at 10 weeks' gestational age presents to the obstetrics clinic with complaints of vaginal bleeding, vomiting, headache, and uterine contractions. The vomiting and headache have been present for 2 weeks, but the contractions and vomiting started over the past 2 days. On physical examination, the temperature is 37°C, the heart rate is 95 bpm, the respiratory rate is 24, and the blood pressure is 150/90 mm Hg. Fetal heart sounds are absent. The cardiac and pulmonary examinations are unremarkable, and there is mild tenderness of the abdomen to deep palpation. Genital examination reveals large grapelike clusters extending into the vagina. Ultrasonography shows a snowstorm pattern with no fetus in the uterus.

90. What is the most likely diagnosis?
   A. Choriocarcinoma
   B. Molar pregnancy
   C. Placental site trophoblastic tumor
   D. Mayer-Rokitansky-Küster-Hauser (MRKH) syndrome
   E. Uterine inversion

ONCOLOGY

A 50-year-old man with a history of peptic ulcer disease and cigarette smoking presents to the primary care clinic with complaints of weight loss and dysphagia of solids. The patient has had abdominal pain and a poor appetite for the past 4 months, during which he has lost 25 pounds. He complains of dull and constant abdominal pain, which is different in quality from the pain he experiences due to peptic ulcer disease. Recently, he has also noted that he experiences reflux and has difficulty swallowing food during meals. A physical examination shows no focal findings other than tenderness to deep palpation and occult blood in the stool. An upper endoscopy is performed, which reveals an ulcer in the proximal stomach that is reported to be consistent with a diagnosis of gastric adenocarcinoma. Subsequent workup shows no evidence of metastases.

91. What is the most appropriate surgical treatment for this patient?
- A. Total radical gastrectomy
- B. Radical distal gastrectomy
- C. Whipple procedure
- D. Ivor-Lewis procedure
- E. No surgery is recommended due to the likelihood of metastatic disease

A 55-year-old woman with a history of cigarette smoking, diabetes mellitus, and alcohol abuse presents to the primary care clinic with complaints of abdominal pain, weight loss, and a rash. The abdominal pain is dull and moderate in severity and has been present for 3 weeks. She has lost 10 pounds during this period. The blood glucose levels have climbed, requiring an increase in insulin dosage. In addition, a rash developed on her ankles and the soles of her feet that began as an erythematous rash and progressed to blistering and ulceration. The rash is pruritic, and the ulcerations are painful. On physical examination, the temperature is 38°C, heart rate is 75 bpm, respiratory rate is 22, and blood pressure is 135/85 mm Hg. No jaundice is noted. The cardiac and pulmonary examinations are unremarkable. The abdomen is nontender and nondistended, with no evidence of hepatomegaly or splenomegaly. The skin of her ankles and soles of her feet displays an ulcerated tender area of skin with ringed erythematous lesions and blisters around the edges. Subsequent workup reveals a suspicious mass in the distal pancreas. Serum glucose is 300 mg/dL.

92. What is the most likely diagnosis?
- A. Insulinoma
- B. Somatostatinoma
- C. Glucagonoma
- D. Mucinous cystic neoplasm of the pancreas
- E. Intraductal papillary mucinous neoplasm

A 67-year-old man with a history of smoking and adenomatous polyps presents to the gastroenterology clinic with complaints of bloody stools. Subsequent colonoscopy detects a 2-cm polypoid mass in the sigmoid colon, which is diagnosed as a well-differentiated adenocarcinoma of the colon.

93. What is the preferred preoperative tumor staging method?
- A. Chest radiograph
- B. Barium enema and abdominal radiograph
- C. CT scan of the bowel with contrast
- D. Serum carcinoembryonic antigen (CEA) level
- E. Endorectal ultrasound

A 55-year-old man with a 40-pack-year history of cigarette smoking presents with complaints of a 20-pound weight loss and progressive dyspnea on exertion over the past 6 months. He complains of gradually worsening anorexia during this period. On physical examination, his temperature is 37°C, his heart rate is 100 bpm, his respiratory rate is 25, and his blood pressure is 110/70 mm Hg. The face and neck show mild edema, and the neck veins are distended. Auscultation of the lungs reveals distant breath sounds bilaterally with dullness to percussion bilaterally up to the eighth rib. The cardiac and gastrointestinal examinations are unremarkable. Subsequent radiography detects bilateral pleural effusions (right > left) and a large mass in the right upper lung extending into the mediastinum. Biopsy of this mass is consistent with a small cell lung carcinoma.

94. What is the most appropriate treatment for this patient?
A. Surgical removal
B. Surgery with irradiation and chemotherapy
C. Neoadjuvant chemotherapy and irradiation followed by surgery
(D) Supportive care with specific management only for brain metastases
E. Intracavitary chemotherapy

A 55 year-old woman presents to her primary care clinic with a palpable mass in the right breast. The physical examination is unremarkable except for a 2 cm firm, irregular mobile mass in the upper lateral quadrant of the right breast. Subsequent mammography detects a stellate mass in this region.

95. Which of the following is the best treatment option?
A. Neoadjuvant chemotherapy with total mastectomy
B. Neoadjuvant chemotherapy with lumpectomy
(C.) Lumpectomy with sentinel node biopsy
D. Total mastectomy with sentinel node biopsy
E. Lumpectomy with axillary lymph node dissection

A 27-year-old woman presents to her primary care clinic with complaints of breast tenderness and straw-colored nipple discharge. She has no family history of breast cancer. She has noticed discharge, swelling, and tenderness of both breasts that varies and appears to coincide with her menstrual cycle. The physical examination is unremarkable except for multiple tender soft masses bilaterally in the breasts. Ultrasound of the breasts reveals multiple cystic structures bilaterally. Fine-needle aspiration performed in the clinic drains serous fluid from two of these cysts.

96. Which dietary change is most likely to improve the breast symptoms?
A. Cessation of alcohol
(B) Cessation of caffeine
C. Increasing vitamin A intake
D. Increasing vitamin B_{12} intake
E. Increasing calcium intake

A 60-year-old man with a history of benign prostatic hyperplasia presents to the primary care clinic for his first screening physical in 5 years. He has had no significant illnesses or hospitalization since the last visit but does complain of pain in the perineal and pelvic region that has gradually increased over the past year. The temperature is 38°C, the heart rate is 80 bpm, the respiratory rate is 20, and the blood pressure is 120/80 mm Hg. Physical examination of the lungs, heart, and abdomen are unremarkable. Digital rectal examination reveals an enlarged and nodular prostate gland. Subsequent workup reveals a prostate-specific antigen (PSA) level of 11 ng/mL and a bone scan consistent with a mass in the L4 vertebral body.

97. Which of the following is the most appropriate treatment?
A. Radical prostatectomy with irradiation
B. Irradiation alone
(C) Orchiectomy with antiandrogen therapy
D. Prostatectomy with antiandrogen therapy
E. Irradiation and antiandrogen therapy

A 3-year-old boy with aniridia presents to the emergency room with abdominal pain and fever. His mother states that his weight gain has been poor for the past few months and that his urine has become amber in color. He has no history of recent infections. On physical examination, his temperature is 38.7°C, his heart rate is 115 bpm, his respiratory rate is 25, and his blood pressure is 120/85 mm Hg. Heart and lung examination is unremarkable. A large mass is palpable on the right side of the abdomen. Ultrasound shows a large mass in the right kidney.

98. What is the most likely diagnosis for this patient?
A. Hydronephrosis
B. Infantile polycystic kidney disease
(C) Wilms' tumor
D. Poststreptococcal glomerulonephritis
E. Renal cell carcinoma

A 65-year-old man with a 30-pack-year history of cigarette smoking, hepatitis B infection, chronic alcoholism, and cirrhosis presents with weakness, abdominal pain, and a 30-pound weight loss over the past 6 months. He attributes the weight loss to a poor appetite but also claims that his diet has not substantially changed. He has had no acute illnesses or hospitalizations for the past year. On physical examination, the temperature is 37°C, the heart rate is 80 bpm, the respiratory rate is 20, and the blood pressure is 130/80 mm Hg. The skin and mucous membranes are moderately jaundiced, and his sclerae are icteric. The cardiac and lung examination are unremarkable. Palpation of the abdomen reveals an enlarged, nodular liver and an enlarged spleen. Subsequent abdominal CT scan demonstrates a suspicious mass in the liver.

99. Which of the following tests will most likely confirm the diagnosis?
A. Carcinoembryonic antigen (CEA)
B. Serum amylase
C. CA-125
D. α-Fetoprotein (AFP)
E. Parathyroid hormone–related peptide (PTH-rp)

A 30-year-old woman presents to the surgical clinic because of a recent diagnosis of hepatic adenoma. The adenoma had been diagnosed from a liver biopsy during a workup for abdominal discomfort during the past 2 months. CT scan of the abdomen shows a 3-cm solid mass in the subcapsular region of the liver. Upon further discussion, the patient also states that she is planning on having at least one child over the next few years.

100. Which of the following is the most significant risk factor for the development of this mass?
A. Hepatitis B infection
B. Hepatitis C infection
C. Schistosomiasis
D. Oral contraceptives
E. Procainamide

PEDIATRICS

A 2-year-old boy with a history of poor feeding and recurrent respiratory infections is brought to the emergency department because of a 2-day history of fever and productive cough. He has had similar respiratory infections several times in the past, which usually resolve only with antibiotic therapy. On physical examination, the temperature is 39°C, the heart rate is 80 bpm, the respiratory rate is 24, and the blood pressure is 100/60 mm Hg. He appears pale and drowsy and periodically coughs, producing thick, green, purulent sputum. Auscultation of the lungs reveals decreased breath sounds in the left lower lung field, a slight wheeze, and a wet-sounding cough. The cardiac and abdominal examinations are unremarkable, but pale, foul-smelling stool is present in the diaper. When asked, the patient's mother states that his stools have always had that appearance.

101. What is the most appropriate diagnostic test to confirm the diagnosis?
A. Sweat chloride test
B. Chest radiograph
C. Abdominal CT scan
D. Barium enema
E. Rectal biopsy

A 1-year-old male is seen at the primary care clinic with irritability and vomiting for the past 3 days. He experiences episodic abdominal pain, during which he cries and draws his legs to his abdomen. His mother has noted dark red stools during this period. He had a similar episode lasting 1 day 2 months ago, but his symptoms improved before being taken to the doctor. On physical examination, the temperature is 38.5°C, the heart rate is 120 bpm, the respiratory rate is 30, and the blood pressure is 95/60 mm Hg. The heart and lung examinations are unremarkable. The patient's abdomen is tender to palpation, with a sausage-shaped mass in the right lower quadrant. Bowel sounds are hyperactive.

102. What is the most appropriate therapy?
A. Barium enema
B. Surgical resection of Meckel's diverticulum
C. Prednisone
D. Dietary changes
E. Enzyme replacement

An 18-month-old female is brought to the emergency department after experiencing an episode of urticaria and wheezing after eating a small amount of egg salad. She has no prior history of such reactions, but has followed a fairly strict diet of formula and baby foods since birth. On physical examination, the temperature is 37.5°C, the heart rate is 100 bpm, the respiratory rate is 25, and the blood pressure is 100/60 mm Hg. A rash consisting of raised bumps and wheals is present on the patient's face, trunk, and limbs. No ulcerations or bullae are noted. Auscultation of the lungs reveals mild wheezing. The cardiac and gastrointestinal examinations are unremarkable.

103. Which vaccinations should be avoided in this patient?
A. Mumps
B. Measles
C. Influenza
D. Varicella
E. Tetanus

A 1-year-old Japanese boy presents with fever, conjunctivitis, swelling, and rash of the extremities for the past 2 weeks. The fever reached as high as 40°C for several days but has decreased recently. The rash started as a diffuse erythematous rash and has recently started peeling on the hands and feet. On physical examination, the temperature is 39°C, the heart rate is 120 bpm, the respiratory rate is 30, and the blood pressure is 90/60 mm Hg. The eyes are erythematous with a dry crust around the eyelids. The throat is erythematous without exudates. The pulmonary examination is unremarkable. Auscultation of the heart detects a pericardial friction rub. The abdominal examination is unremarkable. Examination of the skin displays a maculopapular rash without bullae or vesicles, but with desquamation of the hands and feet.

104. What is the most appropriate treatment?
A. Ibuprofen
B. Prednisone
C. Aspirin
D. Liver transplantation
E. Acetaminophen

A 14-day-old boy delivered at 33 weeks' gestational age from a 40-year-old mother develops vomiting, feeding intolerance, and blood in the stool. He has been in the neonatal intensive care unit since birth owing to respiratory distress at birth. The temperature is 39°C, the heart rate is 145 bpm, the respiratory rate is 35, and the blood pressure is 40/20 mm Hg. The head, heart, and lung examinations are unremarkable. Abdominal examination detects a tender, distended abdomen with hypoactive bowel sounds.

105. Exposure to which of the following substances in utero predisposes to the development of this condition?
A. Heroin
B. Cocaine
C. Marijuana
D. Alcohol
E. Thalidomide

A 13-month-old boy is brought to the primary care clinic because his mother has noticed him "turning blue." Since he started walking a month ago, the patient has had several episodes in which his lips turn blue. During several of these incidents, he assumed a squatting position for several seconds until resuming his activity. The patient's mother had previously noticed his lips turn blue when he cried for long periods of time, but she thought that was a normal response. On physical examination, the temperature is 37.5°C, the heart rate is 120 bpm, the respiratory rate is 25, and the blood pressure is 90/60 mm Hg. He is in the 10th percentile for weight and height. The lips and mucous membranes are moist and pink. A systolic ejection murmur is noted on cardiac auscultation. The pulmonary and abdominal examinations are unremarkable.

106. What radiographic abnormality is most likely present?
A. Boot-shaped heart
B. Egg-shaped heart
C. Absence of a thymic shadow
D. Small heart with increased pulmonary vascularity
E. Heart on the right side of the diaphragm

A 3-day-old girl delivered at 35 weeks' gestational age develops a yellow discoloration of the mucous membranes and skin. The discoloration started at the head and progressed to involve the trunk and limbs. There is no history of infection or intrauterine drug exposure. The patient's blood type is O–. On physical examination, the temperature is 37.5°C, the heart rate is 125 bpm, the respiratory rate is 30, and the blood pressure is 60/35 mm Hg. A mild yellow discoloration of the skin is uniformly present on all skin surfaces. The neurologic, cardiac, pulmonary, and abdominal examinations are unremarkable.

107. Which of the following treatments is most indicated?
   A. Iron supplementation
   B. Phenobarbital
   C. Phototherapy
   D. Plasmapheresis
   E. Dialysis

A 2-week-old boy delivered at 36 weeks' gestational age develops a yellow discoloration of the mucous membranes and skin. The discoloration started at the head and progressed to involve the trunk and limbs. His mother claims that he was breast-feeding poorly during the previous week, but his oral intake has been increasingly steadily for the past few days. There is no history of infection or intrauterine drug exposure. The patient's blood type is O–. On physical examination, the temperature is 37°C, the heart rate is 130 bpm, the respiratory rate is 30, and the blood pressure is 55/30 mm Hg. A mild yellow discoloration of the skin is uniformly present on all skin surfaces. The mucous membranes are pale and dry. The neurologic, cardiac, pulmonary, and abdominal examinations are unremarkable.

108. What is the cause of this child's symptoms?
   A. Dehydration and poor feeding
   B. Immaturity of the neonatal liver
   C. Dysfunction of bilirubin metabolism
   D. Endocrine dysfunction
   E. Hemolysis

Following delivery at 36 weeks' gestational age, a girl presents with tachypnea, cyanosis, and grunting several minutes after delivery. The child had no documented drug exposures or infections in utero. The mother did not receive adequate prenatal care or ultrasound screening after 11 weeks' gestational age. The newborn's vital signs include a temperature of 37°C, heart rate of 140 bpm, respiratory rate of 40, and blood pressure of 30/15 mm Hg. On physical examination, the patient is cyanotic and grunts while breathing. No obstructions are visible in the oropharynx. Breath sounds are absent over the left lung fields. Cardiac auscultation is remarkable only for a displacement of the heart sounds to the right. The abdomen is scaphoid, and tinkling bowel sounds are present that radiate to the left lung field.

109. What is the most likely diagnosis?
   A. Tracheoesophageal fistula
   B. Duodenal atresia
   C. Congenital diaphragmatic hernia
   D. Omphalocele
   E. Gastroschisis

A boy is born at 34 weeks' gestational age with his abdominal viscera protruding through a defect in the abdominal wall. The mother did not receive prenatal care after her first prenatal visit at 10 weeks' gestational age. The patient had no known infections or drug exposures in utero. On physical examination, the temperature is 37°C, the heart rate is 130 bpm, the respiratory rate is 30, and the blood pressure is 50/30 mm Hg. A defect is present in the abdominal wall in the umbilical and supraumbilical region, through which protrudes several loops of intestine encased by a translucent sac. The patient's neurologic, cardiac, and pulmonary examinations are unremarkable.

110. What is the most likely diagnosis?
   A. Tracheoesophageal fistula
   B. Duodenal atresia
   C. Congenital diaphragmatic hernia
   D. Omphalocele
   E. Gastroschisis

PSYCHIATRY

A 75-year-old man with depression complained of insomnia. He requested a medication to help him fall asleep and was given a medication by the on-call intern. At rounds the next morning, the patient is agitated, confused, and unresponsive to questioning.

111. Which of the following medications was most likely prescribed?
A. Trazodone
B. Lorazepam
(C.) Diphenhydramine
D. Haloperidol
E. Risperidone

A 60-year-old man with a 40-year history of alcohol use complains of depressed mood, decreased energy, feelings of guilt, and difficulty sleeping. He started a detoxification program yesterday and appears committed to drinking cessation, and he wonders if he should also be taking medications for his mood.

112. When would be the most appropriate time to start antidepressant therapy?
A. Immediately
B. After 3 days without alcohol intake, and following a reevaluation of his depressive symptoms
(C.) After 2 to 3 weeks without alcohol intake and following a reevaluation of depressive symptoms
D. Do not give antidepressant therapy given the patient's history of substance abuse
E. Prescribe antidepressant medication only if the patient starts drinking again

A 50-year-old man with schizophrenia presents with tremor, restlessness, and involuntary lip smacking. His schizophrenia has been successfully managed in the past with IM injections of haloperidol decanoate every 4 weeks.

113. How would you treat the developing movement symptoms?
A. Discontinue haloperidol, and start chlorpromazine
B. Change the dosing interval for haloperidol decanoate to every 8 weeks
C. These symptoms are a reaction to the decanoate formation of haloperidol. Start the patient on daily oral haloperidol.
(D.) Discontinue haloperidol, and start olanzapine
E. These symptoms are due to a worsening of the patient's schizophrenia. Continue the haloperidol and add an atypical neuroleptic.

A 65-year-old woman with a history of anxiety disorder is undergoing inpatient treatment for a chronic obstructive pulmonary disease (COPD) exacerbation. The patient was unable to remember her home medications upon admission. Although the patient was pleasant and cooperative during admission to the hospital, she has become progressively irritable and agitated over the past 2 days and complains of problems sleeping. The physical examination is significant for a resting tremor and tachycardia.

114. Which of the following medications is most indicated?
(A.) Chlordiazepoxide
B. Trazodone
C. Diphenhydramine
D. Haloperidol
E. Risperidone

An 18-year-old male patient is brought to the ER by his mother because of a 5-day history of reclusiveness, odd speech, poor personal hygiene, and interaction with people who were not present. The patient becomes confused and agitated while in the ER and requires sedation for safety purposes. While discussing the patient's case with his mother, you mention that a possible diagnosis for her son is schizophrenia. Upon hearing this, the mother becomes upset. Her brother was schizophrenic and committed suicide at the age of 25. She knows that psychiatric problems can run in families and is worried about her other son, age 10.

115. What is the likelihood that the younger son will also develop schizophrenia?
A. 0.1%
B. 1%
(C.) 10%
D. 30%
E. 50%

A 7-year-old boy is brought to the primary care clinic because of his mother's complaints about hyperactivity. His early childhood was uneventful, with achievement of his developmental milestones within the normal range. He attended kindergarten for 2 years without any reported behavioral issues by his teachers. Since starting the first grade last year, however, his teachers have consistently commented on his inability to follow directions and his restlessness while sitting in class. He has difficulty staying on-task in class and has been punished several times owing to a lack of consideration for fellow students. He has not been in fights or showed aggressive behavior toward the other students. On physical examination, the temperature is 37°C, the heart rate is 100 bpm, the respiratory rate is 22, and the blood pressure is 100/65 mm Hg. The cardiac, respiratory, and abdominal examinations are unremarkable. Throughout the interview and examination, he is frequently distracted and has difficulty staying seated on the examination table. His mother tells him multiple times not to play with the office equipment, but he persistently disobeys her.

116. What is the most appropriate diagnosis?
A. Oppositional defiant disorder
B. Attention-deficit/hyperactivity disorder
C. Asperger's syndrome
D. Conduct disorder
E. Rett's syndrome

A 3-year-old boy is brought to the primary care clinic because his mother is worried that he is not keeping up with other children his age. He has no history of serious illness, but his mother admits that she has not taken him to the doctor very often since he was born because of the cost. His immunizations have been kept current through community vaccination programs. While his mother is unsure about most of his developmental milestones, she does recall that he did not stand by himself or speak until 18 months of age. He currently speaks in two-word sentences and has recently learned to walk up steps. On physical examination, the temperature is 37°C, the heart rate is 115 bpm, the respiratory rate is 25, and the blood pressure is 100/65 mm Hg. The jaw and ears are disproportionately large. The cardiac, pulmonary, and abdominal examinations are unremarkable. Neurologic function is intact, with 5/5 strength in all limbs, normal reflexes, and intact sensory function.

117. What is the most appropriate diagnosis?
A. Phenylketonuria
B. Trisomy 21
C. Fragile X syndrome
D. Fetal alcohol syndrome
E. Congenital hypothyroidism

A 40-year-old man with a history of depression is brought to the emergency department by his wife because of his increasing confusion over the past 2 days. He has a history of mild depression, which has been well controlled by fluoxetine for the past 2 years. Recently, however, he has become interested in alternative management strategies for his depression, and he altered his diet to minimize snacking and fast food intake, take vitamins, and eat only home-cooked meals during the past 3 weeks. He told his wife last week that he was feeling much better and that he was considering trying to manage his depression through dietary methods alone. For the past 4 days, she has noticed a change in his sleeping patterns, and he has gradually become confused and less responsive to her conversations. On physical examination, the temperature is 37.5°C, the heart rate is 90 bpm, the respiratory rate is 20, and the blood pressure is 140/85 mm Hg. He responds inappropriately to direct questioning and is not oriented to time or place. The cardiac, pulmonary, and abdominal examinations are unremarkable. Strength and sensation are intact, but the patient displays an unsteady gait when asked to walk in a straight line.

118. What is the most likely cause of the symptoms?
A. Overstimulation of serotonin receptors due to dietary intake of tyramine
B. Abrupt discontinuation of a selective serotonin reuptake inhibitor (SSRI)
C. Anticholinergic side effects
D. Interaction between the patient's medication and dietary tryptophan
E. Worsening of the patient's major depressive disorder

A 23-year-old woman presents to her primary care physician with complaints of depressed mood and lack of motivation for the past few months. During this period, she has had poor concentration, a lack of interest in hobbies, and frequent feelings of guilt over her lack of achievement since finishing college. She sleeps for 10–12 hours per day and finds herself snacking frequently, which has contributed to a 20-pound weight gain since last year. She also claims that she has become increasingly sensitive and argumentative about many issues, which has distanced her from her family and friends. On physical examination, the temperature is 37.6°C, the heart rate is 85 bpm, the respiratory rate is 18, and the blood pressure is 120/80 mm Hg. The skin, cardiac, pulmonary, and abdominal examinations are unremarkable. Strength and sensory functions are intact.

119. What is the most appropriate treatment for this patient?
- A. Fluoxetine
- B. Paroxetine
- C. Amitriptyline
- (D) Phenelzine
- E. Buspirone

A 35-year-old man with a recent diagnosis of bipolar disorder returns to the psychiatric clinic with persistent symptoms of hyperactivity, distractibility, and insomnia. He was diagnosed with bipolar disorder 1 month ago and was started on lithium therapy. The patient claims to have taken his medications appropriately, which his wife can confirm. Since starting lithium, both the patient and his wife have not noticed a substantial effect on his symptoms. On physical examination, the temperature is 37°C, the heart rate is 85 bpm, the respiratory rate is 18, and the blood pressure is 125/85 mm Hg. The cardiac, pulmonary, and abdominal examinations are unremarkable. No weakness, tremors, or sensory deficits are present on neurologic examination. A lithium level was drawn last week by a nurse and has returned at a level of 1.0 mEq/L.

120. What is the next appropriate step in therapy?
- A. Increase the dose of lithium until clinical efficacy is achieved
- B. Discontinue lithium, and start paroxetine
- C. Discontinue lithium, and start valproic acid
- D. Discontinue lithium, and treat through psychotherapy alone
- (E) Continue lithium, and add valproic acid

PULMONOLOGY

A 70-year-old man with a history of a myocardial infarction presents to the emergency room with chest pain, shortness of breath, and hemoptysis that started 2 hours ago. He noticed pain and swelling in the right calf yesterday following a 10-hour car trip he took several days ago. He had a mild heart attack 5 years ago but does not have any other history of pulmonary or cardiac disease. On physical examination, the temperature is 38.5°C, the heart rate is 110 bpm, the respiratory rate is 30, and the blood pressure is 140/85 mm Hg. He appears anxious and in moderate respiratory distress. Auscultation of the lungs detects a focal area of decreased breath sounds in the right lower lobe of the lung, but no hyperresonance, dullness to percussion, or egophony. The pulmonary component of the second heart sound is accentuated. The patient's abdomen is nontender and nondistended with normoactive bowel sounds. The right calf shows tenderness, venous engorgement, and 2+ pitting edema.

121. Which of the following is the most appropriate treatment?
- (A.) Anticoagulation with heparin and warfarin
- B. Anticoagulation with warfarin only
- C. Placement of a Greenfield filter
- D. Ceftriaxone and azithromycin
- E. Streptokinase

A 14-year-old boy with a history of seasonal allergies presents to the primary care clinic with complaints of wheezing and coughing when he exercises. The patient is a member of a cross-country running team and has recently experienced wheezing, shortness of breath, and a cough productive of stringy white sputum after running for several miles. He has no history of other pulmonary disease or recurrent infections. On physical examination, the temperature is 37°C, the heart rate is 65 bpm, the respiratory rate is 20, and the blood pressure is 120/80 mm Hg. No erythema or lesions are noted in the oropharynx. The lungs are clear to auscultation, with no expiratory wheezes noted. The cardiac and abdominal examinations are unremarkable.

122. Which of the following is the most effective management?
A. Cessation of strenuous physical activity
B. Pre-exercise use of a β-agonist inhaler
C. A 1-week course of penicillin and azithromycin
D. Bronchoscopy
E. Over-the-counter cough medicine and bed rest

A 70-year-old man with a history of chronic bronchitis requiring home oxygen presents to the emergency department with complaints of increasing oxygen requirements. Chronic obstructive pulmonary disease was diagnosed with 10 years ago, and the patient has required home oxygen for the past 2 years. Until recently, oxygen was necessary only during strenuous activity. He states that he caught a cold 3 weeks ago and has had a difficult time controlling the cough. Currently, he requires oxygen following routine tasks around the house. On physical examination, the temperature is 38.5°C, the heart rate is 70 bpm, the respiratory rate is 24, and the blood pressure is 130/80 mm Hg. The pharynx is mildly erythematous with no exudates. Auscultation of the lungs elicits diffusely decreased breath sounds and hyperresonant lungs, with an occasional rattling cough. The cardiovascular and gastrointestinal examinations are unremarkable. During the course of the examination, the nurse puts the patient on 100% mask oxygen. When returning to the patient several minutes later, he is unresponsive and has stopped breathing. Resuscitation efforts are successful, and the patient is sent to the medical intensive care unit.

123. What was the cause of the respiratory arrest?
A. Pulmonary embolism
B. Fatigue of the diaphragm
C. Increase in the oxygen saturation of the blood
D. Decrease in the HCO_3 concentration of the blood
E. Cardiac arrhythmia

An 18-year-old male is brought to the emergency department after being stabbed in the right posterior shoulder during a knife fight. He complains of shortness of breath and sharp chest pain during inspiration. He has no other history of recent injuries and no significant past medical history. On physical examination, the temperature is 38°C, the heart rate is 110 bpm, the respiratory rate is 30, and the blood pressure is 140/90 mm Hg. He appears to be in respiratory distress. The trachea is deviated to the left. Breath sounds are absent over the right lung fields, which are also hyperresonant to percussion. The cardiac and abdominal examinations are unremarkable.

124. What is the most appropriate initial management?
A. Chest tube placement
B. Needle thoracostomy
C. Aspirin
D. β-Agonist inhalers
E. Intravenous penicillin and azithromycin

For each of the following chest radiographs, select the most likely presentation of the patient.

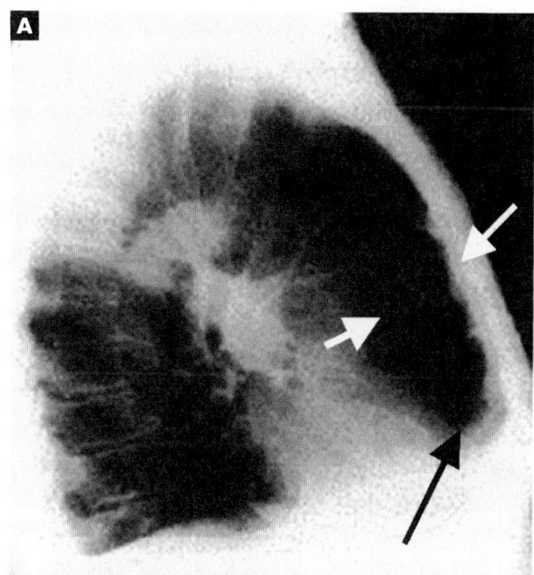

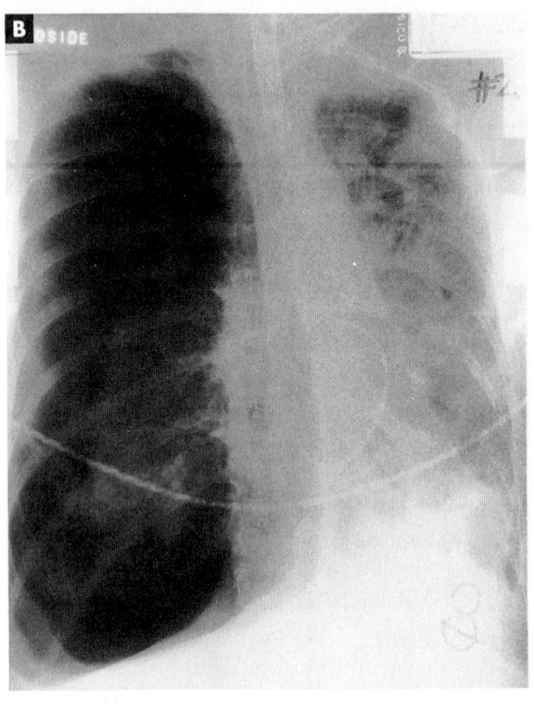

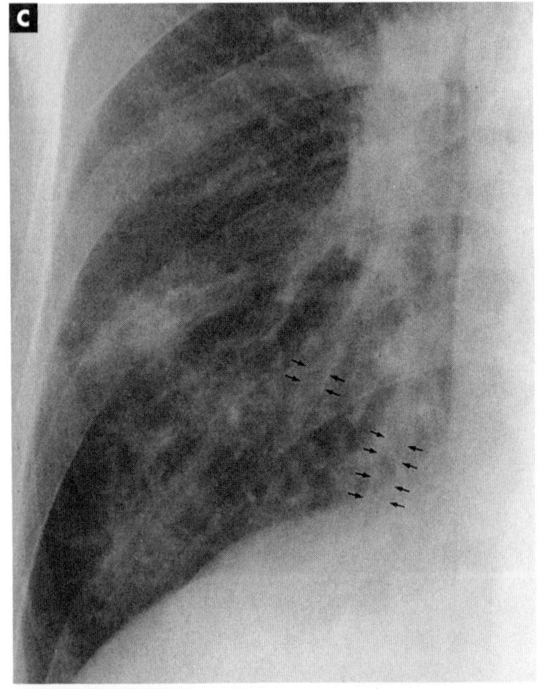

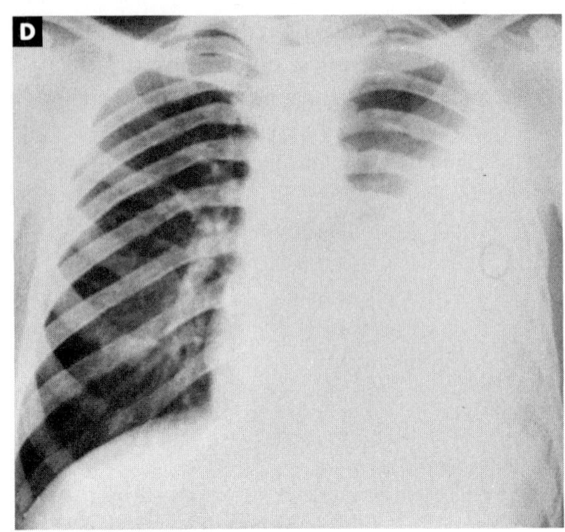

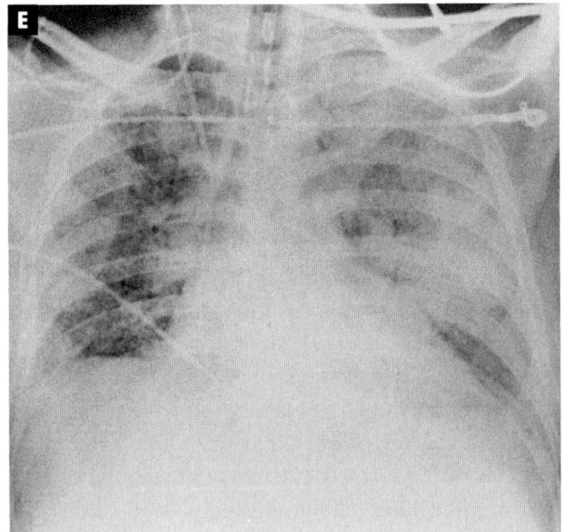

125. A patient with a triad of sinusitis, situs inversus, and infertility.

126. A 40-year-old man with a history of severe burn injury and a complicated hospital course. His current respiratory difficulties are not responsive to supplemental oxygen.

127. An 80-year-old man with a history of heart disease presenting with bilateral pedal edema and crackles in the lungs. The lungs are dull to percussion to the seventh rib bilaterally.

128. A 30-year-old soldier with a bullet wound to the chest.

129. A 70-year-old man with a 40-pack-year history of smoking has an increased anteroposterior chest diameter, dyspnea, and pursed lip breathing.

An 80-year-old man with a history of heart disease and hypertension presents to the primary care clinic with dyspnea on exertion, orthopnea, and shortness of breath that have increased over the past 2 months. The patient notices that he can no longer climb stairs without stopping for rest and that he now needs to prop himself up with two pillows at night to sleep comfortably. He is currently taking simvastatin and metoprolol. On physical examination, the temperature is 37°C, the heart rate is 90 bpm, the respiratory rate is 24, and the blood pressure is 145/90 mm Hg. The neck veins are distended at 45 degrees. Auscultation of the lungs reveals crackles diffusely and distant breath sounds below the eighth rib. The lungs are dull to percussion bilaterally below the eighth rib. The heart beats at a regular rate and rhythm with no murmurs or extra sounds. The abdomen is nontender and nondistended with normoactive bowel sounds. Pitting edema is present bilaterally to the knees. Pleural effusions are noted on a chest radiograph.

130. Which of the following test results are most likely from this patient's pleurocentesis specimen?
A. High pleural protein, high pleural LDH, no atypical cells, marked lymphocytosis
B. Low pleural protein, high pleural LDH, no atypical cells, no lymphocytosis
C. High pleural protein, low pleural LDH, atypical cells present, marked lymphocytosis
D. Low pleural protein, low pleural LDH, no atypical cells, no lymphocytosis
E. High pleural protein, high pleural LDH, no atypical cells, no lymphocytosis

RHEUMATOLOGY

A 21-year-old male college student presents to the primary care clinic with a 1 week history of eye irritation and dysuria. He has also noticed pain in his hips and knees since the onset of these symptoms. He has no prior history of these symptoms and denies any recent injuries. His attempts to relieve the itching and redness in his eyes using moisturizing eye drops have been unsuccessful. On physical examination, the temperature is 38°C, the heart rate is 70 bpm, the respiratory rate is 20, and the blood pressure is 120/80 mm Hg. The conjunctiva appear injected and dry with a tan crust around the eyelids. No oral lesions or facial rashes are noted. The cardiac, pulmonary, and abdominal examinations are unremarkable. No weakness or sensory deficits are noted. There is mild swelling of the fingers, and the sacroiliac joint is tender to palpation with a mildly restricted range of motion due to pain.

131. Which pathogen is associated with the development of this disorder?
A. *Staphylococcus aureus*
B. *Streptococcus pyogenes*
C. *Neisseria gonorrhoeae*
D. *Neisseria meningitidis*
E. *Chlamydia trachomatis*

A 42-year-old woman with a history of arthritis presents with complaints of eye irritation and difficulty in swallowing food for the past month. Her arthritis is present in her hands, knees, and hips and has not worsened recently. She has noticed that her eyes are dry and irritated lately but that they improve markedly with moisturizing drops. She also notices that her mouth is dry and that she has difficulty swallowing food because of the discomfort that it causes. On physical examination, the temperature is 38°C, the heart rate is 90 bpm, the respiratory rate is 20, and the blood pressure is 130/75 mm Hg. The eyes are dry with mild injection of the conjunctiva. The oropharynx is pale and dry with no lesions present. The cardiac, pulmonary, and abdominal examinations are otherwise unremarkable. There is mild tenderness and restriction of motion in her hands, knees, and hips. No rashes are present.

132. Which of the following renal conditions may occur with this disorder?
A. Adult polycystic kidney disease
B. Poststreptococcal glomerulonephritis
C. Minimal change disease
(D) Type I renal tubular acidosis
E. Type IV renal tubular acidosis

A 50-year-old woman with a history of ventricular ectopy, hypertension, hypercholesterolemia, and depression presents to the primary care clinic with complaints of a rash and joint pain that have been gradually worsening for the past 2 months. She first noticed the rash on her cheeks and nose and assumed that it was an allergic reaction to her face soap. The rash has not improved despite changing skin care products and stopping cosmetic use. The rash becomes more severe following exposure to the sun. She notices joint pain and stiffness in her hands, hips, and knees that do not improve with activity. She has no new complaints of headaches, dizziness, or depressed mood. Her current medications include procainamide, metoprolol, simvastatin, fluoxetine, and aspirin. On physical examination, the temperature is 37°C, the heart rate is 100 bpm, the respiratory rate is 20, and the blood pressure is 145/90 mm Hg. An erythematous maculopapular rash is present on the cheeks and nose. Small buccal mucosal ulcers are noted on examination of the oropharynx, and her mucus membranes appear pink and moist. The cardiac and pulmonary examinations are unremarkable. There is mild tenderness to deep palpation of the abdomen, and bowel sounds are normoactive. The joints of the hands, knees, and hips are mildly tender with a mildly restricted range of motion.

133. Which of this patient's medications is responsible for the symptoms?
A. Metoprolol
B. Simvastatin
C. Fluoxetine
D. Aspirin
(E.) Procainamide

A 50-year-old woman with a 30-pack-year history of smoking presents to the primary care clinic with gradually worsening fatigue, weakness, and joint pain for the past 4 months. During this period, she has noticed that her exercise tolerance has decreased and parts of her legs have become numb. Her daily activities are also hampered by pain and stiffness in her hands, hips, and knees that do not improve with activity. She has never experienced these symptoms in the past. She has no history of recent trauma. On physical examination, the temperature is 37°C, the heart rate is 90 bpm, the respiratory rate is 20, and the blood pressure is 110/60 mm Hg. Examination of the oropharynx shows an enlarged tongue, moist mucous membranes, and an absence of ulcerations. The lungs are clear to auscultation. The heart examination is unremarkable. A smooth liver edge is palpated 3 cm below the costal margin, and a small amount of ascites is present. There is mild stiffness and tenderness in the joints of the hands, hips, and knees. Strength of the flexors and extensors in the arms is 5/5 bilaterally. Strength is 3/5 in the plantar flexors right foot and 4/5 in the dorsiflexors of the left foot. There is a loss of pinprick sensation over the right calf. ECG shows a low-voltage QRS complex in all leads with mild right axis deviation.

134. What is the most appropriate therapy?
A. Methotrexate
B. Azathioprine
(C.) Melphalan
D. Hydroxychloroquine
E. Aspirin

A 45-year-old woman presents to the primary care clinic with complaints of pain, stiffness, and deformity of her hands and wrists that has gradually progressed over the past year. She notices that her symptoms of joint pain and stiffness are worse in the morning and are not relieved by activity. She has no history of injury to her hands, and her only current medication is ibuprofen for joint pain. On physical examination, the temperature is 38°C, the heart rate is 85 bpm, the respiratory rate is 18, and the blood pressure is 110/70 mm Hg. The mucous membranes are pink and moist, and no conjunctival injection or oropharyngeal ulcerations are noted. The lungs are clear to auscultation. The cardiac and abdominal examinations are unremarkable. There is no focal weakness or sensory abnormalities. The hands and wrists are tender and stiff bilaterally, especially at the metacarpophalangeal joints. A deformity of the hands consisting of a proximal interphalangeal flexion and a distal interphalangeal extension is present bilaterally.

135. Which of the following synovial fluid findings is most likely present?
A. Increased neutrophils
B. Osteophytes
C. Needle-shaped, negatively birefringent crystals
D. Rhomboid, positively birefringent crystals
E. Myxoid cartilage

A 65-year-old man with a history of poorly controlled type 2 diabetes mellitus and alcohol abuse presents with acute onset of pain, swelling, tenderness, and stiffness in his elbows, feet, and knees. He noticed the onset of symptoms after a 3-day drinking binge last week. He has experienced mild joint pain in the past, but nothing nearly so severe as his current symptoms. His medications include simvastatin, glyburide, metformin, and aspirin. On physical examination, the temperature is 38°C, the heart rate is 80 bpm, the respiratory rate is 20, and the blood pressure is 140/85 mm Hg. He is moderately obese and his face is flushed, but no rashes are noted. The cardiac and pulmonary examinations are unremarkable. Bowel sounds are normoactive and the abdomen is nontender to palpation. A small amount of ascites is present in the abdomen, but there is no evidence of hepatomegaly. There are no focal weakness or sensory deficits. There is marked erythema and swelling of the great toe on the right foot and the left elbow at the olecranon. There is tenderness bilaterally in the feet, knees, and elbows, and moderately limited range of motion due to pain.

136. What is the most appropriate initial treatment?
A. Colchicine
B. Allopurinol
C. Prednisone
D. Indomethacin
E. Acetaminophen

137. The patient improves and is subsequently discharged on several oral medications for long-term control of his symptoms. One week later he returns to the clinic and states that his blood glucose has consistently been greater than 200 mg/dL since he left the hospital, despite adherence to the same diet he used prior to admission. Which of the following medications is most likely causing this problem?
A. Colchicine
B. Allopurinol
C. Prednisone
D. Indomethacin
E. Acetaminophen

A 40-year-old man presents to the emergency department with complaints of hemoptysis for the past day. He has also noticed discoloration of his urine periodically over the past month. He has no prior history of significant urinary or pulmonary disease. On physical examination, the temperature is 38°C, the heart rate is 90 bpm, the respiratory rate is 22, and the blood pressure is 110/70 mm Hg. The eyes are mildly proptotic. Mild crackles are heard in the left lower lung. Coughing elicits bloody sputum. The cardiac and abdominal examinations are otherwise unremarkable. No lesions are noted on the patient's genital examination, but his urine specimen is tea-colored and displayed a 4+ blood on dipstick analysis.

138. This patient is most likely to have which of the following immunologic abnormalities?
A. cANCA
B. pANCA
C. Antinuclear antibodies
D. Anti-Jo antibodies
E. Rheumatoid factor

A 70-year-old man presents to the emergency room with fatigue, malaise, and a severe headache over the past day. He has no history of migraine headaches and has never had a headache similar to his current symptoms. The pain is concentrated in his temples and his eyes and is exacerbated by clenching his jaw. On physical examination, the temperature is 38.5°C, the heart rate is 80 bpm, the respiratory rate is 20, and the blood pressure is 120/80 mm Hg. Mild tenderness is present over the temples. There are no focal neurologic deficits. The cardiac, pulmonary, and abdominal examinations are unremarkable.

139. What is the most appropriate treatment?
A. Aspirin
B. High-dose glucocorticoids
C. Low-dose glucocorticoids
D. Azathioprine
E. Melphalan

A 60-year-old man presents to the primary care clinic with fatigue, malaise, and abdominal pain for the past 2 weeks. During this period, he has also noticed black tarry stools during bowel movements and a tendency to stumble on his right leg while walking. He is not currently taking medications. On physical examination, the temperature is 37°C, the heart rate is 90 bpm, the respiratory rate is 18, and the blood pressure is 150/90 mm Hg. The heart and lung examination are unremarkable. There is moderate tenderness to deep palpation of the abdomen, and bowel sounds are normoactive. Neurologic examination is significant only for 3/5 strength in his proximal right leg extensors and 4/5 strength in his left foot dorsiflexors. In addition, there is a loss of pinprick and vibration sensation over the dorsum of the right hand. No rashes are present. The musculoskeletal examination is otherwise unremarkable. An angiogram is subsequently performed, which shows thrombosis and aneurysm formation in the superior mesenteric artery.

140. Which of the following pathogens is most often associated with this disorder?
A. *Staphylococcus aureus*
B. Epstein-Barr virus
C. Hepatitis B virus
D. *Borrelia burgdorferi*
E. *Streptococcus pyogenes*

ANSWERS

answers

CARDIOLOGY

1. (B) Verapamil is the treatment of choice in this patient for management of his arrhythmia. While both beta-blockers (propranolol) and calcium channel blockers (verapamil) are the first-line therapy for supraventricular tachycardias, the use of beta-blockers is contraindicated in patients with asthma. Quinidine can also be used for supraventricular arrhythmias but has a harsher side effect profile than verapamil. Sotalol and ibutilide can be useful for atrial arrhythmias (atrial fibrillation and flutter) but they can also produce torsades de pointes and ventricular arrhythmias.

2. (A) Indications for stress testing include suspected coronary artery disease, risk stratification following myocardial infarction, and documentation of the progression of coronary artery disease. However, stress tests are contraindicated within 48 hours of a myocardial infarction, so the only patient described for whom a stress test is indicated is the one who had a myocardial infarction 1 week previously. Arrhythmias, unstable angina, and severe aortic stenosis are all contraindications for cardiac stress testing.

3. (D) Of the tests described, the electrocardiogram is the most likely to be abnormal 30 minutes following the onset of a myocardial infarction. Elevations of CK-MB and troponin are found in a myocardial infarction, but usually are not detectable until at least 4 hours after the onset of the event. Chest radiography and CT scan are not useful for the detection of myocardial infarction.

4. (D) The use of ACE inhibitors, such as captopril, is contraindicated in patients with renal artery stenosis, because it can cause renal insufficiency. The other agents listed are safe for use in patients with renal artery stenosis, as long as other complicating factors are not present.

5. (A) This patient has left-sided congestive heart failure, which can be treated with all the agents listed except for verapamil. Calcium channel blockers are contraindicated in congestive heart failure because they have negative inotropic effects that may impair cardiac function.

6. (C) Of the medications listed, only hydrochlorothiazide has been shown to increase patients' LDL levels. Other medications that can increase LDL levels include progestins, estrogens, glucocorticoids, β-adrenergic antagonists, and alcohol.

7. (B) The treatment regimen of choice for acute bacterial endocarditis is nafcillin with gentamycin. Vancomycin with gentamycin can alternatively be used in areas with a high prevalence of methicillin-resistant *Staphylococcus aureus* (MRSA). Penicillin, ampicillin, and rifampin are used in the treatment of other forms of endocarditis. Amoxicillin can be used for endocarditis prophylaxis in patients with prosthetic valves or pre-existing valvular disease.

8. (D) The tracing shows a prominent Q wave and an inverted T wave, which can be found in old myocardial infarctions. Angina might present with ST segment depression. Prinzmetal's angina and acute myocardial infarction will have ST segment elevation. Left bundle branch blocks show notched QRS complexes.

9. (A) Hypovolemia, metabolic acidosis, and electrolyte abnormalities are postoperative complications that can occur following cross-clamping of the aorta. Withdrawal of hormones and bowel strangulation are complications of adrenal tumor removal and hernia, respectively. Postoperative infection and atelectasis usually do not become symptomatic until 1 to 2 days following surgery.

10. (C) The findings here are most consistent with restrictive cardiomyopathy, since they incorporate right-sided heart failure, a powerful point of maximal impulse (PMI), and low-voltage QRS complexes. Hypertrophic and dilated cardiomyopathy usually present with symptoms more consistent with left-sided heart failure (although dilated cardiomyopathy can cause both right- and left-sided heart failure). Constrictive pericarditis presents with symptoms very similar to this case, but the PMI is not palpable. Pericardial tamponade presents with right-sided heart failure, distant heart sounds, and hypotension.

EMERGENCY MEDICINE TOPICS

11. (C) Because this is a superficial burn (not involving the dermis) but is severe enough to cause blisters, the patient has a second-degree burn. Second-degree burns heal without grafting over several weeks. First-degree burns resolve after several days, and third-degree burns do not heal without skin grafting.

12. (B) This patient appears to have carbon monoxide poisoning, as indicated by his history of inhalation injury and cherry red skin and blood. The standard of care for the treatment of carbon monoxide poisoning involves the use of 100% (hyperbaric) humidified oxygen. Some of the other interventions may be necessary in this patient, but they do not directly and immediately address the issues this patient is having with carbon monoxide toxicity.

13. (A) With a history of trauma and physical examination findings consistent with a splenic injury, it is likely that the patient's symptoms of pallor and cool, clammy hands are due to a ruptured spleen.

14. (A) The patient's history is consistent with a cardiogenic shock immediately following a myocardial infarction. Unlike in other forms of shock, volume resuscitation is not always beneficial in cardiogenic shock. Owing to their cardiac insufficiency, patients can develop pulmonary edema if excessive fluids are administered, which may worsen their clinical outcome. The most satisfactory treatment for cardiogenic shock often involves surgery, which can include coronary revascularization, intra-aortic balloon pump placement, or corrective surgery for valvular abnormalities.

15. (B) Nausea, vomiting, delayed jaundice, and hepatic failure within 96 hours are signs of acetaminophen poisoning. N-acetylcysteine is the appropriate antidote.

16. (E) Mania, delirium, dry mouth and eyes, and tachycardia are signs of anticholinergic toxicity. Physostigmine is the appropriate antidote.

17. (F) Miosis, salivation, urination, bronchospasm, weakness, and confusion are signs of cholinergic toxicity. Pralidoxime chloride is the appropriate antidote.

18. (C) Hematemesis, diarrhea, hypotension, and hepatic failure are signs of iron toxicity overdose. Iron pills are visible on abdominal radiographs, which may provide additional evidence for the cause. Deferoxamine is the appropriate antidote.

19. (A) Hypotension and dizziness in a patient who has a history of hypertension is consistent with toxicity related to either beta-blocker or calcium channel blocker ingestion. The appropriate antidote for beta-blocker overdose is glucagon, which is not offered as a choice here. The appropriate antidote for calcium channel blocker overdose is calcium chloride.

20. (D) A history of bruising and bleeding is consistent with warfarin (Coumadin) overdose, especially in a patient who is most likely taking warfarin for anticoagulation (which might be found with chronic atrial fibrillation). Vitamin K is the appropriate antidote.

ENDOCRINOLOGY

21. (B) The symptoms of short stature, abdominal adiposity, and decreased exercise tolerance in a child are most consistent with growth hormone deficiency. Prolactin deficiency would not cause symptoms in a child. GnRH deficiency causes delayed puberty in a child, which is not noticeable by 10 years of age. The weakness and weight problems are consistent with hypothyroidism, but the weight gain is diffuse (rather than a disproportionate distribution of fat in the abdomen) and symptoms of nonpitting edema, and cold intolerance are also present. Adrenal insufficiency causes weakness but is more commonly associated with weight loss than weight gain.

22. (A) Bromocriptine or cabergoline are the medical treatments of choice for hyperprolactinemia. An alternative approach in this case would be to try to change the patient's antipsychotic regimen, but that choice is not given here. The other measures suggested in this question would not affect the secretion of prolactin by the pituitary.

23. (A) Levothyroxine is the treatment of choice for Hashimoto's thyroiditis. Total thyroidectomy is the treatment for thyroid cancer. Thyroid lobectomy is a common treatment for toxic adenoma of the thyroid. Aspirin therapy is useful in patients with subacute thyroiditis.

24. (C) The presentation of radiation exposure and a nontender, firm thyroid mass is consistent with malignancy. Of the types of thyroid cancer, papillary thyroid cancer is both the most common type and the type most frequently associated with radiation exposure. Toxic multinodular goiter and toxic adenoma would cause symptoms of hyperthyroidism. Hashimoto's thyroiditis is more likely to be associated with a tender neck mass than a firm, nontender one.

25. (A) Of the therapeutic options listed, surgery has been shown to allow the most complete resolution of exophthalmos in Graves' disease.

26. (D) The most appropriate surgical intervention for a toxic adenoma is thyroid lobectomy. Subtotal thyroidectomy is the surgical technique indicated for toxic multinodular goiter. Prior to either type of surgery, antithyroid drugs (propylthiouracil or methimazole) and iodine should be administered to return the body to a euthyroid state. Aspirin and prednisone have no role in the treatment of a toxic adenoma.

27. (A) This patient has primary hypoparathyroidism, most likely due to infarction of the parathyroid glands following thyroidectomy. The electrolyte abnormalities found in hypoparathyroidism include low serum calcium, high serum phosphorus, and low serum parathyroid hormone.

28. (D) The most effective therapy for secondary hyperparathyroidism is renal transplantation, since it restores normal kidney function and restores normal intestinal calcium reabsorption. In patients too sick or unable to receive a transplant, dietary management with a low-phosphorus, high-calcium diet is effective in managing secondary hyperparathyroidism.

29. (E) Adrenal adenomas are surgically removed, but removal of aldosterone-secreting tumors is preceded by treatment with spironolactone to suppress aldosterone secretion. The other agents described are useful for controlling hypertension, but they do not affect the circulating levels of aldosterone. Failure to suppress aldosterone secretion presurgically in primary hyperaldosteronism (aldosteronism) can result in an inability of the body to respond to circulating aldosterone following surgery owing to the dramatic and sudden decrease in circulating aldosterone levels.

30. (A) Although the patient's family history of autoimmune disease makes Addison's disease a strong possibility here, treatment with ketoconazole also can produce primary adrenal insufficiency. Other medications that can cause primary adrenal insufficiency include metyrapone, aminoglutethimide, trilostane, and RU486.

GASTROENTEROLOGY

31. (A) This patient's symptoms of postemetic pain, minimal hematemesis, decreased breath sounds (due to left pneumothorax), and mediastinal crunch (Hamman's sign) are most consistent with a diagnosis of Boerhaave's syndrome. In cases of Boerhaave's syndrome, the best management includes surgical repair of the tear, drainage of the mediastinum, and antibiotic therapy. In contrast, a Mallory-Weiss tear is managed by localized stoppage of the bleeding by means of cautery or sclerosing agents during endoscopy. Pneumatic dilation and section of the cricopharyngeus muscle are treatments for achalasia and Zenker's diverticulum, respectively.

32. (B) This patient's symptoms of chest pain, exacerbation of asthma, and an acid taste in the mouth are most consistent with a diagnosis of gastroesophageal reflux disease (GERD). Of the treatments offered, the best choice is omeprazole (a proton pump inhibitor) for pharmacologic therapy. Cimetidine (an H_2 blocker) has numerous drug interactions, which make it less ideal for use. Aluminum hydroxide produces some symptomatic relief but is less effective than omeprazole. Surgery is an option for the treatment for GERD, but the techniques offered in the question are not indicated for this disease. Pneumatic dilation is performed in achalasia, while the Graham patch procedure is used in peptic ulcer disease.

33. (A) This patient's symptoms of epigastric pain that is worsened by eating and relieved by antacids is most consistent with a gastric peptic ulcer. If the history had featured pain that was relieved by eating and antacids, then it would have been more consistent with a duodenal peptic ulcer. Most cases of either type of ulcer are associated with *Helicobacter pylori* infection, and treatment of this organism should be included in the initial therapy. For gastric peptic ulcers, the therapy of choice includes treatment with clarithromycin, omeprazole, and metronidazole. Sucralfate is more useful in cases of duodenal peptic ulcers. Nissen fundoplication is a surgical intervention for GERD, not peptic ulcer disease. Tetracycline is not a component of any regimen used against *Helicobacter pylori* infection.

34. (E) The patient's presentation of sharp epigastric abdominal pain radiating to the back, steatorrhea, a history of alcoholism, and ecchymoses in the flank and periumbilical areas are most consistent with acute hemorrhagic pancreatitis. According to Ranson's criteria, the prognosis of pancreatitis can be predicted on the basis of a variety of factors that might be present at admission to the hospital or within 48 hours of admission. Of the possibilities here, the blood glucose level, lactate dehydrogenase level, and white blood cell count all exceed the values set forth in Ranson's criteria, which indicates a worse prognosis. The criteria state that a drop of 10% in the hematocrit in the first 48 hours is unfavorable prognostically, but the single measurement given in this question is insufficient to evaluate the prognosis. The patient's age (<55) is the only factor here that is prognostically favorable.

35. (D) The patient's symptoms of periumbilical pain that migrates to the right lower quadrant, onset of abdominal pain before the onset of nausea and vomiting, peritoneal signs (including psoas sign), and fever are most consistent with acute appendicitis. The most effective therapy for a nonperforated acute appendicitis is surgical removal of the appendix followed by a single day of antibiotic therapy. If evidence of appendiceal perforation is seen in the operating room, then the duration of antibiotic therapy is extended to a 5- to 7-day course. Aggressive intravenous rehydration, cessation of oral feedings, and observation are acceptable treatment for acute pancreatitis. Débridement with drain and jejunostomy tube placement is a possible treatment for mesenteric ischemia. Pharmacologic therapy with clarithromycin, omeprazole, and metronidazole is an acceptable treatment for peptic ulcer disease.

36. (D) The patient's symptoms of nausea, vomiting, and colicky abdominal pain that is relieved by vomiting (as well as the history of abdominal surgery) are most consistent with small bowel obstruction due to adhesions. Protracted vomiting leads to the development of a hypochloremic, hypokalemic metabolic alkalosis due to the loss of HCl^- in the emesis fluid.

37. (D) The patient's symptoms and signs of hematemesis, melena, hypovolemia, and portal hypertension are most consistent with bleeding esophageal varices. In a patient with portal hypertension and esophageal varices, rupture of the varices can be prevented by lowering the blood pressure with beta-blockers (such as metoprolol). A protein-rich diet, omeprazole, cimetidine, and metoclopramide do not affect the blood pressure enough to have an effect on the development of variceal rupture.

38. (B) On the basis of the patient's history of alcoholism and the liver function test results (AST and ALT are both <500, but the AST/ALT ratio is >2), this patient most likely has alcoholic hepatitis. The most effective management of alcoholic hepatitis is corticosteroid therapy with drinking cessation. Interferon alpha therapy is used for chronic viral hepatitis. Liver transplantation is typically reserved for more severe liver disease. N-acetylcysteine is an antidote for drug-induced hepatitis due to acetaminophen poisoning. Azathioprine is an immunosuppressive agent used in the treatment of autoimmune hepatitis.

39. (C) This patient has symptoms consistent with hepatic encephalopathy, which is caused by ammonia toxicity in the brain. The treatment of choice to lower ammonia levels in patients with chronic liver disease includes dietary restriction of protein and the use of lactulose and neomycin (which will kill ammonia-producing organisms in the intestine). Levodopa is a synthetic form of dopamine that is used in Parkinson's disease. Bromocriptine is an ergot alkaloid that can be used in hyperpituitarism. Acetaminophen is an anti-inflammatory that can cause liver damage when taken in high doses. Sucralfate is used in the treatment of duodenal ulcers.

40. (A) The presentation of fever, right upper quadrant pain, Murphy's sign, nausea, and vomiting is most consistent with acute cholecystitis. Cholelithiasis or choledocholithiasis may also be present in this patient, but they would be insufficient to cause her current symptoms. A Klatskin tumor would present with painless obstructive jaundice. Chronic cholecystitis would have a longer duration of symptoms, and the symptoms would be less severe.

HEMATOLOGY

41. (B) Given the patient's lack of other pertinent medical history, lack of medication or supplement use, and recent onset of anemic symptoms coincident with a heavy menstruation, this patient is most likely suffering from iron deficiency anemia. Thalassemia, sideroblastic anemia, autoimmune hemolytic anemia, and microangiopathic hemolytic anemia are much rarer causes of anemia and much less likely to present in this fashion in an otherwise healthy young female.

42. (C) This patient is receiving both heparin and warfarin at the moment. Heparin enhances antithrombin III, which neutralizes most of the coagulation factors except for fibrinogen, factor V, and factor VIII. Warfarin inhibits activation of the vitamin-dependent coagulation factors (II, VII, IX, and X). Both the PT and PTT are prolonged with either drug; however, the PT is primarily used to follow warfarin therapy and the PTT for following heparin therapy.

43. (C) This patient's symptoms of mild thrombocytopenia (50,000–100,000 μL) and thrombotic complications while on warfarin and heparin are most consistent with heparin-induced thrombocytopenia (HIT). In cases of HIT, it is important to discontinue the heparin and any warfarin that the patient may be receiving. The heparin contributes to the HIT, and patients with HIT who receive warfarin are at risk for the development of catastrophic limb thrombosis. Lepirudin (a synthetic version of a substance produced by leeches) is the best alternative anticoagulant for use in these patients because it directly inhibits thrombin and does not cause HIT.

44. (E) Coagulation factor inhibitors prolong the PTT (or PT) and do not correct to normal after normal plasma is mixed with the patient's plasma in a test tube. This occurs because inhibitors are antibodies that bind vital components for clotting in both the patient's plasma as well as the normal plasma.

45. (D) In hemophilia A, the patient has a prolonged PTT that corrects with mixing of patient plasma with normal plasma in a test tube. This occurs because the deficient clotting factor in the patient's sample is present in the normal plasma.

46. (C) Disseminated intravascular coagulation is usually associated with trauma, malignancy, or obstetric complications (e.g., amniotic fluid embolism). PT, fibrin degradation products, and D-dimer are increased.

47. (B) Vitamin K deficiency may develop owing to warfarin therapy, fat malabsorption, or antibiotic therapy.

48. (A) In von Willebrand's disease, the PT is normal, the PTT is prolonged, the bleeding time is prolonged, and factor VIII activity is decreased. In addition, the von Willebrand factor antigen levels are decreased, and the ristocetin cofactor assay measurements are decreased.

49. (A) The high hematocrit in the presence of recurrent thrombotic disease (a myocardial infarction a year ago and a transient ischemic attack currently) is most suggestive of polycythemia vera. Essential thrombocytosis presents in a similar fashion, but the platelet level is much higher (>600,000). The patient's heart rate is too low for atrial fibrillation (which causes embolism rather than thrombosis), and an irregular rhythm is not mentioned. Myelofibrosis causes anemia, which is not present in this case. Leukostasis shows exceptionally high WBC counts.

50. (C) This patient's anemia, proteinuria, constipation, and bone pain are most consistent with a diagnosis of multiple myeloma. In addition, the presence of a high total serum protein and a low serum albumin (which should account for the majority of serum protein) indicates that there is a significant amount of abnormal circulating protein, which would also be present in multiple myeloma. Monoclonal gammopathy of undetermined significance and Waldenström's macroglobulinemia can also produce large amounts of circulating immunoglobulins, but they do not involve the bones or kidneys. Myelofibrosis would not produce proteinuria. Amyloidosis does not produce lesions in the bone but can cause proteinuria.

INFECTIOUS DISEASES

51. (C) This patient has streptococcal pharyngitis with scarlet fever (the cause of the sandpapery rash). In patients with streptococcal pharyngitis, common complications include abscesses, glomerulonephritis, and rheumatic heart disease. Antibiotic therapy prevents the progression to abscesses or the development of rheumatic heart disease, but it does not prevent the development of glomerulonephritis. Toxic epidermal necrolysis and staphylococcal scalded skin syndrome are not associated with streptococcal pharyngitis. Colitis is not a complication of scarlet fever.

52. (B) This patient has infectious mononucleosis, which is frequently misdiagnosed as streptococcal pharyngitis. Patients with infectious mononucleosis who receive ampicillin or penicillin therapy can develop a rash that is often confused with an allergic reaction. Amoxicillin, clavulanic acid, doxycycline, and tetracycline do not cause this type of reaction.

53. (A) This patient has epiglottitis, which is a medical emergency owing to the possibility of airway closure. The treatment of choice in epiglottitis involves emergent intubation of the child and empiric therapy with intravenous cefuroxime. Penicillin is the treatment of choice if this patient has streptococcal pharyngitis. Ribavirin is the treatment of choice if this patient has respiratory syncytial virus (RSV).

54. (A) This patient has a positive PPD with an otherwise negative workup for tuberculosis. In many countries where tuberculosis is common (such as China), people receive the BCG vaccination, which causes the patient to seroconvert to a positive PPD status. In these cases, it is necessary to determine the likelihood that the patient actually has tuberculosis before starting potentially toxic, long-term isoniazid therapy based solely on the PPD results. In cases where antituberculosis therapy is indicated in a PPD-positive patient without clinical disease, the most appropriate therapy is isoniazid and vitamin B_6 for a period of 9 months. Cases of active TB require combination therapy with pyrazinamide, isoniazid, rifampin, and ethambutol. Bronchial washings can be used to assess TB status in patients who are unable to produce adequate sputum samples.

55. (D) Determination that a child is HIV-negative requires consistent negative tests for the first 2 years of life. The preferred test for the first 18 months of life is the polymerase chain reaction (PCR) test, which detects conserved DNA sequences in the viral genome. After 18 months of age, the ELISA is the preferred screening test.

56. (A) Patients with CD4 counts less than 100 cells/mm^3 require prophylactic therapy that covers both *Pneumocystis carinii* and toxoplasmosis. Trimethoprim-sulfamethoxazole provides coverage against both of these organisms. Clarithromycin is indicated in patients with a CD4 count of less than 75 cells/mm^3 to provide coverage against *Mycobacterium avium-intracellulare,* and isoniazid is required in patients with positive PPD tests or for whom a high suspicion for TB exists but the patient is too immunosuppressed to have a positive PPD test.

57. (B) Pregnant patients who have had more than one outbreak of genital herpes during pregnancy or who have had an outbreak during the last 4–6 weeks should be given acyclovir at 36 weeks. Active lesions at the time of labor are indications for cesarean section, but delivery by NSVD can be performed if no herpetic lesions are noted in the birth canal at the time of delivery.

58. (C) This patient has symptoms of pelvic inflammatory disease and Gram's stain of the cervical exudate shows organisms consistent with *Neisseria gonorrhoeae.* Gonorrhea is effectively treated with ceftriaxone. In addition, she should be treated with azithromycin for a possible coexisting chlamydial infection. Chlamydia is very common and is clinically more silent than gonorrhea, and patients are frequently infected with both organisms. Metronidazole is a treatment for bacterial vaginosis, and antifungal cream is a treatment for candidiasis.

59. (A) This patient's history of tick bite, erythema migrans, and subsequent development of arthritis in the large joints is most consistent with a diagnosis of Lyme disease, which is caused by infection with *Borrelia burgdorferi.* The treatment of choice for Lyme disease in patients over 8 years old is doxycycline. Amoxicillin is the treatment of choice for patients who are under 8 years old because doxycycline can cause discoloration of the teeth in this age group. Chloramphenicol is a treatment of choice for Rocky Mountain spotted fever (doxycycline is an alternative treatment of choice). Penicillamine is a treatment for some rheumatologic causes of arthritis.

60. (A) The patient's history of cellulitis with an ill-defined bluish discoloration of the skin and systemic signs is most consistent with necrotizing fasciitis. Clostridial myonecrosis usually presents in a similar fashion but is more frequently associated with a bronze discoloration of the skin. Toxic epidermal necrolysis and Stevens-Johnson syndrome are associated with allergic reactions rather than cellulitic infections. Staphylococcal scalded skin syndrome is associated with infection and desquamation, but the blue discoloration of the skin is not present.

NEPHROLOGY

61. (A) This patient has nephrotic syndrome, most likely due to membranous glomerulonephropathy associated with chronic NSAID use. The principal abnormalities present in nephrotic syndrome include proteinuria, edema, and hypercholesterolemia and fatty casts in the urine. The patient has no symptoms of electrolyte abnormality (confusion, muscle pain, arrhythmia, constipation, etc.), and the lack of glucose in the urine makes hyperglycemia a less likely option.

62. (B) This patient's history of recent muscle trauma associated with a 4+ blood reading on dipstick testing in the absence of RBCs on microscopic examination is most consistent with rhabdomyolysis. His history does not mention hypotension or other symptoms of hypovolemia, and the absence of RBCs in the urine makes traumatic kidney injury an unlikely cause of his condition. The lack of RBCs on microscopic examination also excludes nephritic syndrome as a cause of his renal failure.

63. (A) This patient's acute renal failure is due to intrinsic renal disease resulting from high levels of myoglobin. The most appropriate treatment is to remove the myoglobin from the blood by means of hemodialysis. The patient's renal disease is less likely to be due to hypovolemia, direct kidney injury, or nephritic syndrome, so blood transfusion, removal of the kidney, immunosuppression, and plasmapheresis are unlikely to be effective.

64. (A) In respiratory acidosis, the patient has a pH of less than 7.35 with a pCO_2 of greater than 45. In acute respiratory acidosis, the expected compensation would involve an increase of 1 mEq/L of HCO_3 (over the normal value of 24) for every 10 mm Hg CO_2 above 40 measured. In this case, the pCO_2 is 50, so the expected increase in bicarbonate in an acute respiratory acidosis is 1 mEq/L. Since the patient's bicarbonate matches this expectation (24 + 1 = 25 mEq/L), this situation is an acute respiratory acidosis.

65. (B) In respiratory acidosis, the patient has a pH of less than 7.35 with a pCO_2 of greater than 45. In chronic respiratory acidosis, the expected compensation involves an increase of 3.5 mEq/L of HCO_3 for every 10 mm Hg CO_2 above 40 measured. In this case, the pCO_2 is 60 mm Hg. In this patient, the measured bicarbonate is 31, which is consistent with the expected compensation for chronic respiratory acidosis (24 + 7 = 31 mEq/L). If the patient were in acute respiratory acidosis, the expected HCO_3 would be 26 mEq/L.

66. (E) In metabolic acidosis, the patient has a pH of less than 7.35 with an HCO_3 of less than 22. Compensation for metabolic acid-base disturbances occurs through ventilatory changes, as indicated by the pCO_2 of 30 in the ABG. You can estimate the pCO_2 expected in compensation for a metabolic acid-base change by using the last 2 digits of the pH measurement. In this case, the patient has a pH of 7.30 with a pCO_2 of 30. These values match the expectations for a metabolic acidosis with respiratory compensation.

67. (C) This patient has hyponatremia, which is most likely due to syndrome of inappropriate antidiuretic hormone secretion (SIADH), as indicated by the euvolemia, hypotonicity of the blood, and hypertonicity of the urine described in the history. SIADH has a variety of causes, but the medications that are most frequently associated with it include antipsychotics, antidepressants, and thiazides.

68. (A) This patient's presentation of hypernatremia with hypertonic serum and hypotonic urine is most consistent with diabetes insipidus. In this patient, the history of cranial surgery in the absence of any prior renal problems makes neurogenic diabetes a more likely cause of the symptoms than nephrogenic diabetes insipidus. The treatment of choice in neurogenic diabetes insipidus is desmopressin (DDAVP). The hypernatremia should be gradually corrected (at a rate no greater than 0.5 mEq/L/hr) to prevent development of central pontine myelinolysis. Sodium restriction and hydrochlorothiazide are treatments for nephrogenic diabetes insipidus. Hemodialysis, calcium gluconate, insulin, and bicarbonate all are treatments for hyperkalemia.

69. (B) This patient has both hypokalemia and hypomagnesemia, which most likely were produced by potassium and magnesium loss in her diarrhea. In cases such as this, it is most appropriate to correct the hypomagnesemia before the hypokalemia, because the correction of the magnesium levels will cause a transcellular shift of potassium and increase the serum potassium levels. If both magnesium and potassium supplementation are attempted simultaneously as the initial therapy, the patient may become hyperkalemic. If the magnesium is corrected and the potassium remains low, then potassium supplementation can be used to treat the hypokalemia.

70. (B) This patient has a presentation most consistent with hyperkalemia, which can cause weakness, small bowel ulcers, and characteristic ECG changes (such as peaked T waves and an increased PR interval). While the other electrolyte abnormalities can produce a variety of generalized symptoms and ECG changes, the peaked T waves are specific for hyperkalemia. Beta-blockers can inhibit potassium entry into cells, which can produce hyperkalemia. Insensitivity to insulin in diabetes (or the lack of insulin in type 1 diabetes) will cause a deficiency in insulin-mediated transport of potassium into cells, so hyperkalemia can develop in diabetes as well.

NEUROLOGY

71. (E) The patient's acute onset of unilateral paralysis and sensory loss of the leg with sparing of the upper extremity and face is most consistent with a stroke involving the anterior cerebral artery on the left side. The patient does not show any signs of increased intracranial pressure (such as headache, lethargy, or papilledema), so the stroke is more likely to be ischemic than hemorrhagic. This patient is mildly hypertensive, but the ischemic nature of the stroke indicates that the blood supply to the brain has been impaired. Given her history of chronic hypertension, lowering the blood pressure at this point may further impair cerebral blood flow and cause additional infarction. This is a more dangerous possibility than allowing her hypertension to continue for a few more days, so it is best not to additionally treat the patient's hypertension for several days following her stroke.

72. (B) The patient's symptoms of hemiparesis and sensory loss involving the face and arm with relative sparing of the leg is most consistent with a stroke involving the middle cerebral artery. The patient does not show any signs of increased intracranial pressure (such as headache, lethargy, or papilledema), so the stroke is more likely to be ischemic than hemorrhagic. A stroke involving the anterior cerebral artery causes unilateral paralysis and sensory loss of the leg with sparing of the upper extremity and face. A stroke of the posterior cerebral artery is associated with homonymous hemianopsia.

73. (B) The patient's symptoms of a loss of consciousness, dream-like state, and repetitive movements (automatisms) without convulsions or postictal confusion is most consistent with a complex partial seizure. A simple partial seizure does not produce a loss of consciousness. A tonic-clonic generalized seizure is associated with convulsions and postictal confusion. A febrile seizure occurs in association with a fever. A myoclonic seizure produces myoclonic jerking of the limbs and should have presented at a much earlier age.

74. (B) The patient's history of confusion and focal neurologic deficit that developed slowly following an injury is most consistent with a subdural hematoma. All the other options would present more acutely, with a quicker progression of symptoms following the injury. In addition, the patient's age predisposes him to subdural hematoma because the bridging veins in the subdural area grow more fragile with increasing age.

75. (C) This patient's symptoms of tremor, bradykinesia, and akinesia are consistent with parkinsonism. Parkinsonism is often caused by Parkinson's disease, but can also be caused by a variety of toxic exposures, such as MPTP. In addition, survivors of carbon monoxide poisoning can develop persistent neurologic deficits that cause parkinsonism. Of the options listed (cyanide, tetrodotoxin, carbon monoxide, botulinum toxin, and mercury), carbon monoxide is the only agent that is capable of causing parkinsonism.

76. (B) The patient's age and symptoms of mood disorder with involuntary limb movements are highly suspicious for Huntington's disease. In addition, his father's history of suicide raises the question of undiagnosed Huntington's disease. The treatment for Huntington's disease is symptomatic. The patient's movement symptoms could best be managed using haloperidol. Fluoxetine could help the patient's mood symptoms but would not improve his movement symptoms. Metoprolol has no usefulness in this case. Levodopa and amantadine could actually worsen the patient's movement disorder owing to their ability to increase dopamine availability.

77. (C) The patient's symptoms of weakness, fatigability, and dysphagia, in the presence of both upper and lower motor neuron signs, are consistent with a diagnosis of amyotrophic lateral sclerosis (ALS). In patients with ALS, only symptomatic management is available. The preferred agent for the treatment of spasticity is baclofen. Levodopa and amantadine are useful in the treatment of Parkinson's disease. Ibuprofen and metoprolol have no effect on spasticity.

78. (A) The patient has symptoms of multiple neurologic deficits that are separated in time and space, which is a classic presentation of multiple sclerosis (MS). In addition, her current symptoms of optic neuritis and her prior history of trigeminal neuralgia are both common in MS patients. Of the options listed (oligoclonal IgG bands, prion proteins, leukocytosis, tau protein, and gram-negative diplococci), the only one that is associated with multiple sclerosis is the presence of oligoclonal IgG bands in the cerebrospinal fluid. Meningococci and leukocytes are present in the CSF of patients with bacterial meningitis. Circulating prion proteins may be present in patients with diseases caused by prions, such as Creutzfeldt-Jakob disease.

79. (A) The patient's symptoms of radicular pain, weakness, and hyporeflexia in the distribution of a single spinal nerve root (C5) are most consistent with impingement of a spinal nerve root. The patient's recent history of trauma, combined with the placement of the injury, make a herniated disk the most likely cause of the compression. Demyelination in the spinal cord would interrupt tracts and cause deficits below the level of injury. Demyelination or dysmyelination of the peripheral nerve causes similar symptoms to those seen in this patient but would tend to be spread throughout multiple peripheral nerves and would not be reproducible by moving the patient's neck. Degeneration of neurons in the anterior horn would not cause sensory deficits.

80. (D) The patient's symptoms of ptosis, fatigability, and weakness in the absence of sensory abnormalities are consistent with a diagnosis of a myasthenic syndrome. The distinction between myasthenia gravis (MG) and Lambert-Eaton myasthenic syndrome (LEMS) depends on the presence of autoantibodies (against the acetylcholine receptor in MG and against a calcium channel in LEMS) and their behavior in response to repetitive stimulation. Repetitive stimulation causes a decrease in muscle responsiveness in MG, which is seen in this case. This is due to a decreasing number of available acetylcholine receptors with each stimulus. MG is associated with thymomas but not with small cell lung carcinoma, colon carcinoma, papillary thyroid carcinoma, or hepatocellular carcinoma.

OBSTETRICS AND GYNECOLOGY

81. (E) This patient has Rh group incompatibility and is currently in her first pregnancy. She has not been exposed to the Rh antigen, so she should not be producing IgG antibodies that bind to the fetal red blood cells during the current pregnancy. The rosette test is positive because it detects extremely low numbers of fetal RBCs in the maternal circulation, but the Kleihauer-Betke test is necessary to quantitate them. On the Kleihauer-Betke test, 20 μg/mL is the threshold for giving Rh_o(D) immunoglobulin, since lower concentrations are not sufficient to promote an immune response.

82. (E) The patient's symptoms of amenorrhea, mood swings, sleep disturbances, and infertility, combined with her response to a progestin challenge test, are consistent with an endocrine cause for her amenorrhea. Amenorrhea caused by endometriosis, adhesions, ovulatory failure, or abnormal cervical mucus would not have responded to a progestin challenge test.

83. (E) Identification of atypical cells on the patient's Pap smear is an indication for a more thorough evaluation of the patient. A cone biopsy of the cervix would be sufficient to evaluate the cervix for possible neoplasia and to characterize the extent of localized lesions.

84. (C) The patient's fibroids are not a particular concern unless the pregnancy is at risk. Most treatment options present a risk to the pregnancy, so the preferred treatment is to remove the fibroids at the time of delivery. In addition, the fibroids can grow during pregnancy and can complicate a vaginal delivery; therefore, the existence of fibroids is an indication for cesarean section. Mifepristone is the generic name for RU-486, which is contraindicated in pregnancy.

85. (A) This patient's development of hypertension, edema, and proteinuria in the third trimester of pregnancy is sufficient for a diagnosis of preeclampsia. Her blood pressure measurement is within the range of mild preeclampsia, which can be treated with $MgSO_4$ (for seizure prophylaxis) and hydralazine (for the hypertension). $ZnSO_4$ does not provide seizure prophylaxis and is not used in preeclampsia. Metoprolol is not used for management of hypertension in pregnancy, because the effects of hydralazine have been much more completely studied. Immediate delivery of the fetus is indicated only in cases where fetal lung maturity is demonstrated and/or when the immediate safety of the mother or the baby is at risk.

86. (C) The patient's hypertension prior to pregnancy is consistent with a diagnosis of chronic hypertension. During pregnancy, it is safer use a medication that has been extensively studied in pregnancy, such as hydralazine, than to continue metoprolol or change to captopril. The presence of hypertension during the physical examination dictates the necessity of treating her with something, since hypertension can cause prematurity, uteroplacental insufficiency, and oligohydramnios.

87. (D) The patient's presentation and ultrasound results are diagnostic for placenta previa. So long as the fetus and mother are not in danger from the extent of blood loss, patients with placenta previa are managed with observation. In some cases, the placental site shifts in the final weeks of pregnancy, and placenta previa is not present at delivery. These cases are delivered by vaginally (NSVD). Cases in which placenta previa still exists at delivery are indications for cesarean section. Blood transfusion and delivery of the fetus are possible therapies for patients who are hemodynamically unstable. Surgical ablation of the placenta is never performed.

88. (E) The patient's history of abdominal trauma, vaginal bleeding, and pelvic pain and the presence of fetal distress and hemodynamic instability are highly suggestive of placental abruption. The advanced stage of the pregnancy makes it likely that the fetal lungs are capable of producing surfactant, which means that betamethasone is not required. In this case, the fetus can be delivered immediately by cesarean section, with additional operative management of any other bleeding sources. Abruption is a contraindication for vaginal delivery.

89. (C) This patient's history of hirsutism, virilism, obesity, and enlargement of the ovaries is consistent with polycystic ovary syndrome. Adult polycystic kidney disease, serous cystadenoma of the ovary, and acromegaly would not produce virilization. 21α-Hydroxylase deficiency (a cause of salt-wasting congenital adrenal hyperplasia) can produce virilization, but it would present in infancy.

90. (B) The patient's symptoms of headache, vomiting, hypertension, uterine contractions, and grapelike clusters extending into the vagina are indicative of molar pregnancy. This is further confirmed by the snowstorm appearance of the ultrasound, which is a classic finding in molar pregnancy. This combination of symptoms, particularly the grapelike clusters in the vagina and the ultrasound findings, are so classic for this entity that they exclude choriocarcinoma and placental site trophoblastic tumor. Mayer-Rokitansky-Küster-Hauser (MRKH) syndrome is a müllerian dysgenesis in which the vagina is present only as a rudimentary pouch. Uterine inversion occurs when the uterus is turned "inside out" following delivery of the placenta and has no role in this case.

ONCOLOGY

91. (A) The patient's symptoms of weight loss, dysphagia, dull abdominal pain, and melena are consistent with a diagnosis of gastric carcinoma located in the proximal stomach. The diagnosis and location are confirmed by upper endoscopy. There is nothing in the patient's history or physical examination that indicates metastasis. The surgical treatment of choice for gastric carcinoma in the proximal stomach is total radical gastrectomy. A radical distal gastrectomy is used for a tumor of the distal stomach. A Whipple procedure (pancreaticoduodenectomy) is used for resection for tumors of the head of the pancreas. An Ivor-Lewis procedure is used for resection of esophageal masses.

92. (C) This patient's symptoms of increasing insulin resistance, weight loss, and abdominal pain suggest that she may have some sort of endocrine neoplasm involving the pancreas. The skin findings are indicative of necrotizing migratory erythema, which is a distinctive presentation associated with glucagonoma. These skin findings are not present in an insulinoma, a somatostatinoma, or a nonendocrine pancreatic neoplasm (mucinous cystic neoplasm or intraductal papillary mucinous tumor).

93. (E) This patient's diagnosis of colonic adenocarcinoma is established in the vignette. For preoperative staging of colonic tumors, endorectal ultrasonography is the preferred technique. A chest radiograph is useful for evaluating metastatic disease to the lungs but is not involved in staging the actual tumor. Barium enemas with radiography are useful in the detection of diverticula but are not the best modality for evaluating tumors. CT scan of the bowel with contrast is useful in tumor staging but is not as sensitive as an endorectal ultrasound. Serum CEA levels are not an effective tumor staging tool but are be useful following treatment in assessing the likelihood of tumor recurrence.

94. (D) The patient's diagnosis of small cell lung carcinoma is established in the vignette. The current symptoms of facial edema, distention of the neck veins, and bilateral pleural effusions are most likely to be caused by compression of the superior vena cava (SVC syndrome), which results in deficient venous return to the heart from the head and upper limbs. Involvement of the SVC renders the tumor inoperable; therefore, surgery is not a realistic treatment option. Intracavitary chemotherapy is useful in other, more anatomically restricted tumors (such as esophageal cancer) but is not useful in this case. Unfortunately, the only useful treatment for this patient is to provide supportive care and provide management of brain metastases in order to preserve the patient's quality of life.

95. (C) The patient's symptoms of a palpable breast mass with a stellate mammographic abnormality are suspicious for breast carcinoma. In this situation, the most appropriate initial operative management is lumpectomy with sentinel lymph node biopsy (biopsy of the first node in the lymphatic drainage chain to evaluate for metastatic spread). Neoadjuvant chemotherapy is not indicated, because it has not been established whether this patient has breast cancer. Total mastectomy with sentinel node biopsy is an excessive procedure for this patient, because the goal is to perform an excisional biopsy and confirm the diagnosis. Similarly, a full axillary node dissection is not performed unless the patient has breast cancer that is demonstrable in the sentinel lymph node.

96. (B) The patient's symptoms of breast tenderness, straw-colored nipple discharge, and symptoms that vary with the stages of the menstrual cycle are consistent with the diagnosis of fibrocystic change. The typical treatment for this disease involves the use of NSAID medications for discomfort and the discontinuation of stimulants (such as caffeine). The cysts can also be drained by fine-needle aspiration.

97. (C) The patient's symptoms of pelvic pain with an enlarged, nodular prostate and a prostate-specific antigen of 11 ng/mL are most consistent with prostate cancer metastatic to bone, which is confirmed by the bone scan. In cases of prostate cancer with metastatic skeletal disease, the most effective therapy involves orchiectomy with antiandrogen therapy owing to the hormone-responsive nature of the tumor. Irradiation alone is used in prostate cancer with local extracapsular spread. Prostatectomy with antiandrogen therapy does not remove the most significant source of endogenous androgens.

98. (C) The presence of aniridia (absence of the iris), abdominal pain, and hematuria, combined with the detection of a solitary solid renal mass on ultrasound in a child, is most consistent with Wilms' tumor. Hydronephrosis causes cystic dilatation of the kidney. Infantile polycystic kidney disease does not appear to be a solitary renal mass. Poststreptococcal glomerulonephritis is not associated with a mass lesion. Renal cell carcinoma produces a solitary renal mass in the kidney but is much less likely than a Wilms' tumor in a patient of this age.

99. (D) This patient's symptoms of weakness, abdominal pain, and weight loss, in association with a history of smoking, hepatitis B infection, chronic alcoholism, and cirrhosis, make hepatocellular carcinoma the most likely cause of the liver mass. Hepatocellular carcinoma increases the serum α-fetoprotein (AFP). Increased carcinoembryonic antigen (CEA) is seen in association with colon adenocarcinoma. Increased amylase is found in association with tumors of the pancreatic head. Increased CA-125 is found in association with surface-derived tumors of the ovary. Increased PTH-related protein is associated with renal cell carcinoma and squamous cell carcinoma of the lung.

100. (D) The development of a solitary liver mass in a young, otherwise healthy woman makes hepatic adenoma the most likely diagnosis. Development of hepatic adenomas has been associated with the use of oral contraceptive pills. Another liver mass that is common in this age group is cavernous hemangioma, but that would appear hypoechoic (rather than solid) on the CT scan. Hepatitis B and schistosomiasis are risk factors for the development of hepatocellular carcinoma. Procainamide is associated with the development of drug-induced lupus erythematosus, which is unrelated to this case.

PEDIATRICS

101. (A) This patient's symptoms of steatorrhea, recurrent respiratory infections, and poor feeding as a child are consistent with cystic fibrosis. Of the tests listed, the most appropriate is a sweat chloride test. The chest radiograph or abdominal CT scan would show nonspecific findings consistent with pulmonary infection. A barium enema is useful for the diagnosis of intussusception but not of cystic fibrosis. A rectal biopsy is useful for the diagnosis of Hirschsprung's disease.

102. (A) The patient's symptoms of abdominal pain, lower gastrointestinal bleeding, and a sausage-shaped mass are most consistent with intussusception. A barium enema provides both diagnostic information and treatment for the problem. Meckel's diverticulum most often presents around 2 years of age (intussusception most often presents between 2 months and 2 years of age) with painless rectal bleeding. Prednisone is not indicated as a therapeutic option. Dietary changes would be sufficient if constipation was the sole complaint. Enzyme replacement is a potential therapy in children with cystic fibrosis.

103. (C) The patient's symptoms are most consistent with a mild allergic reaction to eggs. In patients with a history of egg allergy, the influenza and yellow fever vaccines should be avoided because they contain egg-derived components. The vaccines for mumps, measles, varicella, and tetanus do not contain egg-derived components and should therefore be safe to administer in a patient with egg allergy.

104. (C) The patient's history of fever, swelling, and desquamative skin rash, in combination with Japanese ancestry and a pericardial friction rub, is most consistent with a diagnosis of Kawasaki disease. Kawasaki disease is one of the very few indications for the use of aspirin in children. Another possible therapy for Kawasaki disease is high-dose intravenous gamma globulin. Ibuprofen and acetaminophen are insufficient for treatment. Prednisone is actually contraindicated because it can worsen the aneurysms that can occur in these patients. Liver transplantation is a treatment for Reye's syndrome, which occurs following a viral infection and aspirin ingestion in children.

105. (B) The patient's history of prematurity, vomiting, blood in the stool, fever, and a tender, distended abdomen is highly suggestive of necrotizing enterocolitis. This entity is associated with intrauterine exposure to cocaine. Heroin and marijuana do not produce structural birth defects. Alcohol exposure in utero produces a variety of neurologic, facial, and cardiac abnormalities (fetal alcohol syndrome) but does not cause necrotizing enterocolitis. Thalidomide exposure causes meromelia (partial absence of the limb) but is not a cause of necrotizing enterocolitis.

106. (A) The patient's history of episodic cyanosis that occurs at times of increased activity is consistent with tetralogy of Fallot. The behavior whereby the child squats for a short time to relieve the cyanosis is particularly characteristic of a "tet spell." On a chest radiograph, tetralogy of Fallot shows a boot-shaped heart. An egg-shaped heart is found in patients with transposition of the great arteries. Absence of a thymic shadow is found in DiGeorge syndrome, which can be associated with truncus arteriosus. A small heart with increased pulmonary vascularity is seen in total anomalous pulmonary venous connection. The heart and liver would be on opposite sides of the body in situs inversus.

107. (C) This patient's history as a slightly premature girl who develops mild jaundice several days after birth in a head-to-toe fashion is most likely due to physiologic jaundice. Cases of physiologic jaundice are treated with observation or phototherapy (which works by photoisomerization of bilirubin to more excretable forms). There is no evidence that this patient has an abnormality of iron metabolism. Phenobarbital is not indicated here, but it can be used in jaundice due to Crigler-Najjar syndrome (a disorder of bilirubin metabolism) because it causes hepatic enzyme induction. Plasmapheresis and dialysis are not used to treat neonatal jaundice. If removal of bilirubin is required, an exchange transfusion is performed instead.

108. (A) The child's symptoms of jaundice, poor feeding, and dry mucous membranes are most likely due to "breast milk jaundice," which is caused by dehydration and poor feeding early in life. The other options (immaturity of the neonatal liver, dysfunction of bilirubin metabolism, endocrine dysfunction, and hemolysis) are less likely because of the age of the patient at the time when the jaundice developed and the clear-cut relationship between the jaundice and the period of poor feeding.

109. (C) This patient's history of respiratory distress immediately after birth, in combination with absent breath sounds (but present bowel sounds) over one side of the thorax, is most consistent with congenital diaphragmatic hernia. None of the other listed disorders (duodenal atresia, tracheoesophageal fistula, omphalocele, and gastroschisis) should cause bowel sounds to be present in the lung fields. In addition, omphalocele and gastroschisis should have obvious external malformations in the abdominal wall.

110. (D) The patient's history of an external abdominal wall defect narrows the diagnostic possibilities to omphalocele and gastroschisis. The presence of a peritonealized sac encasing the intestinal contents makes this case an omphalocele. In gastroschisis, there would be edematous loops of bowel visible through (and possibly protruding from) the abdominal defect. Tracheoesophageal fistula, duodenal atresia, and congenital diaphragmatic hernia are not associated with gross defects of the abdominal wall.

PSYCHIATRY

111. (C) The patient is suffering from medication-induced delirium, which is particularly common in elderly patients who have been given drugs with anticholinergic actions. Of the drugs listed (trazodone, lorazepam, haloperidol, risperidone, and diphenhydramine), diphenhydramine (Benadryl) is the most anticholinergic. Of the choices given, risperidone is the least likely to cause delirium in the elderly patient.

112. (C) During the start of a detoxification program, it is impossible to discern whether a patient with depressive symptoms has major depressive disorder or a substance-induced mood disorder. In the case of alcoholism, it is best to evaluate the patient's depressive symptoms for at least 1 to 3 weeks following the patient's last drink to allow resolution of any substance-induced depression. If the patient continues to have depressive symptoms at this point, then antidepressant therapy may be indicated.

113. (D) The patient is suffering from extrapyramidal side effects of haloperidol, a typical neuroleptic. Because extrapyramidal effects can be irreversible, the treatment is immediate discontinuation of the typical neuroleptic and change to an atypical neuroleptic, such as olanzapine. Switching the dosing method, timing, or medication, that is, switching to a lower potency typical neuroleptic (chlorpromazine), is insufficient to prevent the progression of these symptoms.

114. (A) The patient is experiencing symptoms typical of withdrawal from alcohol or a benzodiazepine. Given her history of anxiety disorder, it is likely that she is withdrawing from a fast-acting benzodiazepine, such as alprazolam. In the case of either withdrawal, the treatment of choice for the minimization of withdrawal symptoms and prevention of seizures is the use of a slow-acting benzodiazepine, such as chlordiazepoxide. Trazodone is an antidepressant that is often used when patients have difficulty with mood combined with insomnia. Diphenhydramine is an antihistamine with anticholinergic side effects. Haloperidol and risperidone are antipsychotic drugs that might be used in cases of agitation.

115. (C) The incidence of schizophrenia in individuals with a first-degree relative with schizophrenia is 10%.

116. (B) The child's symptoms of inattentiveness, impulsivity, and hyperactivity, in the absence of defiant or violent behavior, is most consistent with a diagnosis of attention-deficit/hyperactivity disorder. Patients with oppositional defiant disorder show hostility and defiance toward adults. Patients with Asperger's and Rett's syndromes show developmental delay. Patients with conduct disorder show a disregard for others and display hostile and violent behavior.

117. (C) The patient's symptoms of developmental delay, in combination with his physical findings of large ears and jaw, are most consistent with a diagnosis of fragile X syndrome. The patient would also have macro-orchidism if he was past pubertal age. The other options listed (phenylketonuria, trisomy 21, fetal alcohol syndrome, and congenital hypothyroidism) are not associated with these morphologic abnormalities.

118. (B) The patient's symptoms of gait disturbance, sleep problems, and mental status changes shortly after abruptly stopping a selective serotonin reuptake inhibitor (SSRI) are most consistent with SSRI discontinuation syndrome. Dietary intake of tyramine can cause difficulties in patients taking monoamine oxidase inhibitors but not SSRIs. Dietary intake of tryptophan does not affect any psychiatric drugs. SSRI medications have minimal anticholinergic effects. A worsening of the patient's major depressive disorder is possible, but the proximity of his symptoms to his abrupt discontinuation of his SSRI makes an SSRI discontinuation syndrome more likely. In addition, a worsening of the patient's major depressive disorder should not have affected the patient's gait.

119. (D) This patient's symptoms of depression, with the paradoxical findings of excessive appetite and sleeping, are most consistent with atypical depression. The symptoms of atypical depression are often unresponsive to SSRIs or tricyclic antidepressants but instead are often best treated with monoamine oxidase inhibitors (such as phenelzine).

120. (E) This vignette describes a bipolar patient who is unresponsive to lithium, despite having adequate circulating lithium levels. In bipolar patients unresponsive to lithium, the preferred therapeutic strategy is to add an additional medication (such as valproic acid), rather than to change the lithium dose or switch drugs entirely.

PULMONOLOGY

121. (A) The patient's history of chest pain, respiratory distress, and hemoptysis, combined with a recent deep vein thrombosis of the leg, is highly suggestive of a pulmonary embolism. Because the patient is not already taking anticoagulants, the appropriate management is to start heparin and warfarin during his stay in the hospital. Warfarin alone does not provide adequate anticoagulation for at least the first 3 days of therapy. A Greenfield filter is indicated if the patient had recurrent pulmonary embolism or anticoagulation is contraindicated. Antibiotic therapy is appropriate only if the patient has pneumonia. Thrombolysis with agents such as streptokinase are indicated only if the pulmonary embolism is causing hemodynamic compromise in the patient.

122. (B) The patient's symptoms of wheezing and cough productive of white sputum following several minutes of exercise is most consistent with exercise-induced asthma. The treatment of choice is pre-exercise use of β-agonist inhalers. It is not necessary to prevent the patient from physical activity. There is no evidence of infection (fever, malaise, abnormalities on physical examination) in the patient's history, so antibiotics and over-the-counter cough remedies would not be useful in this case. Bronchoscopy would be useful only if an airway obstruction was suspected.

123. (C) This patient has come to the hospital because of an exacerbation of his chronic bronchitis. He has a history of COPD for years, which raises the possibility of carbon dioxide retention due to his chronic disease. Patients who retain CO_2 often do worse with supplemental O_2, because they are predominantly using hypoxemia for their respiratory drive. Acutely increasing the O_2 saturation causes them to lose the stimulus for breathing and leads to respiratory arrest. Although pulmonary embolism and cardiac arrhythmia are additional possible causes of respiratory arrest, the timing of the respiratory arrest shortly after 100% mask oxygen was started excludes these diagnoses.

124. (B) The patient's history of recent thoracic trauma, pleuritic chest pain, absent breath sounds on one side, and tracheal deviation to the opposite side is consistent with a tension pneumothorax. In this situation, the immediate treatment involves needle thoracostomy to allow air to escape from the pleural cavity and allow inflation of the lung. Chest tube placement is also required but requires a greater amount of time and preparation. Aspirin, β-agonist inhalers, and antibiotics are not useful in the management of tension pneumothorax.

125. (C) The triad of sinusitis, situs inversus, and infertility is consistent with a diagnosis of Kartagener's syndrome. These patients frequently develop bronchiectasis. Bronchiectasis displays a "tram track" appearance with thickening of the bronchial walls.

126. (E) A history of severe burn injury and a complicated hospital course, with symptoms unresponsive to supplemental oxygen in a 40-year-old man, is consistent with adult respiratory distress syndrome (ARDS). ARDS presents with pulmonary infiltrates diffusely throughout the lung fields that develop within 24 hours.

127. (D) A history of heart disease presenting with pedal and pulmonary edema and bilateral dullness to percussion in an 80-year-old man is consistent with a pleural effusion. Pleural effusion displays a fluid collection with a visible meniscus denoting the air-fluid level.

128. (B) A 30-year-old soldier with a bullet wound to the chest is most likely to develop tension pneumothorax. Tension pneumothorax displays hyperlucency and diaphragmatic flattening on the affected side, with deviation of the trachea away from the affected lung.

129. (A) An increased anteroposterior chest diameter, dyspnea, and pursed lip breathing in a 70-year-old man with a 40-pack-year history of smoking is consistent with emphysema, a form of chronic obstructive pulmonary disease (COPD). In COPD, patients have clear lung fields with hyperinflated lungs and clear diaphragms.

130. (D) This patient's history of CHF exacerbation with no findings suggestive of infection or malignancy is most consistent with development of a transudative pleural effusion. In this instance, you would expect pleurocentesis fluid to have low protein, low LDH, and no evidence of atypical cells or lymphocytosis. High protein and high LDH are found in an exudative effusion. In addition, lymphocytosis is found in exudative effusions associated with viral infections, tuberculosis, or malignancy. Atypical cells are present in effusions associated with malignancy.

RHEUMATOLOGY

131. (E) The patient's triad of conjunctivitis, arthritis, and dysuria (suggestive of urethritis) is most consistent with Reiter's syndrome. Reiter's syndrome is associated with nongonococcal urethritis, usually due to infection by *Chlamydia trachomatis.*

132. (D) The patient's symptoms of arthritis with dry eyes and dry mouth are consistent with Sjögren's syndrome. A key way to distinguish Sjögren's from the other rheumatologic diseases that cause eye irritation is that the eye symptoms resolve with moisturizing drops in Sjögren's syndrome. Of the disorders listed (adult polycystic kidney disease, poststreptococcal glomerulonephritis, minimal change disease, type I renal tubular acidosis, and type IV renal tubular acidosis), Sjögren's syndrome is associated only with an increased risk of developing type I renal tubular acidosis.

133. (E) The woman's symptoms of a butterfly-shaped facial rash, photosensitivity, arthritis, and oral ulcers are most consistent with a diagnosis of systemic lupus erythematosus (SLE). This disorder develops spontaneously or in response to certain medications, which include quinidine, chlorpromazine, hydralazine, isoniazid, methyldopa, and procainamide (mnemonic—Q CHIMP). Because she is taking procainamide, it is possible that her symptoms were caused by this drug. Drug-induced lupus is usually reversible within 4 to 6 weeks.

134. (C) The patient's symptoms of restrictive cardiomyopathy, neuropathy, arthritis, and macroglossia are most consistent with a diagnosis of amyloidosis. The treatment of choice for amyloidosis is melphalan. Azathioprine and hydroxychloroquine are used in the treatment of SLE. Methotrexate is used in the therapy of rheumatoid arthritis. Aspirin can be used for symptomatic relief of pain in a variety of conditions.

135. (A) This patient's symptoms of joint pain and stiffness that is worse in the morning and not relieved by activity, in combination with the boutonnière deformity present in her hands, are most consistent with rheumatoid arthritis. On aspiration of the affected joints, it is most likely that a large number of neutrophils will be present. Needle-shaped, negatively birefringent crystals are present in gout. Rhomboid-shaped, positively birefringent crystals are present in pseudogout. Myxoid cartilage is abnormal cartilage that can be found in malignant neoplasms involving chondrocytes.

136.(D) The patient's symptoms of episodic arthritis that may be exacerbated by alcohol, diabetes, and arthritis. Swelling of the elbows and toe are most consistent with gout. During an acute attack of gout, the most appropriate therapy of the options given is indomethacin. Colchicine and allopurinol are used in the management of gout but should not be used during acute attacks because they may worsen the patient's symptoms. Prednisone is used in the management of gout but is used with caution in diabetics. Acetaminophen is not particularly effective in the management of gout.

137. (C) Corticosteroid treatments decrease responsiveness to insulin, so they should be used with caution in diabetics. Of the options listed, all could potentially be used in the management of gout or of joint pain, but prednisone is the medication most likely to induce hyperglycemia in a diabetic.

138. (A) The patient's history of hemoptysis (bloody cough), hematuria, and proptosis are consistent with a diagnosis of Wegener's granulomatosis. This disorder is associated with the presence of circulating cANCA (cytoplasmic antineutrophil antibodies). Churg-Strauss syndrome (a small vessel vasculitis associated with asthma and eosinophilic pneumonia) is associated with the presence of circulating pANCA (perinuclear antineutrophil antibodies). Antinuclear antibodies are found in systemic lupus erythematosus. Anti-Jo antibodies are present in dermatomyositis and polymyositis. Rheumatoid factor is found in rheumatoid arthritis. Of these disorders, the only one in which hemoptysis is a common presenting syndrome is Wegener's granulomatosis.

139. (B) The patient's symptoms of severe headache, mild fever, temporal tenderness, and jaw claudication are most consistent with a diagnosis of temporal arteritis. High-dose glucocorticoids are the treatment of choice for this disorder. Low-dose glucocorticoids are used in the management of polymyalgia rheumatica and a variety of other disorders. Azathioprine is a treatment used in Behçet's syndrome and in several other rheumatologic disorders. Melphalan is used in the treatment of amyloidosis.

140. (C) The patient's symptoms of abdominal pain, melena, mild hypertension, and muscle weakness (proximal > distal) are consistent with a diagnosis of polyarteritis nodosa. The diagnosis is further confirmed by the angiographic abnormalities in the superior mesenteric artery (a medium-sized artery). Polyarteritis nodosa is associated with infection with the hepatitis B virus and the presence of antibodies binding the hepatitis B surface antigen. None of the other infections listed (*Staphylococcus aureus,* Epstein-Barr virus, *Borrelia burgdorferi,* or *Streptococcus pyogenes*) have been associated with the development of polyarteritis nodosa.

INDEX

Page numbers followed by f or t indicate figures or tables, respectively.